Stefano Carpani has assembled an incredible num
Jungians" in this two-volume anthology, presenting
on contemporary clinical and theoretical classic
The New Ancestors will no doubt become a highly
anthology for the Jungian community and will most likely be found in the libraries
of most Jungian institutes and societies as well as on the shelves of scholars and
practitioners.

Misser Berg, *Jungian Analyst, Denmark, President-Elect of the IAAP*

In acknowledging Jungian voices from which we are all descended, Stefano Carpani
has put together this marvelous two-volume anthology on theoretical, clinical and
applied depth psychology that will be essential reading for generations of neo-
Jungians to come. From orthodox, post-classical and contemporary perspectives,
these seminal analysts and academics offer a rich compendium of novel ideas that
are harbingers for the future of analytical psychology.

Jon Mills, *Faculty, Postgraduate Programs in Psychoanalysis &*
Psychotherapy, Adelphi University

The *Oxford Dictionary* defines evolution as the appearance or presentation of events
in due succession. This innovative book project sets for itself the rather challenging
goal of exploring the evolution of analytical psychology from its roots and
foundations in the formulations of the founding figures of C. G. Jung, Marie-Louise
von Franz, Jolanda Jacobi etc., to the following generation of post-Jungians (till the
mid 1980's), in order to reflect on the future direction and evolution of these notions
and concepts from the perspective of contemporary neo-Jungians (recent graduates of
analytic training programs). Rather than perpetuating conceptual splits from different
schools of analytic thought, this younger generation of analytical psychologists or
neo-Jungians favors trans-disciplinarian inclusiveness and recognizes the value,
indeed the necessity, of integrating ideas and concepts from different psychoanalytical
schools of thought and perspectives with regard to the very nature of the analytic
relationship, and to the transference and counter-transference as an interactive field
in order to broaden and deepen our understanding of psyche and psychic process.
This expanded perspective also includes the body as a channel for expression of
psyche and makes allowance for the exploration of evolving notions of sexuality and
sexual identity. This perspective includes the psychosocial level as well and gives
credence to and recognition of the very real impact of socio-economic conditions on
psychological development.

The goal of this novel and innovative undertaking is to explore what the current
notions and ideas of the authors in this anthology might portent for the evolution
and future development in our understanding of the mysteries of psyche and of the
individuation process. Each author is a recognized authority in their field of interest
and together they represent perspectives from different training orientations and
different cultures, including Europe, North America, South America and South
Africa.

This anthology would be of great interest to analytical psychologists as well as to the candidates in analytical training programs around the world. In addition, I strongly believe that the inquisitive openness to and novel exploration of the notions presented will also appeal to and help build bridges to psychoanalysts and psychotherapists from different schools of thought and orientation as well as to academics interested in further exploring the underlying notions, concepts and theory. I also believe the articles in this anthology will respond to the curiosity of a large lay audience that has a profound and devoted interest in Jung and in the mysterious and often convoluted process of individuation.

In light of the fact that this anthology seeks to broaden our perspective and to explore avenues for the future development of our understanding of psychological development and of the mystery of the individuation process, it seems very likely that it would rapidly become an essential resource for further discussion among future generations of analysts and therapists of every orientation as well as of academics and students.

Tom Kelly, *Past President, IAAP*

Anthology of Contemporary Theoretical Classics in Analytical Psychology

This anthology of contemporary classics in analytical psychology brings together academic, scholarly and clinical writings by contributors who constitute the "post-Jungian" generation.

Carpani brings together important contributions from the Jungian world to establish the "new ancestors" in this field, in order to serve future generations of Jungian analysts, scholars, historians and students. This generation of clinicians and scholars has shaped the contemporary Jungian landscape, and their work continues to inspire discussions on key topics including archetypes, race, gender, trauma and complexes. Each contributor has selected a piece of their work which they feel best represents their research and clinical interests, each aiding the expansion of current discussions on Jung and contemporary analytical psychology studies.

Spanning two volumes, which are also accessible as standalone books, this essential collection will be of interest to Jungian analysts and therapists, as well as to academics and students of Jungian and post-Jungian studies.

Stefano Carpani, M.A., M.Phil., is an Italian sociologist (post-graduate of the University of Cambridge) and psychoanalyst trained at the C.G. Jung Institute, Zürich, accredited analyst CGJI-Z/IAAP and a Ph.D. candidate in the Department of Psychosocial and Psychoanalytical Studies from the University of Essex. He works in private practice in Berlin (DE) in English, Italian and Spanish. He is the initiator of the YouTube interview series *Breakfast at Küsnacht*, which aims to capture the voices of senior Jungians. Since 2017, he has collected more than 70 interviews. He is among the initiators of *Psychosocial Wednesdays*, a digital salon molded on those Freud's Wednesdays meetings in Vienna and on Jung's meetings at the Psychological Club, and feature speakers from various psychoanalytic traditions, schools and associated fields. He is the author of numerous papers and edited books, including *Breakfast at Küsnacht: Conversations on C. G. Jung and Beyond* (Chiron, 2020—IAJS book award finalist, for "Best Edited Book"); *The Plural Turn in Jungian and Post-Jungian Studies: The Work of Andrew Samuels* (Routledge, 2021); *Individuation and Liberty in a Globalized World: Psychosocial Perspectives on Freedom after Freedom* (Routledge, in print, June 2022); *Lockdown Therapy: Jungian Perspectives on How the Pandemic Changed Psychoanalysis* (Routledge, in print, July 2022).

Anthology of Contemporary Theoretical Classics in Analytical Psychology

The New Ancestors

Edited by Stefano Carpani

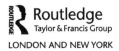
Routledge
Taylor & Francis Group

LONDON AND NEW YORK

Carla Indipendente, cover illustrator

First published 2022
by Routledge
4 Park Square, Milton Park, Abingdon, Oxon OX14 4RN

and by Routledge
605 Third Avenue, New York, NY 10158

*Routledge is an imprint of the Taylor & Francis Group, an informa
business*

British Library Cataloguing-in-Publication Data
A catalogue record for this book is available from the British
Library

Library of Congress Cataloging-in-Publication Data
Names: Carpani, Stefano, editor.
Title: Anthology of contemporary theoretical classics in analytical
   psychology : the new ancestors / edited by Stefano Carpani.
Description: New York, NY : Routledge, 2022. | Includes
   bibliographical references and index. |
Identifiers: LCCN 2021047620 | ISBN 9780367710194 (hardback) |
   ISBN 9780367710200 (paperback) | ISBN 9781003148982 (ebook)
Subjects: LCSH: Jungian psychology. | Psychoanalysis.
Classification: LCC BF173.J85 A68 2022 | DDC 150.19/54—dc23/
   eng/20211216
LC record available at https://lccn.loc.gov/2021047620

ISBN: 978-0-367-71019-4 (hbk)
ISBN: 978-0-367-71020-0 (pbk)
ISBN: 978-1-003-14898-2 (ebk)

DOI: 10.4324/9781003148982

Typeset in Times New Roman
by Apex CoVantage, LLC

To my Jungian ancestors,
To those suffering (and their caregivers),
To Carolina, Ferdinando, Valerio, and Leonardo,
This book is dedicated.

Contents

Epigraphs

Each thing is, as it were, in a space of possible states of affairs.
Ludwig Wittgenstein (Tractatus logico-philosophicus)

Lo duca e io per quel cammino ascoso
intrammo a ritornar nel chiaro mondo;
e sanza cura aver d'alcun riposo,135
salimmo sù, el primo e io secondo,
tanto ch'i' vidi de le cose belle
che porta'l ciel, per un pertugio tondo.138
E quindi uscimmo a riveder le stelle.
Dante Alighieri, "Divina Commedia", *Inferno*, Canto I, vv.1/3–10/12

Acknowledgments

I want to thank all contributors who generously accepted my request to contribute to this anthology. I would like to express my gratitude to Routledge, who supported my idea to create such a book.

Introduction

The New Ancestors and the "Agenda 2050" for Analytical Psychology

Stefano Carpani

"Who exactly are today's Jungian ancestors?" asked Andrew Samuels, when endorsing my book titled *Breakfast at Küsnacht* (Carpani, 2020). "Not really Jung, von Franz, Wolff, Neumann, Jacobi, Hillman, Fordham, etc., etc.," he answered, and continued: "well, of course we all read them, but ancestors change. The analysts who studied under those giants are, if not today's giants, at least already ancestors in their own right."

This is the basis from which I developed the idea for this book,[1] and I asked myself, "Who are the (new) ancestors for my generation of newly certified analysts?" Of course, "ancestors" is a controversial term, and maybe we have to distinguish between mentors and ancestors. I propose that mentors are personal, and that the mentor and the mentored mutually attract each other and benefit from the relationship. Without this precondition, there is no mentor-mentored relationship: take, for example, Plato and Socrates, and Jung and Freud (which was certainly a mentoring relationship while it lasted and became for Jung an ancestral relationship only after Freud's death).

Therefore, ancestors—I propose—are collective and belong to the whole community (family). You cannot choose an ancestor; they are there! But when talking about ancestors, we have to be careful, because if we follow the *Cambridge Dictionary*, we find that an ancestor is "a person related to you who lived a long time ago."[2] I prefer the version from the *Collins Dictionary*: "Your ancestors are the people from whom you are descended,"[3] and there is no doubt that—although our daily lives are so different from those of our ancestors—we could trace our ancestors back a few hundred years. This is exactly what I am trying to do with this book! Synonymous to this are the concepts of forefather and -mother, predecessor, precursor and forerunner; someone who was there before you and had an influence on you and who you have become.

I propose that the ancestors mentioned previously by Samuels[4] are the ancestors of the previous generation [his generation: the post-Jungians (Samuels, 1985)]. Therefore, the question is, who are the ancestors of *my* generation [the neo-Jungians[5] (Carpani, 2021)] and the next generation(s)? Who are the *new* ancestors? This book tries to answer those questions. And hopefully this book will serve as a

DOI: 10.4324/9781003148982-1

guidebook for those venturing into this field, looking for the "new ancestors" as well as to serve future generations of Jungian analysts, scholars, historians and students.

The importance of this book to the Jungian community lies in the overall impact of the work of the individuals contributing to it. The book also plays a role in expanding current discussions on Jung, the post-Jungians and contemporary analytical psychology studies, and some of the important issues addressed by them. Furthermore, the book constitutes a recognition of the generation of post-Jungians who shaped analytical psychology.

Another important consideration, which helped me to advance and shape the idea of an anthology of contemporary classics in analytical psychology, is that fact that, despite the many differences [as Verena Kast underlined in the preface to my book *Breakfast at Küsnacht* (Chiron, 2020)], we should reflect deeper on the figure and symbolism of the "the Jungian analyst" and that, if and when we do so, we can "feel and discern a common basic attitude." I believe there is a truth in what Kast stated. Therefore, there is "a common basic attitude" as well as heterogeneous one. It is also important to underline that Jung should not be taken as a *Messiah* (who already said everything there is to say) and that the *Jungians* are not a cult! This would arm our field.

How were the ancestors included in this anthology chosen? I conducted an informal (international) survey of candidates and colleagues in 2019. I asked them, "Who exactly are today's Jungian ancestors?"

I asked colleagues to name their own "new ancestors" among those analysts and scholars (living) active in analytical psychology from the 1980s onward. This was to avoid confusion with the first generation of Jungians [i.e. the *classical school* as Andrew Samuels (1985) put it, or—as I call them—"the orthodox Jungians"]. Out of this survey, 48 names were suggested. I contacted all 48 suggested contributors via email. Only 29 agreed to take part in the project. One dismissed my invitation with contempt, saying that they did not wish to join a mass grave with those with whom they had lifelong acrimony; all others did not respond.

When contacting each of the contributors, I asked them to provide the following: "a paper which you feel represents yourself, your work, and your intellectual and/or clinical trajectory" and "a detailed and *poetical biography* (written in first person), including as much information about you as you are willing to share." Therefore, I did not choose which papers to publish; they decided! They also decided how much personal information to share about themselves. And we know how little personal information confident analysts are willing to share.

This book, of course, is full of biases. The first bias is that fundamental authors at least as seminal as those included are missing. This is because, for instance, I was not able to include those who were no longer alive by the time I knew I would be doing this book. Some living analysts who influenced my generation, on the other hand, are no doubt not yet ready to regard themselves as "ancestors." And I may not have realised that I should have contacted others. Perhaps a third volume can be published in the future (if a colleague wants to take over this from me) that covers work in analytical psychology as applied mainly in the arts and humanities in the academy and others omitted here.

Right now, a bias can be seen in the balance (or imbalance) of clinical versus academic contributors. There is a reason for this. In thinking of analytical psychology as a clinical field, the people whom I asked to recommend those who they thought of ancestors and who had shaped their understanding of analytical psychology were all accredited analysts and candidates in training. If I had asked the same question of academic scholars, the names supplied would likely have been different.

Apart from celebrating new ancestors within analytical psychology, this book aims to bring a (finalistic) look at the future and ask, "what is the task of my generation?" "What is the 'agenda 2050' for analytical psychology?" I feel the answers lie in the following steps:

1   A Jungian psychosocial-relational model
2   *Kulturkritik*: social critics as much as personal therapists
3   The neo-Jungians
4   Time for extraversion
5   Medicine contra *the soul*

Jungian Psychosocial-Relational Model

Let's look at psychosocial studies and relational psychoanalysis—which have been the models within which psychoanalysis has moved (adapted) in the past few decades—and try to link them with our field.

Jung and the Psychosocial

In my Ph.D. work (unpublished), which employs the pioneering survey of the reach of analytical psychology offered by Progoff (1955: 161), I show the first element that makes Jung a pioneer of psychosocial studies and, thereby, the fact that Jung perceived that "the human psyche cannot function without a culture, and no individual is possible without society." Moreover, Jung "makes it his principle that all analysis must start from the primary fact of the social nature of man" (Progoff, 1955: 161). In the development of analytical psychology, Redman's claim (2014, cited in Frosh, 2014) is that what can be called Jungian psychosocial studies

> have . . . an equal concern for the depth and range of *social* processes that are in play and help constitute the context or phenomenon in question . . . this implies a concern for phenomena over and above those arising from social interaction to include those belonging to large groups and social system and structure.

On this basis, I would claim that Jung's work is by its very nature psychosocial and vice versa. I claim this because Frosh (2014: 161)—when discussing which books would be published as part of Palgrave's *Studies in the Psychosocial*—underlines that "books in the series will generally pass beyond their points of origin to generate concepts, understanding and forms of investigation that are distinctively psychosocial in character" and that "transdisciplinary objects of knowledge are continually invented in ways that demand the blurring of previously disciplinary boundaries" (Frosh, 2014: 167). This is certainly Jung's approach: from medicine to psychiatry to occult phenomena (Ph.D. thesis) to alchemy (beyond drive theory) to myth (collective unconscious) and physics (synchronicity).

This is also confirmed by Redman (cited by Frosh, 2014: 166), who stated that "seeking to investigate how the social is implicated in the psychological, psychosocial studies necessarily pay close attention to psychosocial and emotional states and view these states as lively and consequential, for psychological and social life as well."

Furthermore, Frosh emphasises that psychosocial studies "draw[s] heavily on psychoanalytic studies, but also on various models of social and political theory." In this attitude, I frame Jungians such as Progoff, Samuels and Watkins as well as non-Jungians such as Craib, Orbach and Layton. All of these authors share the common characteristic of transdisciplinarity. In fact, Frosch developed his theory from the core premises of depth psychology, which he linked to different areas of investigation, sometimes giving the impression that his work was about religion or anthropology, ethnology, philosophy, etc., rather than psychology.

Interestingly, both contemporary psychosocial studies and Jung's method of cross-disciplinary survey dovetail with what Freud suggested in 1926 in *The Question of Lay Analysis*, that in

> a college of psycho-analysis, much would have to be taught in it which is also taught by the medical faculty [alongside] branches of knowledge which are remote from medicine . . . the history of civilization, mythology, the psychology of religion and the science of literature.

If we add ethnology, anthropology and alchemy (among Jung's other interests), and take Jung's view that all of these apply to analytical psychology, we will describe the usual curriculum of the C.G. Jung Institute in Zürich since 1948.

Jung and the Relational

As noted by Aron and Mitchell (1999: xii), relational psychoanalysis emerged in the context of early 1980s' American psychoanalysis and now "operates as a shared subculture" that "has stuck deep, common, chords among current clinical practitioners and theorists." Relational psychoanalysis developed thanks to the pioneering effort of psychoanalyst Stephan Mitchell, supported by Robert Stolorow, Jay Greenberg and Aron himself (Aron and Mitchell, 1999: x). The factors contributing to its development were as follows (Aron and Mitchell, 1999: x): (a) the influence of the interpersonal psychoanalysis of Harry Stack Sullivan, Erich Fromm and Clara Thompson from the 1930s and 1940s; (b) object relations theory and the works of Fairbairn, Winnicott and Bowlby from the 1970s; (c) Kohut's "self-psychology" of the late 1970s; and (d) American psychoanalytic feminism and feminist psychoanalysis, including the work of Jessica Benjamin, and social criticism of the late 1970s and early 1980s.

It was in this landscape that, as Aron and Mitchell (1999: xi–xii) noted, Greenberg and Mitchell coined the term "relational" in 1983 to bridge the various strands of psychoanalysis current at that time, which included interpersonal *relations*, object *relations*, self-psychology, social constructivism, psychoanalytic hermeneutics and gender theorisation.[6] From these standpoints, Greenberg and Mitchell worked on a model (Aron and Mitchell, 1999: xiii–xv) that would do the following:

1   Provide an alternative understanding (to classical drive theory)
2   Generate a new understanding of precisely the phenomena that drive theorists have traditionally regarded as foundational: the body, sexuality, pleasure, aggression, constructionality, the patient's free association
3   Argue that mind occurs in "me-you patterns" (see Sullivan) and that the analyst is merely a "participant-observer . . . embedded in the transference-countertransference matrix" (Aron and Mitchell, 1999: xv)
4   Build on Winnicott's (1960: 39n, cited in Aron and Mitchell, 1999: xi) statement that "there is no such a thing as an infant—only the infant-mother unit"
5   Emphasise the emergence of what Ogden calls "the intersubjective Analytic-third" when speaking of "two-person psychology" (Aron and Mitchell, 1999)

Del Loewenthal and Samuels (2014: 4) recently highlighted the "widespread realization that the therapy relationship runs in both directions, is mutual, and involves the whole person of the practitioner," adding that "the 'relational' is most apparent in . . . Freud, Klein and object relations theories as well as Jung." Thus, he (Ibid., 2014: 4–5) reminds us of the mounting research evidence that the analytic relationship is the crucial factor in successful psychological therapy, and in asking why this is the case, he refers to Hargaden and Schwartz's (2007) description of relational psychoanalysis:

6   Emphasise the centrality of the relationship
7   Emphasise that therapy involves a bi-directional process
8   Emphasise that therapy involves both the vulnerability of therapist and client[1]
9   Emphasise the use of countertransference in thoughtful disclosure and collaborative dialogue
10   Emphasise the co-construction and multiplicity of meaning

As noted by Andrew Samuels (2012, unpublished), Jung asserted that because analysis was "dialectical," involving mutual transformation through the therapeutic relationship, its method was necessarily dialogic and would have to include

---

1 I do not like to refer to those coming into analysis with me as "clients." I prefer to refer to them as "patients" (from latin *patiens -entis*), which means to suffer and to bear. In fact, patients, come to us because they suffer emotionally.

"emotionally charged interactions" between therapist and patient. Samuels (2012, unpublished) notes that analysis, according to Jung, is "an encounter . . . between two psychic wholes in which knowledge is used only as a tool" (points 3 and 4 presented earlier). Therefore, with Sullivan's idea "that mind always emerges and develops contextually, in the interpersonal field" (Aron and Mitchell, 1999: xv) and with Greenberg and Mitchell's assertion that "[t]here is not such a thing as either the patient or the analyst—only the patient-analyst unit" (Aron and Mitchell, 1999: xv).

Additional reasons why Jung should be considered a relational *ante litteram* (points 1 and 2) include that Jung (together with Adler) realised the need to move beyond Freud's drive theory and sought an alternative in which Freud's drive theory and sexuality, Adler's inferiority and compensation, and Jung's symbolic life and spirituality could coexist. Such an approach would, as Aron underlines, examine "issues of sex and gender" (Aron and Mitchell, 1999: xi), which in drive theory, with its fixed attitudes toward sexuality and aggression, are obscured with regard to how they take in meaning in the relational context (Aron and Mitchell, 1999: xvi). I think most of the analysts who contributed chapters to these two volumes would agree with this view.

I should mention here that my own Jungian relational-psychosocial model is based on the following pillars:

1   It connects theory and clinical work (therefore helping to prove the accuracy and efficacy of analytical work with patients)
2   It is transdisciplinary
3   It is pluralistic (Samuels, 1989) and demonstrates an attitude of inclusion (to replace the split and separation typical of the history of psychoanalysis)
4   It "starts from the premise that the individual is born into a set of social and psychological circumstances" (Orbach, 2014: 16)
5   It "investigate[s] the ways in which psychic and social processes demand to be understood as always implicated in each other" (Frosh, 2014: 161)
6   It has an "emphasis on affect, the irrational and unconscious process, often, but not necessarily, understood psychoanalytically" (Frosh, 2014: 161)
7   It offers a conflict-relational approach (Orbach, 2014) and stresses the need for continuous adaptation in the process of people becoming who they authentically are
8   Becoming (who people authentically are) is seen as a liberation (Watkins, 2003)
9   Analysis is framed as "accompaniment" (Watkins, 2013) based on "the co-construction and multiplicity of meaning" (Hargaden and Schwartz, 2007)

All of these points are developed in pioneering form in the chapters included in this book. They contextualise the "agenda 2050" for a Jungian relational-psychosocial model that knows how not to disturb the deep process of individuation which is the task of my generation to continue to protect, following the guidelines laid down by our newest ancestors.

Kulturkritik: Social Critics as Much as Personal Therapists

Samuels suggests that within both the microcosm of an individual and the macrocosm of the global village, "we are flooded by psychological themes" and that "politics embodies the psyche of a people" (Samuels, 2001: 5). Thus, he reminds us that "the founders [of psychoanalysis] felt themselves to be social critics as much as personal therapists" (Samuels, 2001: 6), and in this respect, he recalls Freud, Jung, Maslow, Rogers, Perls, the Frankfurt School, Reich and Fromm. He also notes that, in the 1990s, psychoanalysts such as Orbach, Kulkarni and Frosch began to consider society once more, but notes that although "the project of linking therapy and the world is clearly not a new one . . . very little progress seems to have been made."

Thus, he stresses that today "more therapists than ever want psychotherapy to realize the social and political potential that its founders perceived in it" but is aware of the "large gap between wish and actuality" (Samuels, 2001: 7). I argue that the Jungian relational-psychosocial model might fill this gap.

In contrast to Hillman, Samuels actively demonstrated "how useful and effective perspectives derived from psychotherapy might be in the formation of policy, in new ways of thinking about the political process and in the resolution of conflict" (Samuels, 2001: xi), and he claimed that "our inner worlds and our private lives reel from the impact of policy decisions and the existing political culture." In considering why policy committees do not include psychotherapists, Samuels notes that "you would expect to find therapists having views to offer on social issues that involve personal relations" (Samuels, 2001: 2). This is Samuels' most innovative proposition: to see psychoanalysts (as well as individuals) as activists with a fundamental role to play within society.

I propose that we should work both inside and outside the consulting room as successful consultants for politicians, organisations, activist groups, etc., and also work to regain the *quid*—which we inherited, although did not enact—of the founders of psychoanalysis (social critics and personal therapists). Becoming again and anew *Kulturkritik*, we might be able to continue to play (or to play anew!) a role in the development of 21st-century societies.

The Neo-Jungians

The neo-Jungians are the third generation of Jungians [the first generation (1961–1985) being initially called the Zürich School[2] or "the orthodox Jungians" (by me), and the second generation (1985–2011) being called "the post-Jungians" by Samuels].

The *neo-Jungians*[7] (Carpani, 2020) employ Jung (in a new fashion) along with other schools and traditions of psychoanalysis (and beyond psychoanalysis) that mutually contaminate and enrich each other. The neo-Jungians, encompassing

---

2 Also called Classical School by Samuels

eclecticism and integration, aim to restore and enhance Jung's work and analytical psychology at the core of depth psychology by studying the psyche as plural. This new approach is constituted by

> a heterogeneous, international, and multicultural group of scholars who on the one hand base their work on the teachings of Jung (and the post-Jungians), while on the other hand have opened their investigations beyond analytical psychology. Therefore, the *neo-Jungians* are able to balance the teachings of Jung and the post-Jungians with those teachings coming from other schools and traditions (both within and beyond psychoanalysis) in a mutual and plural, enriching exchange. In fact, contemporary *neo-Jungians* can be linked (although not limited) to relational (and post-relational) psychoanalysis, feminist psychoanalysis, the intersubjective approach, psychosocial studies, and cultural studies, to name a few.
>
> (Carpani, 2020)

The *neo-Jungians* find their frame of reference in the aforementioned Jungian psychosocial-relational model. Thus, there are many ways to be Jungian (or to be a Jungian), and this is very good news. It signifies that analytical psychology is alive and reflects the continuing interest in, as well as perhaps even rejuvenation of, Jung's theories at the beginning of the 21st century.

The task of the neo-Jungians is to look at the future and, first,—to honour and preserve the work of the first and second generations of Jungians.

Extraversion Is Not Superficial

Jungians mainly stress introversion in their clinical writings. And this has not always been helpful outside our circle. I hope that, in the next 30 years, some of us (the most extraverted ones perhaps!) will be able to influence society as *Kulturkritik* (outside of our usual circles), by presenting our work at non-Jungian and non-psychoanalytic conferences and talking about our approach (with pride and courage and without inferiority) with different media outlets, policymakers and institutions of different sorts.

Becoming extraverted would be the most innovative aspect. Therefore, to follow Samuels would mean to see psychoanalysts (as well as individuals) as activists with a fundamental role to play within society.

Medicine Contra *the Soul*

Another point, which is of fundamental importance, concerns training analysis, who is to be admitted to train within Jungian Institutes around the world, and how this will be conducted.

Hillman (2010: 156) underlines that "it is up to each individual involved in the analysis to defend their own experience—the symptoms, the sufferings, the neuroses, and also the invisible positive results—in front of a world that gives no credit to these things." And he continues, "the soul can return to being a reality only if it has the courage to take it as the reality before its life, to take sides with it instead of just 'believing' in its existence."

As such, this appears to support the model carried forward by the C.G. Jung Institute in Zürich, where—by tradition—non-MDs and non-psychologists can participate in the training. I am convinced that this approach is the best and that it must be implemented globally. It follows that the title of medical doctor or psychologist should be removed as a criterion for admission. This is because the approaches of medicine and psychology, as Hillman suggests, have nothing to do with working with the soul, while the analysis aims to "facilitate the flow and to reconnect the symbolic fragments in a mythical configuration" (Hillman, 2010: 156). And it is no coincidence that among the best analysts are non-MDs and non-psychologists (e.g. Riedel, Samuels and Zoja).

Mine, like Hillman's (2010: 159), is a campaign in favour of analysis, as "modern medicine imposes a split between doctor and his soul" and as it is fundamental that "the practice of psychotherapy, must leave the medical background behind to proceed independently."

Freud wrote on the subject as early as 1926. Freud intervened in defence of Theodor Reik (an Austrian psychoanalyst and collaborator of the same who, in 1924, was accused of abusing the medical profession because he practised psychoanalysis, but had a degree in philosophy) and helped to exonerate him by defending the legitimacy of the use of psychoanalysis by lay people. Freud, in a letter addressed to Julius Tandler (an influential anatomist and Viennese politician), asserted the legitimacy of practitioners like Reik by writing that "psychoanalysis, whether it is considered a science or a technique, is not a purely matter medical" and, second, "it is not taught to medical students at university."[8]

Hillman observes that

> Freud soon realized that it was necessary to partially abandon medicine because the analyst does not physically examine his patient, does not prescribe him medicine, for organic disorders he refers it to others; in the analyst's office there are no medical devices; you don't see white coats and black briefcases.
>
> (2010: 161)

Then Hillman points out that "Freud's fears have come true: Freudian analysis has become the handmaid of psychiatry" and that "Freudian therapy becomes acceptable by medicine" as a natural science (2010: 163). In fact, most MDs, psychiatrists and psychologists have not been analysed. They have never undergone training analysis.

So, I propose that a degree in medicine or psychology should not be the prerequisite to access psychoanalytic training; instead, the criteria used at the C.G. Jung Institute in Zürich should be adopted: write a ten-page autobiography, go through six interviews with accredited analysts, complete 300 hours of training analysis in parallel with (during the second half of the training) individual and group supervision and—as enantiodromia—internship at a psychiatric institution.

Last, following Andrew Samuels' proposal at the 4th Analysis and Activism Conference San Francisco (online) 2020, I agree that, to be truly egalitarian, training should not require a master's degree (or even a bachelor's degree). Candidates should be interviewed and accepted on the basis of their fulfilment of the aforementioned requirements (see those in the preceding paragraph used by the C.G. Jung Institute Zürich) and their willingness to train (learning the theoretical aspects of this profession) and to undergo self-analysis to become a Jungian psychoanalyst.

Structure of the Book

The book consists of 14 essays introduced by a poetical autobiography written by the new ancestor who wrote the chapter in question. These speak for themselves and need no further introduction here. But this is what the new ancestors have said to me about their individual chapters:

Paul Bishop: "Seeing With the Eyes of the Spirit"

Taking as its starting point a curious incident recorded in Goethe's *Dichtung und Wahrheit*, this paper explores the implications of what Goethe calls "seeing with the eyes of the spirit." We can find this idea in Neoplatonic, Patristic and medieval mystical writings, as well as in various philosophical authors of the eighteenth century and in Goethe's scientific writings, where we find the suggestion that, in addition to our conventional perceptual apparatus, we can use our imagination or "mind's eye." For his part, Jung seeks to integrate intellect and feeling in his approach to the psyche, telling us both are required to offer an adequate explanation of the psyche. The paper goes on to consider how the notion of synthesis is linked with the central Goethean concepts of morphology, that is, with polarity and *Steigerung* (or intensification). In turn, it suggests that in Jungian thought these ideas feed into the notion of a constellation of the self, into a missionary vision of *Kultur*, and into a theory of the symbol. It concludes by arguing that, from the perspective of German classicism and analytical psychology alike, the relationship between culture and the attainment of the self is a reciprocal one. For Goethe and Schiller as for Jung, the significance of culture lies in assisting us to realise the central nodal point at which all faculties are exercised and co-ordinated. At the heart of this thinking lies a notion of the symbolic life, iconographically embodied for Nietzsche in the figure of Goethe, and "the discovery of the world as a symbolic world" (as Vergely has written) is "a journey which procures an infinite joy."

Ann Casement: "A Critical Appraisal of C.G. Jung's Psychological Alchemy"

This paper is an in-depth exposition of one of Jung's major contributions to psychology. The chapter includes a comparison of that model with the ten well-known

Zen ox-herding pictures, followed by an exploration of Wolfgang Giegerich's revisionist thinking on psychological alchemy.

James Hollis: "Narcissus's Forlorn Hope: The Fading Image in a Pool Too Deep"

The essay examines the conventional myth of Narcissus, surveys its usual forms in daily life, its amplification in Doestoevski's *Notes from Underground*, and moves toward an examination of the need for, the resistance to, and the ineluctable human desire to be seen, and concludes with the acknowledgement of the impossibility of any fixed self-imago.

Verena Kast: "Complexes and Their Compensation: Suggestions From Affective Neuroscience"

The author asks, what influence does it have on the understanding of complexes and dreams, and thus on our clinical work, if we consistently assume that the basis of personality is affectivity, as C.G. Jung understood it, and how is it currently understood by Jaak Panksepp, a leader in affective neuroscience? Does Panksepp's idea of enriching or replacing predominant emotions with compensatory emotions bring a constructive dynamic to the stagnation associated with constellated complex episodes?

Stanton Marlan: "Hesitation and Slowness: Gateway to Psyche's Depth"

This paper focuses on hesitation and slowness in the work of Jungian analysis. It emphasises the importance of patience as a way of achieving depth and of avoiding facile and abstract formulations that lack respect for the true otherness of the analysand and for the fundamental enigmas of analytic work. Alongside the techniques of Freud and Jung, and drawing on Alchemy, Renaissance and Eastern wisdom traditions, the author articulates a complex notion of hesitation. The paper deconstructs simple binary pairings of fast and slow and suggests an attitude of purposeless wandering as an important compensation to the overly technologically oriented attitudes and fast-paced culture that have invaded our therapeutic sensibilities and consulting rooms.

Renos K. Papadopoulos: "The Other Other: When the Exotic Other Subjugates the Familiar Other"

In this paper, the theme of the other will be examined and it will be argued that it is important to differentiate between two distinct types of others—the "exotic" other which is distant and very different from the subject, and the "familiar" other which is closer to the subject. The dynamic relationship between these two others will be investigated, and emphasis will be given to the process through which the exotic other tends to subjugate the familiar other. This relationship will then be discussed in its various applied forms, in the contexts of clinical practice and socio-political dimensions. In particular, a new reading of Jung's approach to the "primitive" will be developed on the basis of the subjugation by the "exotic" other of the "familiar" other. A similar line of investigation will be followed to examine the concept of psychological trauma. In addition, Freud's "narcissism of minor differences" and Bion's distinction between "narcissism" and "socialism" will be considered in the light of this differentiation between these two others.

Denise G. Ramos: "Jungian Theory and Contemporary Psychosomatics"

This article sets out to describe the development of Jungian theory in the field of psychosomatics and its application in clinical practice when dealing with patients with somatic symptomatology. A brief historical review of the area of psychosomatics underlines the lack of psychoanalytical resources to enable an understanding of the integrality of the psyche/body phenomenon.

On the other hand, most of the considerable amount of research demonstrating how emotions influence symptoms being formed at the somatic level lack the theoretical reasoning needed to subsidise them. This fact, reflecting as it does the well-known dissociation between psychology and medicine, reinforces a one-sided model of human development.

Although C. G. Jung's association experiments have already provided the foundation to develop a theory applicable to psychosomatics, few analysts perceive their patient's body as a rich source of symbolic material.

The paper addresses the concepts of complex, transduction and symbol as the main axis for understanding the psyche/body phenomenon by resorting to a symbolic view of the somatic symptoms regardless of their causality. Here, all diseases being considered psychosomatic disorders, therapeutic interventions should be evaluated according to the degree to which systems have been altered. The goal is always to find a state of coherence in the organism by means of interventions at various levels, from psychic to cellular. Clinical cases illustrate how the theory can be applied using techniques from the Jungian field.

Susan Rowland: "Feminism, Jung and Transdisciplinarity: a Novel Approach"

Jung's Collected Works can be read as feminist novels. As such they restory the feminine, incarnate Dionysus and anticipate transdisciplinarity. The Collected Works are novels because they foster many voices. Such tricky writing is the new home of animism, a spirituality allied to a goddess of divine earth, sexuality, body, pluralism rather than dualism. Such an expansive feminine includes what Jung calls feeling and connection as Eros, trickster androgynous plurality and nature as "her" complexity creativity that he named synchronicity.

As James Hillman diagnosed, Jung the feminist novelist is Dionysian in enacting dismemberment into parts. These parts are aware of themselves as parts with an emphasis on embodied consciousness. Jung's trickster and animistic writing is here the dispersed corporeality of the ecstatic god. Taking this unlikely feminist Jung further is to consider his writing as proto-transdisciplinary. For the transdisciplinarity of Basarab Nicolescu in From Modernity to Cosmodernity (2014) is written in the (Jungian) symbol.

Above all, the Jungian symbol occupies what transdisciplinarity calls the logic of the included middle between subject and object. Transdisciplinarity adopts Jung's project of restoring what has been excluded as feminine and taking it into a cultural-epistemological project that can provide a trans-religious and trans-cultural future.

Heyong Shen: "The Dao of Anima Mundi: I Ching and Jungian Analysis, the Way and the Meaning"

In this paper, the author is going to discuss the ancient ineffable notion of "Dao" as an archetype, with emphasis on the goal of embracing "the Heart of Dao", together with the meaning pointed to by Confucius in introducing the term "Zhong" ("Equilibrium") as the psychological path to the state of harmony implied by the word Dao. At the same time, goes further to the Chinese term of "Shi" ("Timing", which in a parallel way spans both the Greek notion of Kairos and the Jungian notion synchronicity), and link Zhong to Shi to discuss "Shi-Zhong" (an "equilibrium with time" achieved through a heartfelt influence often best achieved through wu-wei/acting without acting) as we often must as analysts. There are five parts of this paper for discussion: The Mysterious Heart of Dao, the Subtle Words with Great Meaning; The Metaphor of He-Tu, The Image of I Ching; Shi-Zhong and Gan-Ying, Equilibrium with Time and Synchronicity; The Soul Flower, Images of I Ching, and Meaning; and The Mysterious Heart of Dao, Heartfelt Influence and Response.

Sonu Shamdasani: "From Neurosis to a New Cure of Souls: C.G. Jung's Remaking of the Psychotherapeutic Patient"

This paper studies how from the First World War onwards, C. G. Jung reformulated his psychotherapeutic procedure on the basis of his own self-experimentation. It shows how through doing so, he shifted the aims of psychotherapy from being solely the cure of pathology to one of higher psychological and spiritual development, and in so doing, proposed a new notion of humanity. It studies a series of cases of Jung, demonstrating how he reformulated the "offer" of psychotherapy, how individuals took it up, and how this helped to shape the social role of the psychotherapeutic patient.

Thomas Singer: "A Personal Meditation on Politics and the American Soul"

This paper originated in an invitation to write a paper on politics and the American soul, an almost impossible task, which only fools might undertake. The paper eventually took shape in two sections. The first section focuses on the nature of individual soul and collective or group soul. Imagined as a journey in space and time, I posit the discovery of the soul of the individual and the soul of the nation as occurring at an intersection between the two. There is no assumption that the soul of the nation is unitary. As an example, I discuss a journey to the heartland of America that I took with my family to bury the ashes of my beloved mother-in-law. The second section explores the idea that the soul of the nation is forged or dismembered in the crucible of core cultural complexes working themselves out over time and generations in the national and regional psyches. I define seven fundamental cultural complexes of the United States and examine how they express themselves in specific political conflicts.

Murray Stein: "On Jung's View of the Self—An Investigation"

The author underlines that the self is more than conscious identity (i.e., the ego) because it includes and expresses the full range of the psyche. Beyond this, the self concept links Analytical Psychology and religious doctrines of transcendence. This essay explores the complex relation of the self to the transcendent (Divinity), as Jung understood these terms and employed them, focusing especially on a critical passage from his last major work, Mysterium Coniunctionis. The notion of self as imago Dei grasps the paradoxical nature of the self, a coincidentia oppositorum that is at once personal and impersonal. Jung posits, moreover, a dynamic interactive relation between the self and the transcendence it mirrors. Altogether, this combination of features regarding the self sets Jung's psychology apart from humanistic and personalistic psychologies and secular depth psychologies on the one side, and on the other side from pre-enlightenment dogmatic psychologies such as those of religious fundamentalisms. This essay argues that Jung's depth psychology represents a post-Enlightenment, post-secular, post-humanistic vision of the human being whose psyche links earth and heaven, the here and the beyond, the finite and the infinite. It is a radical attempt to break out of modernity without regressing to medievalism.

Mary Watkins: "Seeing From "the South": Using Liberation Psychology to Re-Orient the Vision, Theory and Practice of Depth Psychology"

Standing outside the mainstream canon of depth psychology are liberatory theorists who were schooled in depth psychology but whose experiences and work for justice and peace are nevertheless largely left out of its purview. As depth psychologists struggle to understand the impact of Eurocentrism and colonialism on their theories and practices, a turn to liberation psychology offers a needed set of alternate vantage points. Seeing from the perspectives of liberatory theorists such as Frantz Fanon, Paulo Freire, Ignacio Martín-Baró, Marie Langer and others helps us to better understand the Eurocentrism of depth psychology, including its relationships to colonialism, capitalism and racism. Liberation psychology, rooted in an interdependent paradigm, asks us to mobilise psychology to join struggles for social, economic, racial and environmental justice. To do so, our psychologies must be transformed into more transdisciplinary efforts to meet these challenges. Watkins gives examples of what such a reorientation looks like by addressing the psychosocial accompaniment of forced migrants, illustrating how the orientations offered by liberation psychology can affect both the "private" and the "public" practices of psychologically minded practitioners.

Luigi Zoja: "The Clash of Civilizations? A Struggle Between Identity and Functionalism"

The history of the West has broken the balance between two polarities of the psyche, mania and depression. Mental times are increasingly accelerated: an apparently productive, functional trend. The mind considered "normal" is no longer halfway between those two extremes, but approaches the manic pole. Reject the necessary pauses for reflection and self-criticism. Also favoured by mass communication, hastiness and superficiality then lead to projecting internal conflicts outwards: in this way, we look for enemies to whom we can attribute them. Yes, the Clash of Civilizations theory emphasises undeniable differences, but obtains mass diffusion by exploiting a pre-existing psychological imbalance: our propensity to maniacality and paranoia.

The West was born with Greece, which practised self-restraint and self-criticism, but then conquered the world by making maniacalism the norm. The other cultures weren't necessarily like that. Before Columbus, China's supremacy was such that it could have started a world conquest. China chose to retire behind the Great Wall. Our haste and lack of self-analysis make our identity creak (the nucleus of the personality supposedly stable, identical), putting functionality before it, which looks to immediate results. An example is provided by psychologists who agree to collaborate in the interrogation of detainees in American extrajudicial prisons such as Guantànamo: but in all fields daily concessions are made for commercial reasons. Similar sales of the Faustian soul, due to their fundamental unacceptability, are removed. Like all unconscious contradictions, they are denied and projected externally. The "clash between irreconcilable worlds" is also the transposition of an internal conflict that has long threatened our identity.

Notes

1 This book is part of a two-volume collection (its twin is titled *Anthology of Contemporary Theoretical Classics in Analytical Psychology: The New Ancestors*).
2 https://dictionary.cambridge.org/dictionary/english/ancestor
3 https://www.collinsdictionary.com/dictionary/english/ancestor

4 Jung, von Franz, Wolf, Neumann, Jacobi, Hillman, Fordham.
5 The neo-Jungians are the third generation of Jungians [the first generation (1961–1985) initially was called the Zürich School and later the Classical School (Samuels, 1985), and the second generation (1985–2011) was called the post-Jungians (Samuels, 1985)].
6 It is also worth mentioning that relational psychoanalysis is linked to the rediscovery of Ferenczi's work and mutual analysis, but it is important to underline that Jung was the first to engage in mutual analysis (with Otto Gross in 1908), much earlier than Ferenczi. I, therefore, claim that Ferenczi built on Jung's legacy without recognizing it openly. The same can be said of Rank and his work on individuation.
7 Not to be confused with Robert Moore's *Neo-Jungian Mapping of the Psyche*: https://robertmoore-phd.com/index.cfm/product/122/a-neo-jungian-mapping-of-the-psyche-understanding-inner-geography--our-challenge-of-individuation.html
8 Letter from Sigmund Freud to Julius Tandler (8.3.1925), retrieved from https://www.psicolinea.it/lanalisi-laica-freud-e-il-caso-theodor-reik/

Bibliography

Aron, L., and Mitchell, S.A. (1999). *Relational Psychoanalysis, Volume 14: The Emergence of a Tradition*. New York and London: Routledge.
Carpani, S. (2020). *Breakfast at Küsnacht*. Asheville, NC: Chiron.
Carpani, S. (2021). *The Plural Turn in Jungian and Post-Jungian Studies: The Work of Andrew Samuels*. London and New York: Routledge.
Freud, S. (1926/1990). *The Question of Lay Analysis*. New York: Norton & Company.
Frosh, S. (2014). The nature of the psychosocial: Debates from studies in the psychosocial. *Journal of Psycho-Social Studies*, 8(1).
Hargaden and Schwartz's (2007), cited in Loewenthal, D., and Samuels, A. (2014). *Relational Psychotherapy, Psychoanalysis and Counselling: Appraisals and Reappraisals*. New York and London: Routledge.
Hillman, J. (2010). *Il Suicidio e l'anima*. Milano: Adelphi.
Loewenthal, D., and Samuels, A. (2014). *Relational Psychotherapy, Psychoanalysis and Counselling: Appraisals and Reappraisals*. New York and London: Routledge.
Orbach, S. (2014). Democratizing psychoanalysis. In D. Loewenthal and A. Samuels (Eds.), *Relational Psychotherapy, Psychoanalysis and Counselling: Appraisals and Reappraisals*. New York and London: Routledge.
Progoff, I. (2013 [1955]). *Jung's Psychology and its Social Meaning*. London: Routledge.
Redman, P., cited in Frosh, S. (2014). The nature of the psychosocial: Debates from studies in the psychosocial. *Journal of Psycho-Social Studies*, 8(1).
Samuels, A. (1985). *Jung and the Post-Jungians*. London: Routledge.
Samuels, A. (1989). *The Plural Psyche*. London: Routledge.
Samuels, A. (2001). *Politics on the Couch*. London: Profile Books.
Samuels, A. (2012). *Jung as a Pioneer of Relational Psychoanalysis*. Unpublished.
Watkins, M. (2003). Dialogue, development, and liberation. In I. Josephs (Ed.), *Dialogicality in Development*. Westport, CT: Greenwood.
Watkins, M. (2013). *Accompaniment: Psychosocial, Environmental, Trans-Species, Earth*. Retrieved on 11 November 2018 from: http://mary-watkins.net/library/Accompaniment-Psychosocial-Environmental-Trans-Species-Earth.pdf

Chapter 1

Paul Bishop

Although I had been aware of Jung through the usual undergraduate interest in such vaguely fringe or occult interests as dream interpretation and the *I Ching*, it was, of all people, a politics tutor at Oxford who opened my eyes to the potential of taking Jung seriously. As an avid reader of Nietzsche, I found that Jung joined those other figures such as Heidegger or Klages who were, one way or another, reacting and responding to the cry, "God is dead" – and who all wrote in German. As a student of German (and French) at Oxford, this was good news! Yet strangely enough, I also discovered that, at least within *Germanistik* circles in Britain, being interested in Jung was a bit like the case mentioned in *Memories, Dreams, Reflections* of the old peasant who discovered that, presumably as a result of witchcraft, two cows had got their heads in the same halter, and who replied to his son's question, "How did that happen?" by responding, "One doesn't talk about such things."[1] For some reason, it seemed that "one doesn't talk about Jung," but that only served, of course, to make him more attractive. Embarking on doctoral research into Jung and Nietzsche, I had the good fortune to have a supervisor who cheerfully described himself as working on the dustbin of German literature and was more interested in helping me to write and structure an argument than in petty point-scoring against outsider figures. Time and again, however, I was struck by the marginalization of Jung by the academy: his *Collected Works* (in English) were in the Radcliffe Science Library, but the *Gesammelte Werke* (in German) were in the Bodleian and had to be ordered by individual volume; only isolated copies of single works were in the Modern Languages library, the Taylorian. For this reason, I have appreciated all the more the kind support of Jungian institutions and individual Jungians, who have generously offered bibliographical advice or invited me to speak to their analytic groups or seminars

Having completed my doctorate in Jung and Nietzsche, and having had the extremely good fortune to have secured an academic job at Glasgow, I now felt that the task was clear: to situate Jung firmly in the German intellectual tradition

---

1 Jung, C.G. (1963). *Memories, Dreams, Reflections*, in Aniela Jaffé, trans. by Richard and Clara Winston, London: Collins, Routledge & Kegan Paul. 124.

DOI: 10.4324/9781003148982-2

represented by such figures as Kant, Goethe, and Schiller. These projects were never intended to be a simple "Jung and . . ."; as one colleague caustically remarked, "the next thing he'll be writing about is Jung and the Spice Girls" (actually, now there *is* an idea). For one thing, my approach to Kant and Jung in relation to the concept of synchronicity was largely sceptical (and it remains so: surely, sometimes a beetle is only a beetle); for another, under the influence of a wise, senior colleague at Glasgow, the relationship between Jung and Weimar Classicism turned out to be far more significant than a simple *Quellenforschung* could have possibly imagined. Yet here fate intervened. For while I had hoped to recuperate Jung for the academy by demonstrating his affinities with such central figures as Goethe and Schiller, these figures themselves were gradually losing their centrality. As dead, white males, they were being swept aside in the name of "theory," albeit a theory that was often insufficiently understood (and even more insufficiently taught). So whilst I had tried to bring Jung back into the academic fold, I had unwittingly brought him into a more postmodern form of disrepute.

Within this changed academic context, however, it seemed to me that Jung acquired fresh significance. While I admire (not least because of their brilliant titles) *The Jung Cult* and *The Aryan Christ*, it nevertheless seemed to me that this new, historiographical critique of Jung fell somewhat wide of the actual academic political mark: to be sure, there were difficult questions to be asked about Jung's political views, but when the arts and humanities themselves were under attack, to focus on them increasingly seemed like an irrelevant skirmish. After all, what *is* the problem with Jung? I, for one, feel that I owe him an immense debt of gratitude because I have learned *so much* from his works; to read the *Collected Works* is to undertake an entire course in the liberal arts, civilization studies, and intercultural studies. One *learns* so much from Jung. Could this, then, be the real source of the problem?

After all, analytical psychology places – in contrast to postmodernism – great emphasis on continuity rather than on rupture or fissure. In *Memories, Dreams, Reflections*, the second part of Goethe's *Faust* is described as "more than a literary exercise" and instead as "a link in the *aurea catena* which has existed from the beginnings of philosophical alchemy and Gnosticism down to Nietzsche's *Zarathustra*" – and on, one might add, to *The Red Book* of C.G. Jung, a work which might justly be described, as *Faust* and *Zarathustra* are, as "unpopular, ambiguous, and dangerous . . . a voyage of discovery to the other pole of the world."[2] For not only does Jung, time and again, invoke Goethe as an essential reference point (and this, for me, is the real significance of the legend that Jung loved to hate to relate about his grandfather being an illegitimate child of Goethe) for his own psychological development: *Memories, Dreams, Reflections* records that *Faust* had "struck a chord" in Jung and "struck him" in a way that he could not but regard as "personal," adding that in *Faust* he saw a dramatization of his own

---

2 Jung 1963: 213–214.

"inner contradictions" and that this work had provided "a basic outline and pattern" of his own "conflicts and solutions."[3] But Jung also links the project of analytical psychology as a whole to what, in his view, *Faust* had "pass over," namely, "respect for the eternal rights of humankind, recognition of 'the ancient,' and the continuity of culture and intellectual history."[4] Or, in the famous words written by Thomas Mann in his letter to Klaus Mann of 22 July 1939: "In the end, to inherit something one has to understand it; inheritance is, after all, culture (*Aber schließlich, zu erben muß man auch verstehen, erben, das ist am Ende Kultur*)."

In a lecture of 1932, Jung included hope (along with faith, love, and understanding) among the "four highest achievements of human endeavor" that are "so many gifts of grace."[5] For what, Jung asked his audience, is a doctor meant to do when he sees that a patient has

> no hope, because he is disillusioned by the world . . . no love, but only sexuality; no faith, because he is afraid to grope in the dark; [and] . . . no understanding, because he has failed to read the meaning of his own existence."[6]

Jung was highly critical of what he called a "psychology without psyche," and he would also be critical of an *education* without psyche. For alas! All too often education does not "give enough meaning to life," and "it is only meaning that liberates."[7]

Seeing With the Eyes of the Spirit

Originally published in Bishop, P. (2013). "Seeing with the Eyes of the Spirit" [Guild Paper 313], London: The Guild of Pastoral Psychology, May 2013. Reprinted with permission.

In his autobiography *Dichtung und Wahrheit* (*Poetry and Truth*), Johann Wolfgang von Goethe gives us one quite specific, and strange, instance of what "seeing with the eyes of the spirit" might mean. He speaks about "the sensation of past and present being one," describing it as "a perception that introduces a spectral quality

---

3 Jung 1963: 262.
4 Jung 1963: 262.
5 Jung, C.G. *Collected Works*, in Sir H. Read, M. Fordham, G. Adler, and W. McGuire, London: Routledge & Kegan Paul. Vol. 11, §501.
6 Jung Vol. 11, §499.
7 Jung Vol. 11, §496.

into the present" (*GE* 4, 457).[1] He gives the example of how, after taking leave of one of his early lovers, Friederike Brion, he experienced the past-in-the-present in a case of what one might term "second sight" when, riding along the footpath towards Drusenheim, he was "seized by the strangest premonition":

> I saw myself, not with the eyes of the body, but those of the spirit [*nicht mit den Augen des Leibes, sondern des Geistes*], coming toward myself on horse-back on the same path, and, to be sure, in clothing I had never worn: it was bluish grey with some gold trimming. As soon as I shook myself awake from this dream, the figure vanished.
>
> (*GE* 4, 370)

"Yet it is curious," Goethe added, "that eight years later I found myself on the same path, coming to visit Friederike once more and dressed in the clothes I had dreamed about, which I was wearing not by choice but coincidence." Here we have a particularly curious instance of what Goethe calls *seeing with the eyes of the spirit*: but what are *the eyes of the spirit*, how can one *see* with them, and what sort of vision do they give us?

In several places in Goethe's scientific writings, we find the suggestion that, in addition to our conventional perceptual apparatus, we can use our imagination or what he calls the "mind's eye." When in *On Morphology* (1817–1824), for example, he writes that "we learn to see with the eyes of the spirit" (*WA* II.8, 37), he is drawing attention to the role of the "productive imagination" not just in scientifically determined or artistically formed intuition but in simple empirical intuition as well. This was pointed out by Ernst Cassirer, who also drew a link between what Goethe called "seeing with the eyes of the mind" and the *saper vedere*, "the perfection of seeing," of which Leonardo da Vinci had spoken (Cassirer 1996: 81).

Even further back, we find the idea of the "eye of the spirit" in some of the early fourth-century patristic writers, such as St Ambrose, who writes in his treatise *On the Mysteries* that "what cannot be seen with the eyes, is seen in a higher sense; it is seen with the eye of the spirit," or St Augustine who, in a famous passage from the *Confessions*, turned his gaze inward and discovered "with the eyes of my soul" the Lord within himself. In his *Mystical Theology*, Pseudo-Dionysius the Areopagite distinguished between "the eye of the body or of the mind," and earlier still, we find Plotinus talking in his treatises or *Enneads* about "inner vision," about "the mind's eye" and about "seeing of a quite different kind" (*Enneads*, I.6.9 and VI.9.11). Thus, there is a rich philosophical, theological and spiritual tradition behind this idea.

At the same time, we also find the expression in contemporary philosophical texts of the eighteenth century. For example, the German idealist philosopher Johann Gottlieb Fichte urged his audience that

> just as your sensuous eye is a prism, in which the ether of the sensuous world, which is in itself quite self-identical, pure, and colourless, breaks into

manifold colours on the surface of things [. . . .] so proceed likewise in matters of the spiritual world, and from the view of your spiritual eye'.[2]

Elsewhere in Goethe's writings, in one of his drafts for the introduction to his *Doctrine of Colour*, he emphasizes the uniqueness of the organ of sight in his conclusion that "the totality of the inner and outer is completed by the eye."[3] In the course of the *Doctrine of Colour*, it becomes apparent that Goethe is thinking not just of physical sight but of a particular kind of *schauen* or contemplation, which could be termed "aesthetic perception." In the aesthetic theory of Johann Gottfried Herder, who was part of the wider circle around Goethe and Schiller in Weimar, (aesthetic) seeing is the end product of all the senses working in concert – "the eye is merely the signpost, merely the reason of the hand; only the hand provides the *forms*, concepts of what they *mean*, what *dwells* within them."[4]

Now, in "A Few Remarks" on the botanical theories of Caspar Friedrich Wolff, Goethe draws on Herder's emphasis on the "haptic sense" or the sense of touch, contrasting the "eyes of the body" with what he calls "spirit-eyes." There is a difference, he writes, "between seeing and seeing," and the two different kinds of seeing, with the two different kinds of eyes, are mutually dependent: "the spirit-eyes have to operate in a continuous living union with the eyes of the body, otherwise one runs the danger of looking and looking past something" (*WA* II.6, 156). These "spirit-eyes," he writes in "On the Spiral Tendency in Vegetation" (1831), enable the spectator to gain access to "an inner perception" (*WA* II.7, 54). In the chapter "Meditations on the Doctrine of Colour and Treatment of Colour in Ancient Writers," part of the historical section of the *Doctrine of Colour*, Goethe speaks of the necessity of seeing science in terms of art. He argues here that, "because, in knowledge just as in reflection, no totality can be brought together – since, in the former, there is no inside, in the latter, there is no outside – we must necessarily conceive science as art, if we are to expect any kind of totality from it." At the same time he speaks of the need to understand any given moment within an aesthetic framework. "The abysses of intuition, a certain perception of the present, mathematical depth, physical precision, heights of reason, acuity of understanding, flexible, desiring fantasy, loving delight in the sensuous" – all these matter, for "nothing can be neglected in the living, fruitful seizing of the moment, through which a work of art, whatever its content, can be created" (*HA* 14, 41).

In his essay "Judgment through Intuitive Perception," Goethe seeks to align this mode of perception with the theory of knowledge propounded by Immanuel Kant. Hence, the frequency with which the term *Anschauung*—implying not just visual but intuitive or nondiscursive apprehension of an object—can be found in Goethe's writings, as in, for example, his maxim that "thinking is more interesting than knowing, but not more than intuition" (*HA* 12, 398). Or to put it another way, thinking is not more interesting than seeing – *seeing*, that is, *with the eyes of the spirit*.

According to the British scholar Elizabeth M. Wilkinson, "Goethe developed the technique of *Anschauung* into a methodological discipline and a fine art; it was by means of it that he made the discoveries he did about the forms of animals and plants" (Wilkinson 1962: 178). Such an *Anschauung* is thematized, too, in many of Goethe's poetic texts, the best-known example perhaps being the affirmation in the conclusion of his "Metamorphosis of Animals" of "the delightful utter certainty" that we can *see*, not just fantasize: "Stand where you are, be still, and looking behind you, backward,/All things consider, compare, and take from the lips of the Muse then,/So that you'll see, not dream it, a truth that is sweet and is certain" (*GE* 1, 162–163). And *Anschauung* remains true to Goethe's ambition to see the inner and the outer in mutually reciprocal terms, as the following short text: "Should you succeed in contemplation:—/First see the inside of creation/And then towards the outside turn—/Then from this you will greatly learn" (*WA* I.4, 137).

For his part, C.G. Jung seeks to integrate intellect and feeling in his approach to the psyche, telling us that both are required to offer an adequate explanation of the psyche. For him, the intellectual judgment alone is "at best, a half-truth" and must admit its own inadequacy (*CW* 6, §856). In a typically Goethean gesture, Jung speaks of taking both approaches, the "causal-reductive" and the "constructive-prospective," and using them to create a "higher synthesis." Only by acknowledging the existence of the types and investigating the typical self-representations of the psyche, as he writes in the "Epilogue" to *Psychological Types*, will we be able to gather the material "whose co-operation will make possible a higher synthesis" (*CW* 6, §857). This notion of SYNTHESIS is linked with the central concepts of MORPHOLOGY, that is, with POLARITY and *STEIGERUNG* (INTENSIFICA-TION). In turn these ideas feed into a conception of the SELF, into a missionary vision *KULTUR* and into a theory of the SYMBOL. To these connections we shall, in the rest of this chapter, now turn. But before that, let us consider some aspects of Goethe's own life and experience.

Goethe's Crisis

It is worth noting the personal background of physiological and psychological crises against which Goethe's life developed. These aspects are often overlooked by his biographers, yet they provide important clues as to why Goethe developed the conception of health that he did. In July 1768, just before he turned 19, Goethe suffered a heart complaint aggravated by excess, from which he took over a year to recover. At the time he was a student in Leipzig, and the pulmonary haemorrhage forced him to convalesce at his home in Frankfurt am Main for over a year. During this period, Goethe began to move in pietist circles and, encouraged by a friend of his mother, Susanna Katharina von Klettenberg, he read various works on mysticism, alchemy and theosophy. As a result, he immersed himself in writings on Gnosticism, Hermetics, Kabbalah and Neoplatonism, including Georg von Welling's *Opus mago-cabbalisticum*, the *Aurea Catena Homeri* and several works by Philippus Aureolus Theophrastus Bombastus von Hohenheim (1493–1541), better known as Paracelsus. When he was recovered, Goethe identified as the effect of convalescence a complete psychological change in himself; at least, this is implied when he says, "I also seemed to have become a different person now" (*GE* 4, 248).

In his home, Goethe set up a small laboratory, and when he went back to university in March 1770, this time in Strasbourg, he continued his investigations into what he called "my mystic-cabalistic chemistry" (*GE* 4, 307). Of his time as a student, he wrote in *Dichtung und Wahrheit* that he was "really more familiar with church history than secular history" (*GE* 4, 351), and he completed a dissertation on the history of religion. As a further witness to the persistence of his interest in Biblical matters, in 1772–1773 he wrote about "Two Important but Hitherto Undiscussed Biblical Questions": did the stones Moses carried down from Sinai contain the ten commandments or ritual cult laws? What was the significance of the speaking in tongues at Pentecost? (*GE* 4, 378–379). But on 26 August 1770, he had told Fräulein von Klettenberg in a letter, "Chemistry is still my secret love."

Much later on in his life, shortly before he began work on his late, great poem entitled "Primal Words. Orphic," Goethe evoked, in a letter to Carl Friedrich Zelter of 26 March 1816, the idea that "each of us has something special inside us, that we seek to develop, by letting it continue to work its effect," a "wondrous being that does its best for us day by day, and so one grows old, without knowing how or why." This notion is closely related to Goethe's use of the Aristotelian concept of *entelechy*. According to Aristotle, each organism can be considered in three ways: (i) its power, or its potential as possibility (*dynamis*); (ii) its energy, its actuality in reality (*energeia*); and (iii) its goal as the organism realizes it in itself (*entelecheia*).[5] Several years later, in conversation with Eckermann on 3 March 1830, Goethe affirmed the Aristotelian concept of *entelechy* and a related idea, the Leibnizian concept of the monad. He remarked that "the obstinacy of the individual and the fact that man shakes off what does not suit him" was "a proof" that something like Aristotle's *entelechy* exists, and he added that Leibnitz had had "similar thoughts about independent beings, and indeed what we term an entelechy he called a monad."

From his personal experience, Goethe understood the function of a physiological or psychological crisis, and his understanding of the individual's biography was essentially a developmental one. As we shall see, his morphological theories are based around notions of change, process and transformation.

Jung's Psychological Understanding

In a paper published in 1914 called "On Psychological Understanding," Jung articulates the difference between his approach and Freud's – between, as he calls them, an "analytic" approach and a "synthetic" approach. He makes this distinction, significantly enough, with reference to the problem of interpreting *Faust*.

According to Jung, although "the analytical-reductive procedure" (as he calls Freudian psychoanalysis) may work well with some cases, such as hysteria, it is less successful at dealing with others, such as schizophrenia (*dementia praecox*). As an example of his feeling "that this method does not altogether do justice to the almost overpowering profusion of fantastic symbolization," Jung cites the case of *Faust* – a text that is truly an overwhelming profusion of fantastic symbolization!

When an academic or a scholarly commentator on *Faust*, as Jung puts it, "traces back all the multifarious material of Part Two to its historical sources," or when he

> gives a psychological analysis of Part One showing how the conflict in the drama springs from a conflict in the soul of the poet and how this subjective conflict is itself based on those ultimate and universal problems which are not strange to us because we all carry the seeds of them in our own hearts,

our response, Jung says, is one of gratitude. (He is being too kind; one suspects that, deep down, his own response was one of boredom). "Nevertheless," Jung adds, "we are a little disappointed" – because such an approach risks being too reductive. After all, he notes, "we do not read *Faust* just to discover that things everywhere are 'human, all-too-human'" (*CW* 3, §391). So why do we read *Faust*? And why should we read *Faust*?

At this point in his paper, Jung reintroduces the opposition between, on the one hand, "retrospective understanding," that is, the "analytic-reductive" approach, which reduces "the unknown to the known and the complicated to the simple," and on the other what Jung calls "prospective understanding," that is, a "constructive" or "synthetic" method. There are echoes in all this of the German philosopher Wilhelm Dilthey (1833–1911), who argued that what distinguishes the humanities from natural science is the reliance of the former on *Verstehen* ('understanding' – or interpretation *from within*) and of the latter on *Erklären* ('explanation' – or interpretation *from outside*), but in Dilthey himself there are also echoes of Goethe and clear references to him.

Jung describes Freud's method of psychological explanation as "strictly scientific" (*CW* 3, §392). Yet this "scientific" method is, Jung argues, inadequate to explain something as complex as *Faust*:

> When we apply this method to *Faust*, it becomes clear that something more is required for a real understanding. We realize that we have completely missed the deepest meaning the poet strove to express if we see in it *only* the universally human—for we can see the universally human wherever we look. What we really want to find in *Faust* is how this human being redeems himself as an individual, and when we have understood that, we have understood Goethe's symbolism.
>
> (*CW* 3, §393)

To use the terminology deployed by Jung in his lecture, we need to aim for understanding that is "objective" – and an understanding is "objective," he continues, when it "connects with life." Such an "objective understanding" is, Jung emphasizes, *not* the same as "causal understanding" (*CW* 3, §416, n.15). This kind of "objective" thinking is, rather, close to the "objective thinking" – or *gegenständliches Denken* – espoused by Goethe.

In "Significant Help Given by an Ingenious Turn of Phrase," Goethe welcomes the commendation afforded his work by the Leipzig professor of psychiatry and anthropology Johann Christian Heinroth, and specifically his praise in his *Textbook of Anthropology* for how Goethe's thinking "works objectively." What this means, Goethe explains, is that "my thinking is not separate from objects; that the elements of the object, the perceptions of the object, flow into my thinking and are fully permeated by it; that my perception itself is a thinking, and my thinking a perception" (*GE* 12, 39). This is precisely the kind of thinking in which Jung is interested – a kind of thinking which corresponds to this (Goethean) kind of "objective" thinking; it is a form of thinking that relates the object to the subject and vice versa. We could call it, in fact, *seeing with the eyes of the spirit*.

What is at stake in this distinction is explained by Jung as follows:

> Anyone who understands *Faust* "objectively",[6] from the causal standpoint, is—to take a drastic example—like someone who tries to understand a Gothic cathedral under its historical, technical, and finally its mineralogical aspect. But—where is the *meaning* [*der Sinn*] of the marvellous edifice? Where is the answer to that all-important question: what goal of redemption did the human being of the Gothic period seek in his work, and how have we to understand his work subjectively, in and through ourselves?
>
> (*CW* 3, §396)

For Jung, the essential precondition of understanding something psychological was the awareness that all knowledge is subjectively conditioned: that is to say, "the world is not 'objective' only; it is also as we see it" (*CW* 3, §397). And so Jung opens up the possibility of a reading of *Faust* that is not "causal" or "reductive" but rather "synthetic" or "constructive":

> A causal understanding of *Faust* tells us very clearly how it came to be a finished work of art, but it does not show us its living meaning created by the poet, which is only alive because we experience it in and through ourselves. Insofar as our actual life, the life we live here and now, is something essentially new and not just a continuation of the past, the main value of a work of art does not lie in its causal development but in its living effect. We should be depreciating a work like *Faust* if we regarded it merely as something that has come to be, and is finished and done with. *Faust* is understood only when it is apprehended as something that becomes alive and creative again and again in our own experience.
>
> (*CW* 3, §398)

Moreover, such a style of interpretation can and must also be applied, Jung suggests, to the interpretation of the human psyche. For "the human soul" is, only in one respect, "something-that-has-come-to-be" and, as such, subject to the causal standpoint. In other respects, it is "something-in-the-process-of-becoming," which "can only be grasped synthetically or constructively" (*CW* 3, §399).[7] (What this means is that we should, Jung believes, read *Faust* as we would "read" the psyche, and "read" the psyche as we would read *Faust*. Equally, might a careful reading of *Faust* put us in a position to "read" the psyche?)

For, in Jung's terms, the psyche occupies the point of intersection between the past and the future because it provides us with "a picture of the remnants and traces of all that is past," and yet in this picture it also gives us "a picture of the burgeoning knowledge of all that is to come, insofar as the psyche itself creates the future" (*CW* 3, §404). Only the "prospective"-"constructive"-"synthetic" method can, Jung argues, understand the psyche as something that is, to use a Goethean term, "something-in-the-process-of-becoming." The subtlety, allusiveness and resonance of Goethean thinking in this passage from Jung is, even in English translation, quite extraordinary:

> What has become is on the one hand the result and culmination of all that has been — this is how it appears to the causal standpoint — and on the other it is an expression of what is to come. Since what is to come is only apparently like the past, but in its essence always new and unique — (the causal standpoint likes to reverse this proposition) — so the present expression of what has become is incomplete, germlike, as it were, in relation to what is to come. Insofar as we regard the present content of the psyche as a symbolic expression of what is to come, the need arises to apply a constructive interest to it. I almost felt tempted to say a "scientific" interest. But our science is identical with the causal principle. As soon as we regard the present psyche causally, that is, scientifically, the psyche as *something-that-is-becoming* eludes us.
>
> (*CW* 3, §405)

Later, in 1929, Jung returns to this dialectical synthesis of the past in the present and the present in the past, and the present in the future and the future in the present. In a short essay published in the *Kölner Zeitung*, Jung again contrasts his own position with Freud's. Here he speaks of the libidinal drives as coming into collision with the spirit (or, to use that scintillating, puzzling German word, with *Geist*) (*CW* 4, §776). Although Jung does not shy away from the fact that he cannot say precisely what *Geist* is, he clearly regards it as a liberating force, as a means of escaping what he calls "the inexorable cycle of biological events" or, as he more strikingly describes it, "the fleshly bond leading back to father and mother or forward to the children that have sprung from our flesh"—from "'incest' with the past and 'incest' with the future," from "the original sin of perpetuation of the 'family romance'" (*CW* 4, §780).

From such shackles, Jung writes, only *Geist* can free us, and he insists on the need for an "authentic-experience-of-the-primordial," for *Urerfahrung*, as he calls it. "We moderns are faced with the necessity of rediscovering the life of the spirit: we must experience it anew for ourselves," he declares, for "it is the only way," he insists, in which we can break "the spell that binds us to the cycle of biological events" (*CW* 4, §780). Thus, Jung raises the tantalizing prospect that a return to the "archaic" and to the "primordial" is also, paradoxically enough, a way forward to the future.

The vocabulary of *Urerfahrung* is redolent of Goethe's famous terminology of the *Urphänomen* (the "primordial" phenomenon), the *Urpflanze* (the "primordial" plant) or the *Urtier* (the "primordial" animal), which brings us to the role of synthesis in Goethe's system of morphology.

Morphology

In a fragmentary text entitled "Polarity," we find a comprehensive list of the opposites in which Goethe is interested: subject(s) and object(s); light and dark; body and soul; the "two souls" that live, alas, in the breast of Faust (*zwei Seelen wohnen, ach! in meiner Brust*); spirit and matter; God and world; thought and extension; ideal and real; sensuality and reason; fantasy and practical thought; being and yearning; the two halves of the body; right and left; breathing (in and out); and magnetism (positive and negative) (*GE* 12, 155).

Polarity is, Goethe says, "a state of constant attraction and repulsion," "a property of matter insofar as we think of it as material" (*GE* 12, 6). According to this principle, the tension between polar opposites provides the mechanism by which life develops. This tension, or *Spannung*, is "the apparently indifferent state of an energetic entity that is on the brink of manifesting itself, differentiating itself, and entering into polarity," as Goethe formulates the idea in an aphorism (*HA* 12, 369).

This dynamic, polaristic conception of nature is even more vividly expressed in another of his *Maxims and Reflections*, in which Goethe writes that the "basic characteristic of an individual organism" is

> to divide, to unite, to merge into the universal, to abide in the particular, to transform itself, to define itself, and, as living things tend to appear under a thousand conditions, to arise and vanish, to solidify and melt, to freeze and flow, to expand and contract.
>
> (*GE* 12, 303–304)

Through the very structure of this sentence, we can see how dynamic – how pullulating with energy – Goethe's conception of organic life is.

In his "Introduction" to *The Propylaea*, the journal he founded to further his aesthetic views, Goethe speculates that

> perhaps the supposition will be proven that all colour effects in nature — like magnetic, electric or other effects — are based on reciprocity, on polarity, or whatever name we may give to the phenomena of duality or indeed multiplicity within one distinct unit.
>
> (*GE* 3, 83)

In fact, a short poetic saying by Goethe reveals, so to speak, the metaphysical ramifications of the magnet: ' "The secret of the magnet, explain that to me!"/No greater secret than love and enmity' (*HA* 1, 306) (here Goethe is tapping into an ancient idea, stretching back to Empedocles). Polarity constitutes, then, a global rhythm, a universal beat to which the entire organic world moves. "All organic movements manifest themselves through diastoles and systoles," as Goethe puts it in his fragment on a "Theory of Tone": "it is one thing to raise the foot, another to put it down," and in rhythmics we find both "weight and counterweight: . . . arsis, upbeat; thesis, downbeat" (*GE* 12, 301).

Polarity alone, however, is insufficient: whilst it provides the dynamic motor for development, that development relies on another principle, dubbed by Goethe *Steigerung*, or "intensification," and described in 1828 as a property of matter "insofar as we think of it as spiritual," as "a state of ever-striving ascent" (*GE* 12, 6). In a note titled "Problems," published in *On Morphology* in 1823, Goethe explains that whilst "the idea of metamorphosis deserves great reverence," it is also "a most dangerous gift from above," because it "leads to formlessness," it "destroys knowledge, dissolves it," and it is "like a *vis centrifuga*, and would be lost in the infinite if it had no counterweight." This counterweight is provided by "the drive-for-specific-character, the stubborn persistence of things which have finally attained reality . . . a *vis centripeta*," as he calls it, which remains basically untouched by any external factor (*GE* 12, 43).

As Goethe makes clear in his text on "Polarity," intensification arises out of polarity: "whatever appears in the world must divide if it is to appear at all," but "what has been divided seeks itself again, can return to itself and reunite," and this happens "in a lower sense when it merely intermingles with its opposite, combines with it" (here the phenomenon is "nullified or at least neutralized"). But *Steigerung* goes beyond *Polarität*, for the union may occur "in a higher sense if what has been divided is first intensified," and then, "in the union of the intensified halves," it will produce "a third thing, something new, higher, unexpected" (*GE* 12, 156). [We might well compare this statement with the principle enunciated by Jung in the "Epilogue" to "Paracelsus as a Spiritual Phenomenon," that "analysis is always followed by synthesis, and what was divided on a lower level will reappear, united, on a higher one" (*CW* 13, §238).]

For Goethe, a tangible example of intensification was provided in the plant world by the leaf, the petal and the fruit, so that "the same organs fulfil nature's laws throughout, although with different functions and under different guises." If these "laws" of morphology apply to all organisms, then they also apply to the self.

Self

Goethe's view of the self takes as its starting point the notion of the plural self, a conception that later greatly interested Friedrich Nietzsche (1844–1900), not to mention Jung. As Goethe writes in "The Purpose Set Forth" in *On Morphology*, the self has to be conceived as a multiplicity. For "each living thing is not unitary in nature, but a plurality," and "even insofar as it appears to us as an individual, it remains a collection of independent living beings." As these beings unite, diverge and unite again, so they bring about an unending process of production (*GE* 12, 64). The plural self, however, needs to be unified towards a central nodal point (or *Mittelpunkt*), even though, as Goethe noted in his journal entry for 14 July 1779, "to find the point of unification of the manifold always remains a secret."

That the realization of such a central nodal point in the individual human being is the goal of a Goethean project becomes even clearer if we turn to his review of a book called *Psychology in Clarification of Phenomena from the Soul* written by Ernst Anton Stiedenroth, professor of philosophy in Berlin and Greifswald. In this review, Goethe criticizes the doctrine of the rationalist philosophers Gottfried Wilhelm Leibniz and Christian Wolff, who divided the human being into "upper" – that is, rational and intellectual – and "lower" – that is, sensuous and physical – functions. Following the principles of Alexander Gottlieb Baumgarten in his *Aesthetica*, he argues that all of the faculties of the human being should be developed – *and* integrated and organized around a unifying nodal point. "In the human spirit, as in the universe," he writes, "nothing is higher or lower; everything has equal rights to a common centre [i.e., *Mittelpunkt*] which manifests its hidden existence precisely through this harmonic relationship between every part and itself' (*GE* 12, 45).

In his review of Stiedenroth, Goethe goes on to argue that four different faculties – the senses and reason, the understanding and the imagination (in German: *Sinnlichkeit und Vernunft, Einbildungskraft und Verstand*) – can be coordinated into a single totality, "a coherent whole" (*GE* 12, 45–46). Here, we find another echo of Herder who, in his treatise *On Knowing and Sensation of the Human Psyche*, had written that "the healthiest human beings of all ages excluded nothing: knowledge and sensation blended *together* in them into human life, into action, into happiness" (Herder 1985–2005: Vol. 4, 374).

In one of his last letters, written on 17 March 1832 to Wilhelm von Humboldt, we find Goethe insisting on the possibility of forging, through their proper use, all human faculties into a totality. "The organs of the human being," he writes, "by means of practice, theory, reflection, success, failure, support and resistance and ever-repeated reflection, link, unconsciously and in free activity, the acquired with the inborn, so that the result is a unity which astonishes the world." It would be hard to find a more concise statement of the project of analytical psychology. And how exactly do we bring about this unity? Through what Goethe calls (in his review of Stiedenroth) an "exact sensory imagination" (*GE* 12, 46) – in other words, through *seeing with the eyes of the spirit*.

Now, in the light of these texts by Goethe, we can see how Jung's comments on the self, particularly in *The Relations between the Ego and the Unconscious*, are saturated with Goethean notions. In this work, he uses the image of a nodal point – or what he calls *ein "Mittelpunkt der Persönlichkeit"* – to describe how the "self" is constellated:

> If we picture the conscious mind, with the ego at its centre, as being opposed to the unconscious, and if we now add to our mental picture the process of assimilating the unconscious, we can think of this assimilation as a kind of approximation of conscious and unconscious, where the centre of the total personality no longer coincides with the ego, but with a point midway between consciousness and the unconscious. This would be the point of new equilibrium, a new centering of the total personality, a perhaps virtual centre which, on account of its focal position between consciousness and the unconscious, ensures for the personality a new, more certain foundation.
>
> (*CW* 7, §365)

In the conclusion to his lecture on "Psychological Aspects of the Mother Archetype," Jung places a strong emphasis on the multiplicitous and conflictual state of the psyche. "Far from being a homogeneous unity," he writes, the psyche is quite the opposite, "a boiling cauldron of contradictory impulses, inhibitions, and affects" (*CW* 9/i, §190). And Jung speaks of "the unity of consciousness" or the personality as something not real or actual but as virtual and as something to be desired.

In his earlier formulations in *The Relations between the Ego and the Unconscious*, Jung speaks of the concept of the self in terms of a "transcendental postulate," as a necessary "hypothesis" which, "although justifiable psychologically," cannot be "proved scientifically" (*CW* 7, §405), and in a lecture in 1932 called *"Vom Werden der Persönlichkeit,"* he concedes that "personality," inasmuch as it is "the complete realization of our whole being," is "an unattainable ideal" (*CW* 17, §291). So the "self" is a form, a *Gestalt*, precisely in the sense that Goethe uses the word in *On Morphology* as "the idea, the concept, or an empirical element held fast for a mere moment of time" (*GE* 12, 64).

Elsewhere in *The Relations between the Ego and the Unconscious*, Jung describes "the desired 'mid-point' of the personality" as "that indescribable something between the opposites, or else that which unites them, or the result of conflict, or the product of energic tension: the coming to birth of personality, a profoundly individual step forward, the next stage" (*CW* 7, §382). In this formulation, we see once again the proximity of Jungian psychology to Goethe's concept of polarity, as well as to his "synthetic" concept of becoming. For Jung, the psyche is an energic, emergent entity, characterized by forces of polarity in a way that Goethe would have completely understood.

Now, the Jungian equivalents to the four faculties of which Goethe speaks in his review of Stiedenroth are the psychic "functions": thinking, feeling, sensation and intuition. Although these psychological functions do not map directly onto the faculties as classically understood, his distinction between "rational" and "irrational" functions corresponds extremely closely to the distinction between "upper" and "lower" faculties (*CW* 6, §983). And Jung, like Goethe, is insistent upon the need to coordinate all such drives, faculties or functions.

For Jung, as well as for Goethe, another image for this combination of the upper ('noble') and lower ('ignoble') faculties can be found in the esoteric tradition of alchemy.[8] (To a certain, if qualified, extent, we can also read *Faust* as an alchemical text.) In *The Relations between the Ego and the Unconscious*, Jung describes the "secret" of alchemy as "the fact of the transcendent function" and its unifying effect as "the transformation of personality through the blending and fusion of the noble with the base components," the union of "the differentiated with the inferior functions," the *coniunctio oppositorum* of "the conscious with the unconscious" (*CW* 7, §360).

But how is this fusion to take place? And how are these human faculties to be coordinated? For German classicism, the means by which the faculties are to be coordinated is aesthetic contemplation. In the aesthetic mode, all faculties are equal, but the coordinating faculty is the imagination, referred to in the eighteenth century as *Einbildungskraft, Imagination*, or *Phantasie*. Jung shared this view of the importance of the imagination or, as he called it, *Phantasie*. In *Psychological Types*, he describes "fantasy" (or *das Phantasieren*) precisely as "a particular form of activity that can manifest itself in all four basic functions" (*CW* 6, §731). Emphasising the visual aspects of fantasy, he defines it as "imaginative activity," as "the immediate expression of the vital activity of the psyche," and as "identical with the course of the psychic energy process" (*CW* 6, §722).

According to *Memories, Dreams, Reflections*, Jung developed his concept of the "self" in the years following his own mental collapse, that is, between 1918 and 1920. During these years, Jung began to understand that "the goal of psychic development is the self." The pattern of this psychic development is important: it is not a "linear development" but "a circumambulation of the self" (*MDR*, 222), a spiral movement, then, uniting the twin Goethean dynamics of "polarity" and "intensification" in an ever closer approximation to a virtual centre that arises from a coordination of all of the drives and all of the psychic functions.

Jung takes the traditional scholastic definition of God – "God is a circle whose centre is everywhere and the circumference nowhere" (*Deus est circulus cuis centrum est ubique, circumferentia vero nusquam*) (*CW* 11, §92 and §229) – and applies it to the self in the formula, "the self is not only the centre but also the whole circumference which embraces both conscious and unconscious" (*CW* 12, §44).

Drawing on the age-old imagery of the centre and the circle, Goethe uses the image of rotation in one of his maxims to express the living nature of the self. "The greatest gift that we have received from God and Nature," so runs this aphorism, "is life, the rotation of the monad around itself, which knows neither rest nor peace; and the impulse to cherish life dearly is in-born and imperishable in each of us" (*HA* 12, 396).

Kultur

Goethe once noted, in the context of Islamic monotheism, that "belief in one, single God always has an elevating effect on the mind, inasmuch as it refers the individual back to the unity of his own interior nature" (*HA* 2, 148). Writing to Goethe on 17 August 1795, Schiller had stated that, "Christianity virtually contains the first elements of what is highest and noblest," by virtue of which he described it as "the only *aesthetic* religion." And we might recall Goethe's remark on Schiller in a letter to Zelter of 9 November 1830: "Schiller was born with an authentic Christ-like tendency, he touched nothing that was common without ennobling it" (*Schiller war eben die echte Christustendenz eingeboren, er berührte nichts Gemeines, ohne es zu veredeln*, as the sentence runs in German).

In his lecture "Psychotherapy Today," Jung insists on the link between attitude and *Anschauung*, claiming that someone's "way of looking at things" is of "enormous importance" for his or her "psychic health," so much so, indeed, that one might almost say that "things are less what they are than how we see them" (*CW* 16, §218). Or, as Goethe once put it, "There is nothing unimportant in the world. It all depends on how you look at it" (or, as the passage runs in German, *Es gibt nichts Unbedeutendes in der Welt. Es kommt nur auf die Anschauungsweise an*) (*WA Gespräche* 4, 59).

As far as Jung is concerned, religions are not just "therapies for the sorrows and disorders of the soul" but they also offer, as he pointed out in 1929, a way to "a higher level of consciousness and culture" (*CW* 13, §71). Similarly, in his lecture on "The Aims of Psychotherapy" (1929/1931), Jung emphasizes the importance of the therapeutic value of the religious attitude and, mutatis mutandis, of historical continuity, for "it is precisely for the religious function that the sense of historical continuity is indispensable" (*CW* 16, §99). In other words, Jung's interest in religion is primarily concerned with its historical and, above all, its *cultural* functions.

For the instrument, by means of which we move towards self-fulfilment, is – for Goethe, for Schiller, for Jung, and for the tradition they represent – called culture.[9] In *Memories, Dreams, Reflections*, we learn that Jung came to understand the necessity of holding to a set of precepts which, he believed, were expounded in *Faust*, albeit negatively, for the text shows us the consequences of ignoring these precepts. Jung, we read, "consciously linked" his work to "what Faust had passed over" – respect for everlasting human rights, recognition of "the ancient," and the continuity of culture and intellectual history (*MDR*, 262).

For his part, Goethe, writing to Herder from Rome on 10 November 1786 – after a day spent visiting the pyramid of Cestius and the archeological remains of the emperors' palaces on the Palatine, and with the ruins of ancient grandeur all around him – reflected on the importance of an awareness of continuity.

> When one contemplates such an existence, which is more than two thousand years old, which through the changes of time has altered in so many varied and in such fundamental ways, and yet still it is the same soil, the same hill, indeed, very often the same pillar and wall, and in the people one still finds traces of an ancient character . . . then one becomes a contemporary of the great decisions of destiny.

Even what is "unworthy and tasteless," things that are *Scheltenswertes und Abgeschmacktes*, can, he added, be recuperated within this historical vision; so there is even room in this perspective for popular culture.

Likewise, Goethe places great emphasis, in his conversation with Eckermann of 1 April 1827, on the importance of the awareness of tradition for the development of the individual. "Study Molière, study Shakespeare; but, above all things, the old Greeks, and always the Greeks," he urges. By way of reply to Eckermann's observation that for "highly-endowed natures the study of the authors of antiquity may be invaluable; but in general it appears to have little influence upon personal character," Goethe responds that, "a worthless man will always remain worthless; and a little mind will not, by daily intercourse with the great mind of antiquity, become one inch greater." For, he continues,

> a noble man, in whose soul God has placed the capability for future greatness of character and elevation of mind, will, through acknowledgement of and familiar intercourse with the elevated natures of ancient Greeks and Romans, develop to the utmost, and every day make a visible approach to similar greatness.

Why do the classics – why does classicism – matter? Because they contain within themselves the material for a cultural programme.[10]

This sentiment is well summarised in the quatrain from the *West-östlicher Divan*: "Those who cannot draw conclusions/From three thousand years of learning/Stay naïve in dark confusions,/Day to day live undiscerning" (*Wer nicht von dreitausend Jahren/Sich weiß Rechenschaft zu geben,/Bleib im Dunkeln unerfahren,/Mag von Tag zu Tage leben*) (*HA* 2, 49; Goethe 1998: 189). What clearly emerges, then, from the sum of Goethe's life and works is a *cultural imperative*.

From this point of view, Jung's range of learning and cultural sophistication makes him, in so many ways, a figure to be envied today. In practical terms, Jung acknowledges the role played by self-knowledge in the process of becoming conscious and participating in culture. For Jung, the solution to contemporary problems lies in the attainment of self-knowledge (or *Selbsterkenntnis*). "The individual who wishes to have an answer to the problem of evil, as it is posed today," we read in *Memories, Dreams, Reflections*, "has need, first and foremost, of *self-knowledge*, that is, the best possible knowledge of his own wholeness" (*MDR*, 362). As Jung makes clear in *Mysterium coniunctionis*, however, such knowledge is not easy to attain. "Self-knowledge is an adventure that carries us unexpectedly far and deep," he writes here, and "even a moderately comprehensive knowledge of the shadow can cause a good deal of confusion and obscurity, for it produces problems of the personality, which one had previously never remotely imagined" (*CW* 14, §741). For this reason, and "since the earliest times," human beings have had recourse to "artificial aids, ritual actions such as dances, sacrifices, identification with ancestral spirits," and so on, in order to engage with and bring back to memory "those deeper layers of the psyche" which "the light of reason and the power of the will" cannot reach (*CW* 14, §743). And Jung specifically makes the point that, although such ideas or *représentations collectives* are always "true," inasmuch as they "express the unconscious archetype," their cultural manifestation – "their verbal and pictorial form" – is "greatly influenced," as he says, by "the spirit of the age" (*CW* 14, §743).

According to Jung, self-knowledge or *Selbsterkenntnis* lies in extending the range of human consciousness whilst simultaneously acknowledging the power of the unconscious – the way that "the life, that has been repressed, forces its way into the open through all the cracks" (*CW* 14, §742). And this kind of self-knowledge is what Jung understood by culture, a position summed up in the aphoristic formula that "attainment of consciousness is culture in the broadest sense, and self-knowledge is therefore the heart and essence of this process" (*MDR*, 356). This emphasis on the link between understanding and culture is comparable with the remark made by another, more prominent, inheritor of the literary tradition of German classicism – Thomas Mann – in his letter to Klaus Mann of 22 July 1939: "But in the end, to inherit something one has to understand it; inheritance is, after all, culture."

From the perspective of German classicism and analytical psychology alike, the relationship between culture and the attainment of the self is a reciprocal one. For Goethe, Schiller and Jung, the significance of culture lies in assisting us to realize the central nodal point at which all faculties are fully exercised and co-ordinated. In this sense, self-knowledge is not a state but rather an activity. For the Enlightenment, the inscription on the Temple of Apollo at Delphi, "know thyself," a topos of the pre-Socratic Western tradition, was a well-known commonplace. In keeping with the Goethean dynamic of INNER and OUTER, however, we should perhaps also recall that the inscription continues: "Know thyself—and thou shalt know all the mysteries of the gods and of the universe." Yet, Goethe memorably voiced his suspicion of the oracle's command, writing the following in "Significant Help Given by an Ingenious Turn of Phrase":

> I must admit that that I have long been suspicious of the great and important-sounding task: 'know thyself'. This has always seemed to me a deception practised by a secret order of priests who wished to confuse humanity with impossible demands, to divert attention from activity in the outer world to some false, inner speculation.
>
> (*GE* 12, 39)

Might Goethe's suspicion of the oracle, over a century-and-a-half later, be extended to a suspicion of psychoanalysis and the narcissistic preoccupation of the modern self with itself? Can we be so preoccupied with our own well-being that we forget the need for political and social engagement? Goethe is often categorized as being a conservative thinker, but his conservatism is not one that excludes an activity in the public sphere!

For Goethe, self-knowledge is based on a recognition of the reciprocity of the inner (self) and the outer (world), according to the dictum that "the human being knows himself only insofar as he knows the world; he perceives the world only in himself, and himself only in the world." The importance of this insight is summarized in the aphoristic remark that "every new object, clearly seen" – i.e., *seen with the eyes of the spirit* – opens up a new organ of perception in us (*GE* 12, 39).

Similarly, the essential reciprocity of self and world runs like a *leitmotif* throughout Jung's writings, and to align the subject(ive) and the object(ive), the self and the world, is what Jung – and Goethe – mean by "the symbolic life."

The Symbolic Life

Read from a Goethean perspective, then, and from the perspective of German classicism, what Jung meant by the "symbolic" is far removed from the comparatively impoverished conception of this term found in, say, the works of Jacques Lacan. In an early letter (10 December 1777) to Charlotte von Stein, Goethe told her, "you know how symbolic my existence is"; and many years later, he told Eckermann in a conversation of 2 May 1824, "I have always regarded all I have done solely as symbolical." Jung's quest for "the undiscovered self" (thus the title of his work of 1958) has its counterpart in Goethe's admission in his conversation with Friedrich Theodor Müller on 28 March 1830: "I have in fact always studied nature and art egoistically, namely to educate myself" (*WA Gespräche* 7, 282).

And it is Nietzsche, aware of his debt to Goethe and a major influence on Jung, who formulates exactly what is at stake in this classical conception of the self. In this passage of powerful literary encomium from *Twilight of the Idols*, Nietzsche offers a portrait *avant la lettre* of the Jungian "self," which brings out the classical values embodied, iconographically, in the figure of Goethe. This portrait remains a compelling evocation of the archetype of the fully individuated "self":

> *Goethe*—not a German event but a European one. . . . What he aspired to was *totality*; he strove against the separation of reason, sensuality, feeling, will (—preached in the most horrible scholasticism by Kant, the antipodes of Goethe); he disciplined himself to a whole, he *created* himself. . . . A spirit thus *emancipated* stands in the midst of the universe with a joyful and trusting fatalism, in the *faith* that only what is separate and individual may be rejected, that in the totality everything is redeemed and affirmed—*he no longer denies*.
>
> ("Expeditions of an Untimely Man," §49, in Nietzsche 1968: 102–103)

"Such a faith," Nietzsche proclaimed, is "the highest of all possible faiths"; a faith that he baptized "with the name *Dionysos*." And it is a vision that continues to inspire today, so that the contemporary French philosopher and Orthodox theologian, Bertrand Vergely, can write of "the symbolic life" (or *la vie symbolique*) without specific reference to Goethe nor to Nietzsche nor to Jung yet in terms highly redolent of all three. "The discovery of the world as a symbolic world," Vergely writes, "is a journey which procures an infinite joy." And he goes on: "The world was silent, insignificant. Now, suddenly, it begins to resonate with thousands of meanings, which in turn bring into motion an entire interior life unknown up this point" (Vergely 2002: 184).

So the tradition continues into our own day, for can we *see with our own eyes of the spirit* how a vast continent of thought opens up: to the list of Goethe, Herder,

Schiller, Nietzsche and Jung, we can add Vergely – and, or so remains to be seen, Rudolf Steiner too.[11]

Abbreviations

CW = Jung, *Collected Works*, ed. Sir H. Read, M. Fordham, G. Adler, and W. McGuire, 20 vols. London: Routledge & Kegan Paul. Cited in the text with volume number plus paragraph number.

GE = Goethe Edition = Goethe's Collected Works, ed. V. Lamge, E.A. Blackall, and C. Hamlin, 12 vols. Boston, MA: Suhrkam/Insel; New York: Suhrkamp, 1983–1989.

HA = Hamburger Ausgabe = Werke, ed. E. Trunz, 14 vols. Hamburg: Wegner, 1948–1960; Munich: Beck, 1981.

MDR = C.G. Jung, *Memories, Dreams, Reflections: Recorded and edited by Aniela Jaffé*, tr. R. Winston and C. Winston. London: Fontana, 1983.

WA = Weimarer Ausgabe = Werke, ed. J.L.G. von Leoper, E. Schmidt, and P. Raabe, im Auftrage der Großherzogin Sophie von Sachsen, four parts, 133 volumes in 143. Weimar: Böhlau, 1887–1919.

Notes

1 The following abbreviations are used in this chapter: *CW* = Jung, *Collected Works*; *GE* = Goethe Edition, Suhrkamp; *HA* = *Goethe, Werke* [Hamburger Ausgabe]; *MDR* = Jung, *Memories, Dreams, Reflections*; *WA* = *Goethe, Werke* [Weimarer Ausgabe].
2 Instruction for a Blessed Life, or Religious Doctrine (1806) (in Fichte 1962: Vol. I.9, 100).
3 Zur Farbenlehre (in *WA* II.5, 12).
4 Sculpture (1778) (in Herder 1985–2005: Vol. 4, 280).
5 According to the anthroposophically oriented literary critic Friedrich Hiebel, these three aspects can be mapped, respectively, onto three different stages of life, namely, (i) childhood as the age of possibility, of artistic potential; (ii) youth as the age of educative energy, the mastering of artistic skills; (iii) maturity, in which the artistic entelechy can reveal itself in full (Hiebel 1961: 15).
6 In the sense of *objektiv*, that is, Freudian, scientific objectivity, not Goethean objectivity (*gegenständlich*).
7 In English, these phrases sound quite clumsy; in German, however, they are elegant simplicity itself (*ein Gewordenes, ein Werdendes*).
8 For further discussion, see Gray (1952) and Hartlaub (1954).
9 For an overview of this conception of culture, which embraces the sciences and the humanities, I recommend Watson (2010).
10 For an admittedly polemical, or refreshingly frank, discussion of this issue, see V.D. Hanson and J. Heath 2001.
11 This chapter was originally presented at an event titled Seeing with the Eyes of the Spirit: Carl Jung and Rudolf Steiner on a Theme of Goethe, an event held at the Guild of Pastoral Psychology on 20 October 2012. I am grateful to the Guild for the original invitation and for permission to reproduce the text.

References

Cassirer, E. (1996). *The Philosophy of Symbolic Forms*, vol. 4, *The Metaphysics of Symbolic Forms*, ed. J.M. Krois and D.P. Verene, trans. J.M. Krois, New Haven and London: Yale University Press.

Fichte, J.G. (1962). *Gesamtausgabe der Bayerischen Akademie der Wissenschaften*, ed. R. Lauth and H. Gliwitzky, Stuttgart: Formmann (Holzboog).

Goethe, J.W. (1998). *Poems of the West and East: West-Eastern Divan — West-Östlicher Divan: Bi-Lingual Edition of the Complete Poems*, trans. J. Whaley, Berne, Berlin, Frankfurt/Main: Lang.

Gray, R. (1952). *Goethe the Alchemist: A Study of Alchemical Symbolism in Goethe's Literary and Scientific Works*, Cambridge: Cambridge University Press.

Hanson, V.D. and J. Heath (2001). *Who Killed Homer? The Demise of Classical Education and the Recovery of Greek Wisdom*, New York: Encounter Books.

Hartlaub, G.F. (1954). 'Goethe als Alchemist', *Euphorion* 48, 19–40.

Herder, J.G. (1985–2005). *Werke*, 10 vols, Frankfurt am Main: Deutscher Klassiker Verlag.

Hiebel, F. (1961). *Goethe: Die Erhöhung des Menschen: Perspektiven einer morphologischen Lebensschau*, Munich and Berne: Francke.

Nietzsche, F. (1968). *Twilight of the Idols and The Anti-Christ*, trans. R.J. Hollingdale, Harmondsworth: Penguin

Vergely, V. (2002). *Petite philosophie du bonheur*, Toulouse: Éditions Milan.

Watson, P. (2010). *The German Genius: Europe's Third Renaissance, the Second Scientific Revolution, and the Twentieth Century*, London, New York, Sydney, Toronto: Simon & Schuster.

Wilkinson, E.M. (1962). 'Goethe's Conception of Form', in E.M. Wilkinson and L.A. Willoughby, eds., *Goethe: Poet and Thinker*, London: Arnold. 166–184.

Chapter 2

Ann Casement

I was brought unwittingly to Jung in 1964, at which time I was struggling with a recurring situation. An enlightened GP referred me to someone I "could talk to", who turned out to be a Jungian analyst—most unusual in those days. I took to analysis immediately and went thrice weekly to discuss dreams, smoke a few cigarettes, and drink coffee. In that first cozy analysis, I started on the painful process of working through the greatest loss of my life—India, my motherland, and being brought, aged 13, to live with my father in London. He was (overtly) a highly successful architect helping to rebuild our part of London, Knightsbridge, where the devastation wrought by the Blitz was still in evidence. He was also (covertly) seriously damaged from fighting in World War II and suffering from PTSD—thus began my early initiation into trying to manage severe mental trauma.

Six months into my first analysis, it was suggested I might be interested in reading some of Jung's books—I have photographs of myself holding a copy of *Answer to Job*, not a word of which I understood at the time. It was also suggested I might like to attend lectures at the Analytical Psychology Club, which I duly did and soon became aware of tensions between senior analysts. The leaders of these antagonistic factions were, of course, Gerhard Adler and Michael Fordham, which signaled the outbreak of the "Jung Wars" of the 1970s in London and the beginnings of in-depth experiences for me of witnessing shadow projections. I have since written and lectured on the topic of shadow, each time finding something new to learn from that old devil.

In the course of that first analysis, I was astonished to have it suggested to me that I might start to train as a "therapist" myself. In due course, I embarked on training that was located in Central Hall across the road from Westminster Abbey and the Houses of Parliament, where I used to time sessions with "clients" according to the chimes of Big Ben.

I was not impressed by the training and so went back into academe for a few years, which I found much more intellectually stimulating, but the psychoanalytic bug was firmly lodged in my psyche and would not let go. I began training again, starting with an internship in psychiatry, which I loved so much I stayed working there for several years. Simultaneously, I was training as a Jungian psychoanalyst at one of the London IAAP societies, though I was tempted to apply to the British Society as my work in psychiatry was supervised by a senior IPA member of the

DOI: 10.4324/9781003148982-3

BP-AS. The main reason I did not do so was because I have always felt that it is important to stay with and work through wherever life brings. Alongside this, Hella and Gerhard Adler, who were then hugely significant and charismatic figures in the analytical psychology world, wanted me to work with them. In the event, I couldn't resist training with people who had been so close to C.G. and Emma Jung.

It was a wrench leaving psychiatry, as I was offered a consultancy, but I realized I wanted to devote my life to functioning as a psychoanalyst not as a therapist working mainly with psychosis. I had grown to love the work and the patients, but life does present difficult choices from time to time.

For decades, I have been practicing as a psychoanalyst in the developmental tradition pioneered by the great Michael Fordham. I am also drawn to the archetypal approach, which I combine with the more clinical one and which I began to learn in the course of having my work supervised by an IPA psychoanalyst. These different approaches have merged to inform my own way of functioning as a psychoanalyst, with Jung's thinking on psychological alchemy ever present. Like Michael, I feel I can never repay Jung for what his work has contributed to every area of my life except by being my own individual self.

Three dyads have been my guides through life—Vishnu/Ganpati, Gandhi/Nehru, and Freud/Jung—and, synthesizing all three, my grandmother.

Professor Ann Casement, London, 2020

A Critical Appraisal of C. G. Jung's Psychological Alchemy

Originally published in Casement, A. (2021). "A Critical Appraisal of C.G. Jung's Psychological Alchemy." In *Jung: An Introduction*. Phonix Publishing House. Reprinted with permission.

Preamble

Psychological alchemy as theorized and practiced by Jung was an important contribution to psychology and has its roots in the ancient art of alchemy, a cross-cultural practice in various parts of the world, including Arabia, China, Egypt, England, France, Germany, Greece, India, Japan, Persia, and Spain. The founding father of *Eastern* alchemy appears to have been Wei Po-yang, who produced the earliest known Chinese treatise on alchemy in 142 CE.

Western alchemy originated in Hellenistic Egypt in approximately 300 BCE; its purported originator, named Hermes Trismegistus (Thrice Great) by the Greeks, is associated with the Egyptian scribe god Thoth, the personification of wisdom, and with the Greek god of communication, Hermes. *Hermetics*, the body of knowledge that grew out of alchemy and that incorporates the physical, astral, and spiritual disciplines over which Hermes or *Mercurius* rules, is the highest knowledge one can attain. The term *hermetic*, meaning tightly sealed, relates to the secure alchemical *container*. "As above, so below" (Jung, 1967**a**, 1967b, p. 140) is the saying from the Emerald Tablet of Hermes Trismegistus associated with this body of knowledge. From 1300 to 1600 CE, *Hermetics* was an important source of knowledge for scientists, as it incorporated a way of influencing and controlling nature.

"As above" indicates the macrocosm, namely, the universe or God. "So below" points to the microcosm, namely, the physical world of human beings. This has been linked theoretically to the *global* and *local* that are inextricably mixed in *chaos theory*, a branch of mathematics that studies the behaviour of dynamical systems which are highly sensitive to initial conditions, for instance, a butterfly flapping its wings in New Mexico at the right point in space and time can cause a hurricane in China—referred to as the *butterfly effect*.

Alchemy's heyday in Europe was during medieval and early modern times, the latter period spanning the late fifteenth century, when printing was invented, to the eighteenth century. One of its best-known practitioners, Paracelsus, the sixteenth-century Swiss physician and alchemist, is often referenced by Jung. Three main aims in the practice of alchemy were to turn base metals into gold; to search for a panacea (the *elixir* or *philosopher's stone*) that would prolong life; and to attempt to produce various substances that would increase the production of vegetation. In early modern Europe, alchemists were mostly concerned with creating pharmacological concoctions, though most attached some religious significance to their work as they were dealing with God's creation—nature.

The pre-eminent seventeenth- to eighteenth-century scientist Isaac Newton spent up to 40 years experimenting on alchemy in his laboratory; apart from any other outcome, this helped to inform his treatise on light called *Opticks*. Newton had to keep secret his alchemical experiments ("chymistry") as they would have been considered heretical by the Christian Church. He was well aware that science advances through effort accumulated over centuries when he acknowledged that if he had seen further, it was by standing on the shoulders of giants. I dare speculate that although this well-known sentiment is usually interpreted as referring to his forerunners in science such as the polymath, Descartes, he was also alluding to the mysteries unraveled in his alchemical quest.

Jung's interest in alchemy was presaged by dreams, culminating in a crucial one in 1926 that showed him and a little coachman in danger on the Italian wartime front with shells exploding all around them. They arrive at an idyllic landscape with a manor house, and as they drive into the courtyard, the gates clang shut behind them. Jung thought they were now trapped in the seventeenth century (Jung, 1963, p. 194).

"The Secret of the Golden Flower"

A dream that preceded this one depicted him in a large house where he discovered a wonderful library dating from the sixteenth and seventeenth centuries. It contained a number of books full of symbols, which he realized many years later were alchemical symbols. At the time Jung was mystified until, in 1928, the Sinologist Richard Wilhelm, sent him a Chinese alchemical text "The Secret of the Golden Flower", though the original Chinese title of this text was "The Mystery of the Golden Light of the Supreme Unity." Jung and Wilhelm published this text in the November 1929 *Europäische Revue,* Volume 2/8, which Jung titled "The Secret of the Golden Flower."

In this text, Jung claimed he had discovered a parallel to the analytical process, namely, the alchemical *opus* of extracting gold from base metals which, in *psychological* terms, is the extraction of the gold of *consciousness* from its source deep in the base matter of *unconsciousness*, ultimately leading to the higher union of two *psychic* realms.

Jung's commentary on "The Secret of the Golden Flower" contains the following:

> What we have left behind are . . . not the psychic facts that were responsible for the birth of the gods. We are still as much possessed by autonomous psychic contents as if they were Olympians. Today they are called phobias, obsessions, and so forth; in a word neurotic symptoms. The gods have become diseases.
>
> (1967b, p. 37)

Why Alchemy?

In order to address this question, we shall return to some of the salient points in the foregoing dream. Although World War I had ended eight years before, Jung deduced that the conflict continues to be fought *intrapsychically*, ergo he had to turn his vision "inwards" to find the solution to the problems represented by the dangerous exploding shells. Jung concluded that they were missiles from the realm of *collective unconsciousness*, primordial inherited structures of the brain from whence everything irrational proceeds. When *archetypal* contents erupt into *consciousness*, they have a highly charged emotional impact and bring with them an experience of *psychic reality*.

Another point of note from the dream is "[n]ow we are caught in the seventeenth century" (Ibid.). That century was the heyday of alchemical experimentation in transmuting lead, or base matter, into gold. Furthermore, the *little* coachman puts one in mind of the *homunculus,* an important figure in *Faust*, Part 2. He is the creation of Faust, the alchemist, who acts as a *psychopomp*, that is, a guide to the inner world. It is the homunculus that realizes Faust needs to develop his feminine side, leading him to the land of mythological Greece and an encounter with Helen. The Italian landscape in the dream may stand for an idyllic pastoral vision, say, a Garden of Eden, wherein lies the *noble savage* uncorrupted by civilization, namely, the trappings of *ego*.

In the sixteenth-century alchemical text we shall be studying, Jung registered the fact that certain words or phrases reappeared throughout: *Mercurius, vas, lapis, prima materia, philosopher's stone*. Thus, Jung came to realize that the alchemists were expressing themselves in symbols through their oft-repeated saying that their gold was *not* the common gold. As symbols are key components of Jung's *psychological* approach, this led to his conclusion that analytical psychology and alchemy overlap. He went on to speculate—a key stance in *psychological alchemy*—that the alchemists preferred to be thought of as gold-makers rather than to be accused of heresy, a serious charge at that time.

Finding this historical link gave credence to the archetypal psychic contents that Jung had discovered in working with patients. Furthermore, the earthy, erotic images of alchemy were compensatory for the sexless imagery of Christianity. Above all, what Jung claimed to be the true opus of the more serious-minded alchemists was equated with his own work. In addition, the archetypal transmutation at work in alchemy gave Jung insight into his inner relationship to Goethe and, in particular, to the latter's magnum opus, *Faust*. We have already touched on the homunculus, though the figure of *Mephistopheles* from that work bears a striking resemblance to Mercurius, the trickster ruler of alchemy. For Jung, alchemy was above all a metaphor for working with unconscious material in analysis.

Mercurius is the central figure in alchemy associated with mercury—slippery, difficult to get hold of—which appears to be all things to all people. Furthermore, Mercurius consists of all conceivable opposites: that is, feminine-masculine; matter-spirit; the alchemical process itself that transmutes the lower into the higher and vice versa; and the devil's as well as God's reflection in physical nature. It is the dialectical work of psychological alchemy to release the mercurial spirit from the base matter of unconsciousness, namely, nature, through a recursive process of *fermentation, corruption, putrefaction, mortification, refinement*, and *distillation*—alchemical terms—in the laboratory of the mind. The hypothesis upon which we focus in this chapter, however, stems from a deeply personal reason for Jung's undertaking this work, namely, *incest*.

Transference-Countertransference

The conjoined term, *transference-countertransference*, is central to the *psychological alchemical* process. In psychoanalytic terminology, *transference* applies to *projections* from the *analysand* onto or, more intrusively, *into* the analyst. On one level, these projections are made up of *shadow* contents, along with those of *complexes*, feeling-toned autonomous subpersonalities present in *personal unconsciousness*. These complexes generally link back to the patient's past life, of which a simple example would be if the patient had a negative relationship with the personal father, this could result in a *negative father complex* being constellated and projected onto the analyst, who is experienced as a negative paternalistic authority figure. This kind of transference, activated by unresolved childhood deprivations and desires still alive in the adult analysand, needs to be worked through by way of *regression* to infantile states.

The term *countertransference* applies to the feelings *introjected* by the analyst as a result of the analysand's *transference projections*. This may be termed the *personal transference-countertransference*; when the analyst is largely in control and the *analysand* is being analyzed *by* the analyst is known as the *transference work*.

The emphasis in this chapter is on another kind of transference-countertransference which is not aimed at helping the analysand to "grow up." This is a dialectical process which involves both analysand and analyst in an immersion in unconscious contents that can bring about the *mutual* transformation of both. This transference process arises from a psychologically *incestuous* relationship between analyst and analysand, who are linked through kinship.

The alchemical process is not a once and for all experience but may be constellated in the course of in-depth analysis, with both analyst and analysand becoming increasingly aware that alchemical processes not only are to be found in analysis but are recurring experiences throughout life. In working through these, the analyst and analysand discover their own paths in life. These incestuous relations must not be concretized or acted in, but recognized and valued for what they are and worked through in the psychological alchemical processes of *corruption* and *distillation* until they can be symbolized.

It is this tortuous process of symbolization depicted in the sixteenth-century alchemical text that this chapter will explore.

> This does not mean that the adept ceased to work in the laboratory, only that he kept an eye on the symbolic aspects of his transmutations. This corresponds exactly to the situation in the modern psychology of the unconscious: while personal problems are not overlooked (the patient himself takes very good care of that!), the analyst keeps an eye on their symbolic aspects, for healing comes only from what leads the patient beyond himself and beyond his entanglements in the ego.
>
> (Jung, 1967**a**, **1967b**, p. 302)

Sabina Spielrein

Jung's intense preoccupation with alchemy led to his insistence that the first English translation of the *Collected Works* should be *Psychology and Alchemy* (personal communication, Gerhard Adler). Jung was particularly interested in the affinity between the ideas expressed in alchemy and his thoughts about archetypal transference-countertransference, which he went on to explore in the 1946 work "The Psychology of the Transference." In order to do this, he undertook a lengthy analysis of what he saw as symbolic transformation in ten woodcuts from a 1550 alchemical text called "The Rosarium Philosophorum", rendered in English as "The Rosary of the Philosophers" or "The Rose Garden."

Jung claimed that there was an analogy between these ten woodcuts and the analytic situation, wherein an *incestuous* attraction may arise between analyst and analysand when archetypal processes are activated in the course of an in-depth analysis. The *libido* that is released as a result may flow simultaneously in a variety of directions, leading to states of great confusion. At these times, the analytic relationship is tested to the full and may, indeed, break down if the powerful energies are not contained but, instead, are acted in.

"The Psychology of the Transference" may be viewed as a final working through of the powerfully erotic encounter Jung had as a young psychiatrist working at Burghölzli Hospital in Zürich with Sabina Spielrein, a nineteen-year-old Russian Jewish patient admitted in 1904, who was diagnosed as suffering from hysteria. Jung had read Freud's *The Interpretation of Dreams* (1976) and was so impressed by it that he adopted the new technique of psychoanalysis in his work with Spielrein, his first psychoanalytic patient. She was discharged from Burghölzli Hospital in 1905 still under Jung's care, and from that time, their joint erotic transference-countertransference feelings began to emerge as set forth in her diaries and letters. The intensity of their relationship peaked in the years 1908–1911, during which time both were in touch with Freud seeking his help. Jung was afraid of jeopardizing his marriage and professional career, and they eventually went their separate ways, though according to the Jungian psychoanalyst Aldo Carotenuto:

> It is reasonable to suppose that whenever Jung touched on the subject of the analyst's relations with the patient, his thought, both conscious and unconsciously, was nourished by his former experience, and in *The Psychology of the Transference* the memory of one of the first intense relationships in his life may well have reappeared with renewed ardour.
>
> (1982, p. 207)

Let us look more closely at what was taking place in the transference-countertransference between Spielrein and Jung. The patient's symptoms included tics, grimaces, and gestures of abhorrence, accompanied by severe headaches. The patient's premature sexuality, compulsive masturbation, and anal eroticism initially remained hidden but, once they manifested, were linked by Jung to the physical punishment her father inflicted on her, often hitting her on her bare buttocks in front of her brothers. Jung was regularly reporting the case to Freud, so it seems extraordinary that neither psychoanalyst diagnosed her illness as having its origin in the *incestuous* relationship with her father.

One may speculate that, for Freud, this oversight related to his relinquishing in 1897 of his earlier hypothesis of *actual* incest between father and daughter. Instead, he substituted *incestuous fantasies* on the part of the daughter for the father and of the son for the mother. This represents a vital turning point in Freud's theorizing that gave birth to psychoanalysis, with the situating of the universal *Oedipus complex* at the core of individual development, as Freud substituted the *reality* of fantasy for the *actuality* of physical incest. The omission of a diagnosis of incest on Jung's part may relate to the fact that he was always ambivalent about Freud's *libido* theory, though his notes contain the following about the beatings: "even though the peak of the experience was that her father was a *man*" (Graf-Nold, 2001, p. 87). This chapter aims to show that the abundant references to incest that

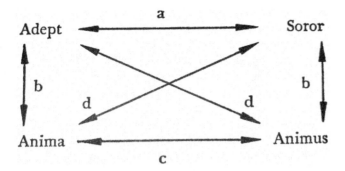

Diagram 2.1 Illustration of Transference-Countertransference

appear on almost every page throughout "The Psychology of the Transference" may be Jung's way of making reparations for his previous oversight in dealing with the incestuous transference-countertransference—both literal and symbolic: "the fatal touch of incest and its 'perverse fascination' symbolizes union with one's own being as a psychic reality, i.e., *individuation* through the endlessly recurring *uroboric* process" (Jung, 1954, p. 217). This incestuous relationship with oneself is fundamentally what Jung was exploring through psychological alchemy.

Jung's reference to Nietzsche's *Thus Spoke Zarathustra* may equally apply to the way in which he experienced working on the transference-countertransference in "The Rosarium": "*Zarathustra* is one of the books that is written with blood, and anything written with blood contains the notion of that subtle body the equivalent of the somatic unconscious" (Jarrett, 1988, p. 443).

For Jung, this reached its culmination in "The Psychology of the Transference", in which *anima* and *animus*, twinned archetypes, are central to the transference-countertransference process of working through affectively laden incestuous longings that are present in archetypal transference-countertransference, the instigator of which is, inevitably, familial. Jung's emphasis on the fact that analysis is a relationship, albeit a special kind of relationship which needs to be contained in the *alchemical retort*, is an important discovery for psychoanalysis.

The series of triangles in Jung's economical diagram (shown in Diagram 2.1), which appears at the beginning of "The Psychology of the Transference", expresses the various directions that transference-countertransference can take in the course of in-depth analysis. The straight line (a) at the top is the relatively uncomplicated personal relationship which helps create the *treatment alliance*. The straight, downward line (b) on the left side indicates the analyst drawing on her *unconscious* and being in touch with her inner *wounded healer* for an understanding of the patient's suffering. The straight, downward line (b) on the right represents the patient's initial awareness of the problems but also *resistance* to that awareness. The two diagonal lines (d) indicate the unconscious impact of the analytical relationship on the two participants, while the bottom straight line (c) points to a direct *unconscious* communication between them, which underpins the core of Jung's approach to archetypal transference-countertransference.

Particular attention should be paid to line (c), as it describes the phenomenon of *psychic contagion* or *projective identification*. All of the preceding were present over the course of the erotic relationship that existed between Jung and Spielrein, as evidenced in her letter to Freud in 1909: "Four and a half years ago Dr Jung was my doctor; then he became my friend and finally my 'poet,' i.e., my beloved. Eventually he came to me and things went as they usually do with 'poetry'" (Carotenuto, 1982, p. 93). Freud initially thought that with a bit more analysis everything could be resolved, including Spielrein's fantasy that "poetry" would lead to the birth of an actual child, Siegfried. Jung, who was Christian, and Spielrein, who was Jewish, fantasized about having an Aryan-Semitic love child. In this regard, Jung eventually wrote to Spielrein in a letter dated 21st January 1918: "You are always trying to drag the Siegfried symbol back into reality, whereas in fact it is the bridge to your individual development. . . . That is, individuation" (Carotenuto, 1982, p. 54).

Jung finally worked through these turbulent emotions in his 1946 paper "The Psychology of the Transference" exemplified by the symbolic "*coniunctio*", namely, the union of anima and animus depicted in line (c) of the diagram. This indicates the culmination of the alchemical process, namely, the birth of the symbolic "*divine child*", that is, Jung's notion of *individuation* as the longed-for Siegfried. Furthermore, Spielrein was an inspiration for Jung's concept of anima and his experience of countertransference. This diagram (shown in Diagram 2.1) succinctly illustrates Jung's view that alchemy was a metaphor for archetypal transference-countertransference, which results in an incestuous attraction not only between the two participants but, more importantly, *within* the analysand and the analyst, which Jung termed *kinship libido*. The latter stems from what Jung refers to as the "numinous idea, the archetype of incest" (1967a, 1967b, p. 301). He claimed it was through the *symbolization* of incestuous libido that the psychological alchemical work comes to its fruition.

"The Rosarium Philosophorum"

Figure 2.1 contains much alchemical symbolism: the sun and moon as opposites; the four elements depicted by four stars; the mercurial fountain and vessel (*vas*); and the *alchemical retort* as an analogy of the psychoanalytic container wherein transmutation takes place. The rise and flow of the water in the fountain characterize Mercurius, ruler of alchemy, as the serpent endlessly fertilizing and devouring itself until it gives birth to itself again, the *uroboros* that is the recursive work of alchemy. Even at this early stage one sees the recursive nature of the alchemical process. The aroused energy of transformation is depicted by the image of the water flowing from the fountain, underlining the fact that psychoanalysis is not an intellectual exercise but one that is driven by *affect*, which must be *distilled* and *contained* in the *vas*.

As previously mentioned, Jung saw alchemy as connecting him in a deep way to Faust, the scholar and alchemist of Goethe's well-known text already mentioned,

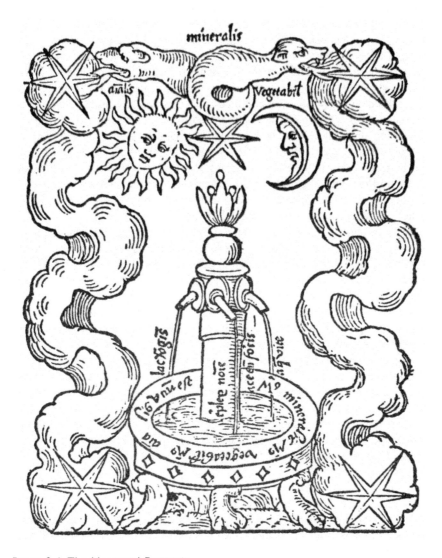

Figure 2.1 The Mercurial Fountain

who projected his own unredeemed dark side into alchemy until Mephistopheles, the devil (Mercurius/Trickster), manifested in his life.

> I regard my work on alchemy as a sign of my inner relationship to Goethe. Goethe's secret was that he was in the grip of that process of archetypal transformation, which has gone on through the centuries. He regarded his *Faust* as an *opus magnum*.

> (1963, p. 197)

Figure 2.1 may be applied to actual analysis between two people. One has to bear in mind the fact that the alchemical process is not a once and for all experience but is a dialectical recursive process. This means that, in the course of a long, in-depth analysis, there are likely to be repeated experiences of an alchemical nature, for instance, when a new or recurring problem presents itself in the patient or analysand's life. This may be signaled by a dream about a family member from the analysand's early life who continues to be particularly problematic for the analysand. This will usually be accompanied by an increase in affect, with corresponding anxiety levels likely to go up as consciousness once more descends to its source in unconsciousness. In this way, the dialectic of the alchemical process may be seen as a spiral, whereby the analysis keeps coming back to the same place but each time with a slight increase in awareness into the problem. The pair are garbed in royal clothes to underline their archetypal nature. The quintessential star in the picture represents transcendent wholeness.

Figure 2.2 brings out into the open the element of incest, an essential component of archetypal transference-countertransference. The king and queen, bridegroom and bride, are depicted standing on the sun and the moon, these latter pointing to the *incestuous* relationship of Apollo and Artemis, the brother and sister from Greek mythology. This is emphasized by the left-handed contact between the two—that is, from the sinister or *unconscious* side. Further associations with the left side are to do with the heart, which is related to love, but also to do with all of the moral contradictions that are connected with *affective* states.

The couple are holding a stem of two flowers in their right hands, which represents the criss-crossing of the analytic relationship as set out in the preceding section. This depicts the multiple relations that may be constellated between analyst and analysand in the course of in-depth analysis. The stems are further crossed at their meeting point from above by a flower held in the beak of a bird descending from the quintessential star representing the dove of the Christian Holy Ghost or the point at which opposites are reconciled.

> Imagination is the star in man, the celestial or supercelestial body. This astounding definition throws a quite special light on the fantasy processes connected with the *opus*. We have to conceive of these processes not as the immaterial phantoms we readily take fantasy-pictures to be, but as something corporeal, a "subtle-body", semi-spiritual in nature.
>
> (Jung, 1953, p. 277)

This is a vital message to take on board, as what Jung is pointing to here is that, in an age before empirical psychology, this kind of concretization was inevitable because everything unconscious, once it was activated, was projected into matter—a hybrid phenomenon, half spiritual and half physical. The act of imagining was a physical activity, and the alchemist related himself not only to unconsciousness but directly to the very substance which he hoped to transform through the power of imagination. In that way, an intermediate realm existed between mind

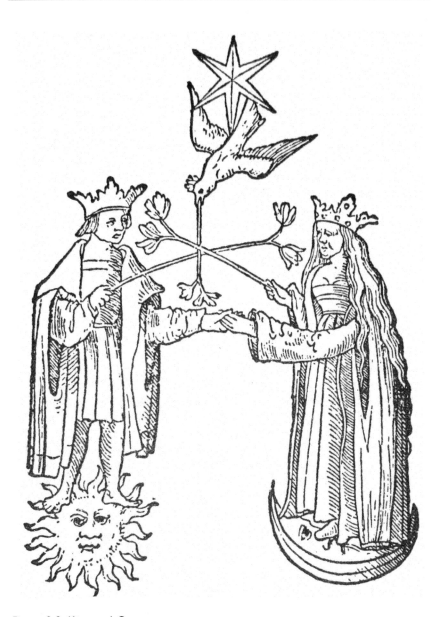

Figure 2.2 King and Queen

and matter, that is, a *psychic* realm of "*subtle bodies*", whose characteristic is to manifest itself in a mental as well as a material form.

According to Jung, the *incest* that is portrayed in Figure 2.2 is a central characteristic of the alchemical approach to analytical work, though he is not advocating *actual* incest between analyst and analysand but pointing to the kinship libido that has been constellated between them and being lived symbolically in the incestuous transference-countertransference. What this means analytically is that to become one's own person entails a symbolic re-entry into the mother, that is, a regression back to an incestuous state in order to be reborn. Symbolic incest, therefore, represents a coming together with one's own being, a union of like with like, which is why it exerts an unholy fascination, as actual incest is seen as sinister and perverse but also fatally attractive—hence the taboo against it in conventional society. The intervention of the dove (the Holy Ghost) depicts the hidden message of this mystical union.

In Jung's own writing about anima and animus, the former stood for a man's inner femininity, while the latter represented a woman's inner masculinity. We will stay with Jung's original configuration as it results in an interesting reversal of what is depicted; in other words, the king is the animus of the female analyst or analysand, and the queen is the anima of the male analysand. This results in a counter-crossing of the sexes with the male analysand represented by the queen and the female analyst represented by the king, thus representing the contra-sexual sides of the analysand and analyst.

Figure 2.3 shows the king and queen in naked confrontation, with the dove once again between them. The eroticism of the picture is mediated by the dove as a symbol of the *soul*, which provides the relational aspect between the king, who personifies spirit, and the queen, who personifies body. In this way, the spiritual and instinctual archetypal duality of the psyche is depicted. The nakedness of the king and queen at this stage points to the fact that the *persona* has dropped away and the naked truth or *shadow* material is becoming constellated, at which time, the analysand reveals his shadow in the course of analysis. The analyst, on the other hand, keeps her shadow concealed from the analysand, though at some point in the analysis, through an error of judgement or being late for an appointment, this will inevitably reveal itself. When that occurs, the analysis may break down if the analysand cannot cope with the shattering of his idealized transference onto the analyst. This would apply to the first kind of transference that was alluded to earlier when personal, unresolved issues to do with childhood are being worked through. If the analysand can accept the less than perfect analyst, namely, the idealized parental figure who was needed at the initial reparative stage of the work, then the analytic couple are able to enter fully into the incestuous kinship libido.

Figure 2.4 shows the two figures naked in the alchemical bath, with the dove again between them. The psychology of this stage centres on a descent into unconsciousness, the path taken in all heroic endeavours leading to symbolic rebirth. There is increased transparency on the part of the analysand, which facilitates a further descent into shadow realms in the psyche, which also involves the analyst. Both Figures 2.3 and 2.4 depict times in the analysis when it is in danger of breaking down as the analysand may not be able to accept that the analyst has weaknesses. Even if this happens, the analysand will leave the analytic container freer of his or her initial complexes and be able to relate more authentically.

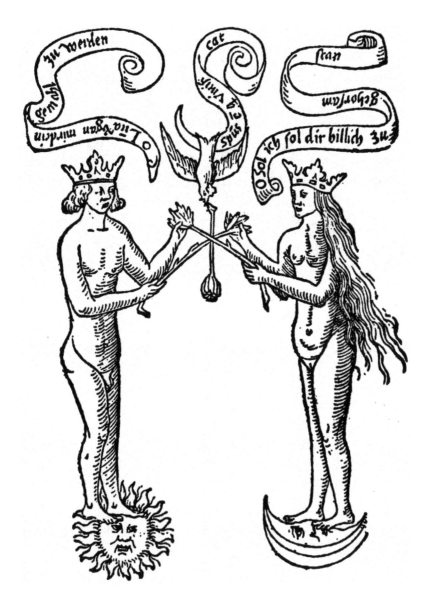

Figure 2.3 The Naked Truth

"The unrelated human being lacks wholeness, for he can achieve wholeness only through the soul, and the soul cannot exist without its other side, which is always found in a 'You'" (Jung, 1954, p. 244). In saying this, Jung is talking not about the synthesis of two individuals but about the union of *ego* with everything that has

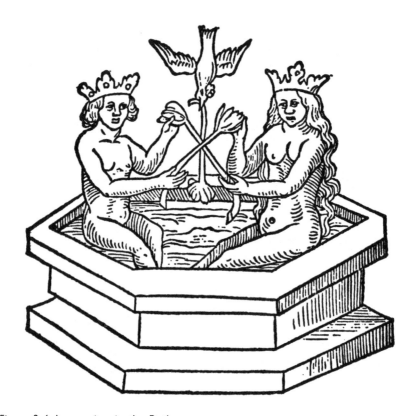

Figure 2.4 Immersion in the Bath

been projected into the "You." The true meaning of the *coniunctio* is that union on a biological level is symbolic of union on the highest level. The analytic relationship paves the way for individuation, where wholeness is an *intrapsychic* process.

Figure 2.5 illustrates the *coniunctio* wherein the passionately embracing pair are enclosed by the water, a "night sea journey", as they have returned to the chaotic beginning, which at first glance looks as if instinct has triumphed. The union depicted here, however, denotes the symbolic union of opposites and of instinctive energy being transformed into symbolic activity. The dove, as the uniting symbol, has disappeared as the pair, in coitus as natural process, has been transformed into a symbolic union.

That is a summary of Jung's interpretation, though it is necessary to add that this is the stage at which the erotic transference-countertransference is heightened and may be enacted between analyst and analysand. This would amount to actualizing the incestuous content of the analytic relationship where, instead, the alchemical container of analysis needs to be able to contain these powerful emotions and let them continue to work themselves through in *uroboric* fashion. It is

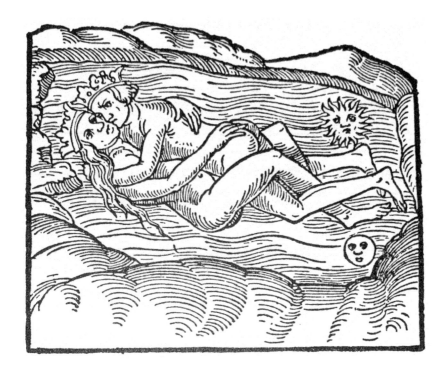

Figure 2.5 The Conjunction

salutary, at this stage, to remind oneself that the philosopher William James called psychoanalysis "a most dangerous method."

Figure 2.6 shows the death or *nigredo* stage that follows from the conjoining of the pair, which is the cessation in the flow of energy once opposites unite. Death means extinction of consciousness and stagnation of psychic life at the stage when the two are united in one body with two heads. "The situation described in our picture is a kind of Ash Wednesday" (Jung, 1954, p. 260). This annual lamentation, which takes place in many cultures, corresponds to an archetypal event. This is linked to the incestuous theme which runs through "The Rosarium" and the resulting dilemma that confronts anyone undertaking a confrontation with unconsciousness. Either way, nature will be mortified, as to commit incest goes against nature, but so is not yielding to ardent desire. With the integration of the powerful contents in unconsciousness into ego, an inevitable inflation results that has a serious impact on ego, which experiences it as a kind of death. This is the *putrefaction* stage, as the conjunction was incestuous and therefore sinful and has to be punished, but also no new life can come into being without the death of the old.

Figure 2.7 shows the *soul* mounting to heaven out of the decaying unified body of the king and queen. Psychologically, this corresponds to a dark state

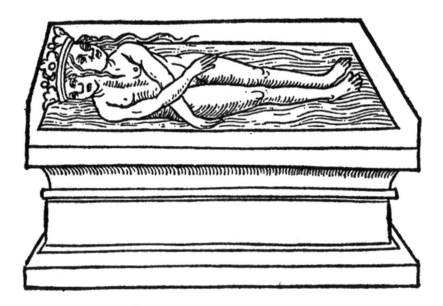

Figure 2.6 Death

of disorientation and the collapse of *ego-consciousness*. When the ego is over-whelmed by unconscious contents, it is experienced as a loss of *soul*—the dark night of the *soul* that is depicted in the works of religious thinkers such as St John of the Cross. Both Figures 2.6 and 2.7 depict states of *depression*, which are experienced as deathlike, underlining necessary states of regression for the analysand. These pictures show the *putrefaction* and *mortification* stages of the alchemical process, when the soul leaves the conjoined analysand-analyst, shown as an empty shell, and re-enters heaven from which it originates. This stage depicts a difficult time for the analysand, and the analytic container needs to be able to contain this despair and pain arising from the loss of the *soul*. It is necessary to withstand this dark night of the soul without intellectualizing it so that it has to be felt deeply. Feeling is necessary to bind one to the reality and meaning of symbolic contents and to their ethical meaning. This is where the analysand needs sufficient ego strength so as not to descend into *psychosis*.

Figure 2.8 shows the dead couple sprinkled with falling dew from heaven. The previous stage of the darkness of death, when the union of opposites reaches its nadir, now begins to lighten. This is a psychological law whereby everything eventually transforms into its opposite, which underlies Jung's notion of the self-regulating propensity of the *psyche* and the related one of *compensation*. This brings renewed life to the analytic relationship with the dawning of new con-sciousness on the part of the analysand as well as the analyst.

Figure 2.9 shows the *soul* returning from heaven and unifying with the puri-fied body. It is this unification which, according to Jung, is the goal of perceptive

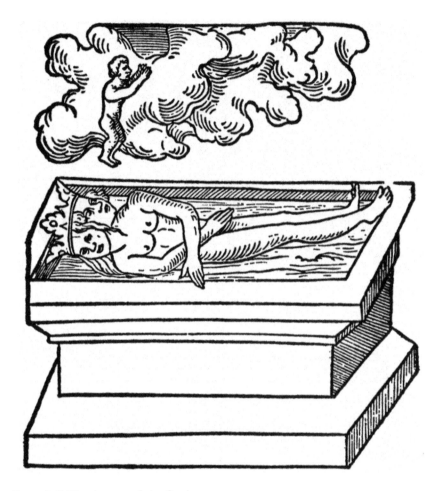

Figure 2.7 The Ascent of the Soul

alchemists and depth psychologists alike. Relationship is at the centre of alchemical transformation in analysis for both analyst and analysand. The soul that has been reunited with the body is the one born of the two, and the anima, as the result of a long analysis, has become a function of relationship between consciousness and unconsciousness.

Two birds at the bottom left of the picture represent the dual nature of Mercurius as a chthonic and a pneumatic being. The presence of these is a sign that, although the *hermaphrodite* in Figure 2.9 appears to be united, the conflict between the two realms has not yet disappeared but is relegated to the bottom left of the picture, that is, the sphere of unconsciousness, further exemplified in the theriomorphic appearance of the birds.

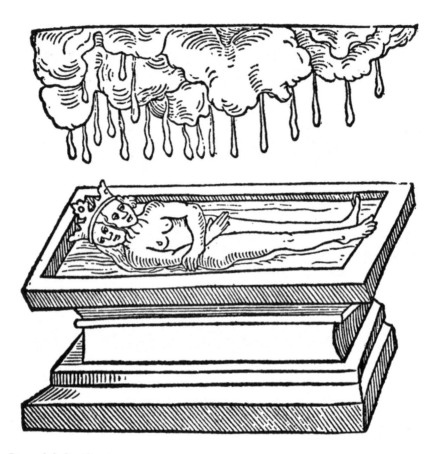

Figure 2.8 Purification

Figure 2.10 depicts the birth of the hermaphrodite, the symbol of wholeness, with the right side of the body being male and the left female. This signifies that the individual has reached the stage of consciousness where the opposites, represented by sun and moon, are held in a balance different from the earlier figure, which represents the state of primordial (unconscious) union. In Figure 2.10, the hermaphrodite stands on the moon, the feminine principle, and holds a snake, the principle of evil connected with the work of redemption. Jung writes of the hermaphrodite that it is a "monstrous and horrific image", as alchemy was compensating for the cleaned-up images of Christianity, "the product of spirit, light and good", whereas alchemical figures are "creatures of night, darkness, poison, and evil" to do with matter (Jung, 1946, p. 316).

At this point, it hardly needs stating that Jung's vision of the psyche was a highly eroticized, even incestuous one, though this was with a view to the goal

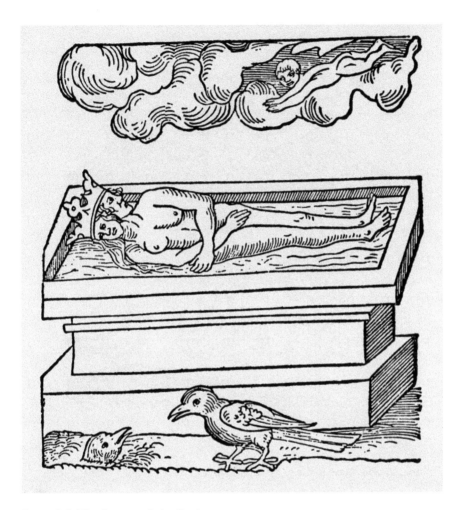

Figure 2.9 The Return of the Soul

of achieving the *higher marriage.* To summarize, this is the relationship to the *syzygy*, the yoked anima-animus developed through the course of a lengthy analysis, culminating in a bisexual being that has integrated consciousness and unconsciousness.

The union of opposites personified by the hermaphrodite symbolizes nothing less than the philosopher's stone or what Jung terms individuation. This, he claims, is the end product of a lengthy alchemical process when the libido is slowly distilled from the alluring fascination of the eroticized transference-countertransference. As Jung states: "The symbol of the *hermaphrodite*, it must be remembered, is one of the many synonyms for the goal of the art" (1954, p. 316).

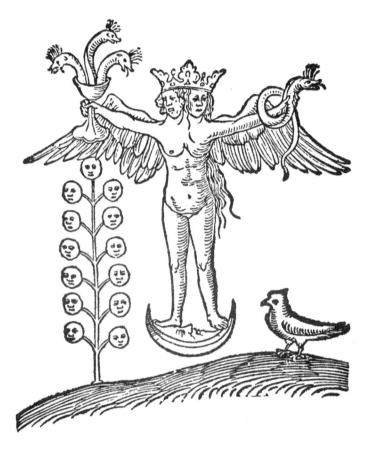

Figure 2.10 The New Birth

As stated at the beginning of this chapter, the alchemical process is a recursive dialectical one, not a once and for all event. During in-depth analysis, this recursive process brings increased awareness with each turn of the spiral of the dialectical process. These are everyday life experiences that are lived only unconsciously but, when worked through in the alchemical process of analysis, allow for the distillation of problems and difficulties until a solution arrives that brings with it increased awareness. Every reader of this chapter has experienced problems and knows that immediate action, namely, reacting to situations, is seldom an effective way of resolving them. The capacity to contain the strong affect that accompanies problems is a hugely important step in travelling on the path to self-awareness. The latter is "a becoming of the self . . . the total, timeless man . . . who stands for the mutual integration of conscious and unconscious" (Ibid., p. 313). A point worth reiterating is that the alchemical process is not a linear one, but a dialectic one.

Concluding Remarks on Jung's Psychological Alchemy

The great lesson of psychological alchemy points to the path along which one may lead one's life without seeking easy solutions—there are none. Ultimately, a final resolution awaits every living being in what Heidegger calls *being-unto-death*, the path of *dasein*—his philosophy taking on increasing vitality for the later stages of life. As already claimed earlier, the discovery of Jung's realization of the psychological potential in the alchemical process is his great contribution to his own discipline. As he himself put it: "there is an eminently psychological reason for the existence of alchemy" (1959, p. 344). As with most other Jungian concepts, it is open to criticism, as exemplified by what follows, but the essential discovery by Jung of the potential for individual development through alchemical processing leads this writer to conclude that alchemy is good *to think with*, a telling phrase from the twentieth-century discipline of *structuralism*. One can ask for nothing more in life than the stripping away of what is extraneous to existence until one is left with the ultimate attainment, namely, a Heideggerian icy, cold logic, the antidote to drowning in affect.

Wolfgang Giegerich's Critique of Jung's Approach to Psychological Alchemy

The material featured in this section is taken from articles written in collaboration with Wolfgang Giegerich himself, which I contributed to *The Journal of Analytical Psychology*. The Berlin-based Jungian psychoanalyst, Giegerich, is the foremost critic of Jung's psychology and who, until 1984, was an uncritical admirer of Jung and an adherent of the archetypal school of analytical psychology. The latter's central tenets spring from imagery and myth. Before we go into Giegerich's model of psychological alchemy, it is important to note some of his general criticisms of Jung.

Whilst being aware that many readers may well be familiar with Giegerich's thinking, I shall spell out some of his main concepts for those who are not. For the latter, I would like to add a word of encouragement because his ideas are not easy to grasp in one reading, as I discovered many years ago when I first started to grapple with his profound thinking. Another vital point is that consciousness as the *hard problem* is being widely researched by neuroscientists, physicists, philosophers, and psychoanalysts such as David Chalmers, Daniel Dennett, and Mark Solms, but it is beyond the scope of this chapter to expound on that here.

Giegerich's critique of Jung is aimed at the latter's reification of concepts such as *the* unconscious and *the* collective unconscious, the latter deemed to be full of content, namely, archetypes. Thus, in Jung's model, the mind is the product of a substrate of archetypes, myths, and *gods*. This is in contrast to the lack of ontic existence of the *objective psyche* that is a key feature of Giegerich's thinking. Furthermore, Jung's notion of individuation and his constant quest for meaning is dismissed as seeking wish-fulfilment rather than truth. In his emphasis on meaning, and in the famous quote about God's existence, "I do not believe, I know", Jung reverts to pre-Kantian metaphysics as the statement runs contrary to the latter's categorical denial that anything could enter consciousness without being pre-organized by the mind. Instead, Kant had to deny knowledge in order to make room for faith. He had already demonstrated that the human mind is inherent in outer reality which, prior to his *transcendental idealism*, had been seen as independent of humans. Alchemy has objectively reached a similar level of reflection as the subject is becoming conscious of itself as observer as well as active participant. With the advent of alchemy, humans have superseded the mythological stage as the whole of mythology, the imaginal is being worked on in the alchemical retort, and the *adept* has risen to a new stage of consciousness.

> It is ("implicit"), i.e., structurally it *is* already thought, even if thought that is still deeply immersed and enveloped in the imaginal form of presentation . . . it provides the *real* bridge upon which the soul could pass from its former status (mythologizing) to its new, modern status of (psycho-) logic, the status of the Concept.
>
> (Giegerich, 2008, p. 138)

To summarize what has been said in the preceding quote: Giegerich's focus is on the "logical" to be found in the alchemical opus, which may appear surprising at first because alchemy expresses itself through imagery, as evidenced in the early part of this chapter on "The Rosarium." For Jung, medieval alchemy was the historical link between Gnosticism and Neoplatonism from the past to the present time, wherein to deal with soul or psyche occurs through the workings of Jungian psychoanalysis. Giegerich, for his part, rejects this and sees alchemy as the historical link between the imagination and dialectical logic.

To further clarify this key point, the alchemical opus gives rise to the objective psyche that is without concrete existence but is, instead, the result of the alchemical processes of distillation, fermentation, sublimation, corruption, mortification, and purification of feelings, emotions, images, and dreams. Giegerich's further critique of Jung's psychology is that it remains largely at the *semantic* level, that is, focusing on content, and has not reached the *syntactical* level where the focus is on form and structure.

Furthermore, Jung's psychology is a-historical rather than historical as it takes no account of the developmental stages of the Western mind from the Reformation, the Industrial and French Revolutions, or, perhaps above all, the Enlightenment. These were some of the foremost ruptures of time in Western history that brought in their wake increasing secularization, which led to the objective psyche emptying itself out of mythical and religious ways of being. At the end of the nineteenth and beginning of the twentieth century, these developmental stages resulted in a new psychological consciousness. "This *psychological* focus is 'objective' to the personal standpoint of both patient and analyst and is comprehended as 'other,' because the standpoint comes from a shift in *perspective*, it is not a literal or hypostasized other" (Hoedl, 2018, p. 126).

In this way, psychology evolved conceptually from a person-to-person realm to a transpersonal logic of whatever is presenting itself—symptom, dream, or interpretation—which enabled the move from a personalistic stance to objective psyche's self-reflection. In practice, this means that though Giegerich meets his patients in the consulting room on a human personal level, giving them the emotional support they need to be in touch with their repressed affects, his *psychological focus* is not on the person but on the concept.

In this way, Giegerich tries to penetrate *thinkingly* into psychological phenomena and bring out their internal dialectic. This may be thought of as the dynamic developmental process in which nothing is discarded or destroyed. Instead, it is *sublated* or overcome while, at the same time, being preserved not lost. *Negation* in the dialectic is the negation of positive, tangible, demonstrable reality, a taking off deeper into the interiority of the phenomenon itself. *Absolute knowledge* is one freed (absolved) from the difference between the absolute and the empirical, the infinite and the finite; it is freed from the endless repetition of binary opposition culminating in a speculative stance that overcomes the alienation of subject and object.

A psychology informed by alchemy would have the task of freeing the spirit Mercurius, which is the thought that is imprisoned in matter, namely, image, emotion, bodily symptom. The true laboratory of the mind in the alchemical opus is the real historical process whereby the contradictory life of itself and its own other will have disappeared as something in their own right and been reduced to sublated moments of unity. Dialectical movement is structurally akin to that of the alchemical opus expressed in its language of decomposition, fermentation, corruption, and solution. In both instances, the recursive process of negation is expressed as the sublimating, distilling, and refining of the prime matter in the work.

According to Giegerich, *psychogenic* bodily symptoms and affects are essentially thoughts that are submerged into the natural, physical medium of body or emotion: "body symptom is submerged emotion, emotion is submerged image, image is submerged thought, and conversely, thought is sublated image, image is sublated emotion, emotion is sublated body reaction" (Giegerich, 2007, p. 255). Giegerich emphasizes that abstract thinking is what today's psychology needs in the shape of more intellect—not more feelings, emotions, or body work. He dismisses the latter as "ego-stuff."

In Jung's exploration of psychological alchemy, he at times spells this out, as follows:

> This does not mean that the adept ceased to work in the laboratory, only that he kept an eye on the symbolic aspect of his transmutations. This corresponds exactly to the situation in the modern psychology of the unconscious; while personal problems are not over looked [*sic*] (the patient himself takes very good care of that!), the analyst keeps an eye on the symbolic aspects, for healing comes from what leads the patient beyond himself and beyond his entanglements in the ego.
>
> (1967a, 1967b, p. 302)

In the preceding, Jung is demonstrating that the more insightful alchemists were moving away from working with concrete physical matter in their laboratories—"our gold is *not* the vulgar gold—*aurum non vulgi*" (Ibid., p. 166)—towards symbolic ideas. Despite this, Jung often stays with ontic images and outgrown myths. Giegerich, on the other hand, has moved away from the imagery Jung depicts in his analysis of "The Rosarium" to the logic of actually lived life at a given historical locus. Psyche's main alchemical laboratory is history, the history of culture and consciousness.

In Giegerich's view, by remaining in the mythological mode of conceptualizing, Jung was stuck in a past of gods and superheroes where humans are mere recipients of divine knowledge, whereas the alchemical opus is an active work by adepts creating knowledge themselves. This is why Mercurius cannot be a full-fledged God as it has the adept's subjectivity in itself; it is thus objectivity and subjectivity at the same time. "With the advent of Alchemy, we could say, it begins to dawn on consciousness that the life of the soul is *logical* life, is thought" (Giegerich, 2008, p. 137).

Today we live in a scientific and technological age, which is where psyche is located and where psychology must be also. The latter should be, as its name implies, a psychology of *logos*, that is, reflective thinking. "We have to think from within our own historical situation and on our own responsibility" (Giegerich, Miller, & Morgenson, 2005, p. 9). Instead, Jung advocated the following: "we are best advised to remain within the framework of traditional mythology, which has already proved comprehensive enough for all practical purposes" (1954, p. 270). This represents a regression on Jung's part, though from time to time he does show awareness that psyche's work is noetic or reflective thought. For instance, the following statement by Jung appears in "The Psychology of the Transference": "the Original Man (Nous) bent down from heaven to earth and was wrapped in the embrace of physis—a primordial image that runs through the whole of alchemy" (1946, p. 246). Further on in the same piece, this statement appears: "It restores the vanished 'man of light' who is identical with the Logos in Gnostic and Christian symbolism" (Ibid., p. 248).

The following quotation succinctly encapsulates Giegerich's approach to psychological alchemy as a dialectical process:

> The work of alchemy is *contra naturam* in displacing human existence from the biological sphere to the slow path to *mindedness*, the relation to or openness for the truth, i.e., the logic of actually lived life at a given historical locus, the freeing of the Mercurius imprisoned in the physicalness of the matter. What is at work here is *not* just the alchemical distillation of the *semantic* contents of ego, for instance, *images* into the logical form of *syntax* of soul; it is the *absolute negation* of the logical form of the content from within itself which arrives back at the starting point but at a transformed starting point.
>
> (Casement, 2011b, p. 716)

This may best be illustrated by the following simple progression: Starting position "A", from which the contradictions inherent in "A" lead to position "non-A", but the contradictions in position "non-A" lead to a new position "not-non-A." The contradictions in that position lead back to the starting point "A", but the latter is not exactly the same naïve "A" that existed at the beginning of the dialectic, as "A" has gone through several *negations* on the way and is enriched and refined by the history of all the negations. The superseded stages are not lost but are still there as sublated moments within the new position "A." This spiraling dialectical movement is structurally akin to the alchemical opus, which also proceeds via negations. In both cases, the recursive process of negation is, in itself and simultaneously, the process of sublimating, distilling, and refining the prime matter here and the consciousness or the logic of the world there.

The simple equation in the previous paragraph will resonate with anyone who has been in analysis and/or practiced as an analyst. Let us turn to a common enough presenting problem for an individual seeking help in dealing with a problematic marriage. This would represent starting point "A." The analysand considers leaving or even divorcing the spouse as a way of resolving the contradictions as well as the tensions in the relationship, which then results in a shift to position "non-A." The contradictions in that position lead to "not-non-A", wherein contradictions continue unabated, so there is a reversion back to position "A", but the analysand is not back at exactly where he started from as position "A" has been through various negations in its progression. If all of this can be contained within the analysis and not *acted out*, the dialectical process has a chance to do its work on the problem at hand.

The concept of the *container* is central to the alchemical process, indicated in the material already presented, as it is within the boundaries of the container that the alchemical work can take place without intrusion from the outside or leakage from within it. This has obvious applicability to the psychoanalytic container. Giegerich contributed a description of his way of practising analysis to an article I wrote up on his work in which he alludes to "going for a walk" with a patient during a session (Casement, 2011a, p. 540). This would be leaking from the alchemical container as opposed to keeping everything *hermetically* sealed within it as the recursive process continues with its refining of the *prima materia*. In psychoanalytic language, it would represent a form of "acting out" of the transference-countertransference, which Giegerich also appears to misinterpret, as in the following: "I do not systematically invite transference reactions. I do not offer myself as a kind of guru or so" (Ibid., 2011a, p. 540).

This depiction of transference is alien to the understanding of transference-countertransference as practiced by this writer, which is not to serve the analyst's self-aggrandizement but, rather, is in the service of the patient or analysand's need to work through unresolved relationships with parents, siblings, and other figures from childhood, which also acts as a source of invaluable information for the analyst. The recursive action of alchemy that has been alluded to previously is what slowly though surely refines all of the base matter, namely, raw sensations and emotions, that are distilled into thought. This central feature of analytic work helps the analysand even after the analysis has terminated, as it becomes internalized as a way of containing and working through the problems and difficulties that are an inevitable part of life.

Final Remarks

Jung stressed the *mutuality* of the alchemical process, underlining his notion that the analyst and analysand are in an equal relationship. This is illustrated in the diagram already presented which emphasizes symmetry in order to express the idea that the analyst is as much in analysis as the analysand, leading to the assumption that the analytic relationship is equal in every way. While fully supporting the notion of the essential mutuality of the two participants in the analytic container, I contend that the analytic relationship is, nevertheless, asymmetrical in the following respects: the analyst has been through analysis and training and has analyzed previous patients or analysands. Furthermore, the analyst's relation to anima and animus is more firmly established and ego is stronger. As a result, the analyst's perception of the analysand is greater, leading to the capacity to use *projection* and *introjection* in ways that give the analyst information about the analysand's *resistances* and helps the analyst not to act out.

Nevertheless, the potential for mutual transformation through the alchemical process is an important contribution of Jung's to psychology. In addition, Jung's emphasis on the importance of the relationship inherent in the analytic encounter is another major contribution to the psychoanalytic community, as is Giegerich's alternative mode of thinking. It has to be said that although Jung did not live up to his claim of mutuality between analyst and analysand, as I hope to have demonstrated in my critique of his analysis of Kristine Mann, which appears in *Jung: An Introduction*, it does not undermine the notion of mutuality as one important difference between the Jungian psychoanalytic approach and that of mainstream psychoanalysis. One small but telling instance of this is the following: it is usual for a patient or analysand in Jungian psychoanalysis to talk of analyzing *with* a particular analyst; in mainstream psychoanalysis, it is customary to talk of being analyzed *by* a particular analyst.

Finally, I would like to add address the question of whether an experience of the alchemical process is possible through the use of technology in conducting analysis. From my long experience over many years of using Skype, Zoom, and/or the telephone for sessions, also known as *tele-analysis*, there has been no difficulty whatsoever in experiencing alchemical transformation by these means. In other words, alchemy and tele-analysis are completely compatible as technology is no hindrance to the production of regression, incestuous longings, or transference-countertransference.

Acknowledgements

"A critical appraisal of C. G. Jung's Psychological Alchemy" was originally published in *Jung: An Introduction* by Ann Casement in 2021. It is reproduced here by kind permission of the publisher, Phoenix Publishing House Ltd. A first version was presented at Gakushuin University, Tokyo.

References

Carotenuto, A. (1982). *A Secret Symmetry. Sabina Spielrein between Jung and Freud.* Foreword by William McGuire. New York: Random House, Pantheon Books.

Casement, A. (2011a). *The Interiorizing Movement of Logical Life: Reflections on Wolfgang Giegerich.* In *The Journal of Analytical Psychology.* Volume 56, No. 4, September 2011. Oxford: John Wiley & Sons.

Casement, A. (2011b). Review of W. Giegerich *The Soul Always Thinks: Collected English Papers.* In *The Journal of Analytical Psychology.* Volume 56, No. 5, November 2011. Oxford: John Wiley & Sons

Freud, S. (1976). *The Interpretation of Dreams.* Harmondsworth: Penguin Books.

Giegerich, W. (2007). Psychology: The Study of the Soul's Logical Life. In A. Casement (Ed.). *Who Owns Jung?* London: Karnac.

Giegerich, W. (2008). *The Soul's Logical Life.* Peter Lang: Frankfurt am Main.

Giegerich, W., Miller, D.G., Morgenson, G. (2005). *Dialectics & Analytical Psychology: The El Capitan Canyon Seminar.* New Orleans: Spring Journal, Inc.

Graf-Nold, A. (2001). *The Zürich School of Psychiatry in theory and practice. Sabina Spielrein's Treatment at the Burghölzli Clinic in Zürich.* In *The Journal of Analytical Psychology.* Volume 46, No. 1, January 2001. Oxford: John Wiley & Sons

Hoedl, J. (2018). *The alchemical 'not' and Marlan's stone that remains a stone. A response to his critique of Giegerich's 'psychology proper'.* In *The Journal of Analytical Psychology.* Volume 63, No. 1, February 2018. Oxford: John Wiley & Sons

Jarrett, J.L. [Ed.] (1988). *C.G. Jung: Nietzsche's Zarathustra. Notes of the Seminar given in 1934–1939. Volume 1.* Princeton: Princeton University Press.

Jung, C.G. (1946). *The Practice of Psychotherapy.* Vol. 16. London: Routledge & Kegan & Paul.

Jung, C.G. (1953). *Psychology and Alchemy.* London: Routledge & Kegan Paul, Ltd.

Jung, C.G. (1954). *The Psychology of the Transference.* In Vol. 16. *The Practice of Psychotherapy.* London: Routledge & Kegan Paul, Ltd.

Jung, C.G. (1959). *The Archetypes and the Collective Unconscious.* Part 1. London: Routledge & Kegan Paul.

Jung, C.G. (1963). *Memories, Dreams, Reflections.* London: Collins and Routledge & Kegan Paul.

Jung, C.G. (1967a). *The Philosophical Tree.* In Vol. 13. *Alchemical Studies.* London: Routledge & Kegan Paul, Ltd.

Jung, C.G. (1967b). *Commentary on 'The Secret of the Golden Flower'.* In Vol. 13. *Alchemical Studies.* London: Routledge & Kegan Paul, Ltd.

Chapter 3

James Hollis

How shall the heart be reconciled to its feast of losses?
                                        Stanley Kunitz, "The Layers"

In the final paragraphs of his memoir, *Memories, Dreams, Reflections*, Jung, who had traveled so far, studied so much, and discerned such depths, found he had no grand pronouncements to make and only a few summary statements to make about his life:

> I know only that I was born and exist, and it seems to me that I have been carried along. I exist on the foundation of something I do not know. In spite of all uncertainties, I feel a solidity underlying all existence and a continuity in my mode of being.

As I finish my 80th year, I find Jung's modest claims resonant with my own conclusions. So much fortuity, so many contradictions, so many false starts and correctives, and so many hurtful and helpful people along the way, and, through it all, a profound gratitude for the journey, an abiding sense that some similar force has carried me all the way, and that, for all the disparate settings and scene changes, I experience a deep continuity with that child who is now in his last years.

A brief word of background is necessary. My parents, while both bright, came from uneducated backgrounds and dire economic circumstances. My father, for example, was pulled out of the eighth grade and sent to work in a factory to support the family. He spent his life there. My mother never knew her Swedish father as he was killed in a coal mine cave-in the New World, and she grew up impoverished. My parents' experience of traumatic diminishment, the impact of the Great Depression, and World War II were understandably engulfing and oppressive forces. Neither felt worthy or entitled to dream. Their message to me was "stay home. We will try to protect each other. Don't expect anything you haven't

DOI: 10.4324/9781003148982-4

earned. And above all, don't go out there; it's too dangerous." This message was both verbal and exemplary, and it dominated my early life.

While I was wholly safe in America's Midwest, my own experience of the war was fraught with communal anxiety, which I picked up from around me, and a pervasive sorrow for the many grieving in the world. As a child, I remember going on a corner and singing sad ballads, and weeping for the world. My peculiar ritual was a private service of identification with the world's woe.

The messages of both diminished expectation and possibility and the Weltschmerz have stayed with me through the years. Only the fortuity of a child's right to an education in America, and the kindness of teachers who saw something in me, kept me from the circumscription of my parents' world. Reading allowed me to travel wider imaginal circumferences, and ultimately education allowed me to travel distant lands. That someday I would wind up studying depth psychology in Zürich was inconceivable. But it happened. And I thank all of them for somehow facilitating that child to read, to learn, to travel, to claim a larger journey.

Having traveled these many years and places, having been blessed with many who loved me beyond my merit and gifted me beyond my capacity, I can also say that there was some driving presence in that child, some daimon one might say, that was seeking expression through me in the world.

Other than our children whom I love, I consider nothing of whatever I personally achieved to be of transcendent value, but I can say that, despite my many flaws, I have served that daimon—as if I had a choice!

The combination of compassion for the suffering souls of this world and the attraction to reading and writing has led me to a rich journey of teaching, writing, and therapy, which somehow paid the bills. Through them, that "continuity" in one's mode of being has been manifest, and the "solidity" coursing beneath supported an abiding curiosity toward the mysteries in which we swim. Through it all runs a deep gratitude for the privileges of being here, of being blessed by the kindness to me of so many, and of getting to explore a larger world. My present state of mind and spirit is similar to that of the poet Stanley Kunitz in his poem "The Layers:"

> Though I lack the art
> to decipher it,
> no doubt the next chapter
> in my book of transformations
> is already written.
> I am not done with my changes.

James Hollis, Ph.D. Washington, DC 2020

Narcissus's Forlorn Hope

The Fading Image in a Pool too Deep

Originally published in Buser, S. and Cruz, L. (eds.) (2017). *A Clear and Present Danger: Narcissism in the Era of President Trump*. Asheville, NC: Chiron. Reprinted in 2021 in *Prisms: Reflections on this Journey We Call Our Life*. Asheville, NC: Chiron. Reprinted with permission.

What seest thou else
In the dark backward and abysm of time?

Shakespeare, *The Tempest*

The deep is the unsayable.

Ludwig Wittgenstein, *Philosophical Investigations*

We all know the outline of the ancient story of Narcissus, and from afar we have judged the self-absorption of the youth transfixed by his own image in the pool. We, who might pause for a moment in the restaurant's mirror, straightening the tie, fluffing the hair, freshening the makeup, can afford such largess, for are we not all above such self-absorption as sank this ancient soul?

Narcissus was cursed to have been "seen in his flaw" as we, perhaps, are not, and Nemesis chose to catch him up on his one-sidedness. Jung's simplest definition of neurosis was the one-sidedness of the personality, a trait for which we are well rewarded today and often handsomely paid. Catching his image in the pond, he was captivated, possessed. Again, Jung's term for the experience of a complex was *Ergriffenheit*: seizure or possession.[1] So captivated by his own beauty, Narcissus's libido turned inward and fed on itself, and he lost the vital erotic vector of life. Life is served by the desire for, the encounter with, the dialogue with the other. This self-absorption is a form of hell. As poet Gerard Manley Hopkins (1916) put it in his poem titled *I Wake and Fell the Fell of Dark*, to be one's own sweating self is to be irredeemably mired in stasis without possibility of movement, dynamism, or growth through the other.

Nemesis is not a god, but one of those impersonal forces—like Dike and Sophrosyne —which course through the cosmos and to which even the gods seem to bend. To the degree that any of us feels insecure, that insecurity will show up over and over and over in venue after venue. Nemesis is a harvest of consequences, consequences which flow from our numerous gaps in consciousness. And wherever we are unconscious, the play of possibility is immense. All cultures, for example, amid their carnival of possibilities, have an archetypal presence called "the trickster." The trickster is that figure, god, animal, or human-oid *jongleur* whose purpose seems to be to upset our apple carts, to remind us that we are not gods, that we are not as knowing, not as much in charge, and not as omnipotent as we might think we are. So, Nemesis enchants Narcissus and he falls into the sickness unto death, the *mortificatio*, the stultification of libido which occurs whenever the dialectic is replaced by one-sidedness, ambiguity by certainty, probing enquiry by fundamentalism, democracy by fascism, and so on.

The first "modern" to really explore narcissism was Fyodor Dostoevsky in his 1863 *Notes from Underground*. This perverse, countercultural analysis explored the collective phantasy of meliorism, the doctrine of "progress," and the phantasy of moral improvement toward which the nineteenth century believed it moved so confidently. On the collective level, the underground man mocks the narcis-sistic self-congratulation of the first world's exhibition, the Crystal Palace outside of London, a hall of glass in which could be seen not only the tools of the new, progressive epoch but the self-congratulatory genius that procured them. But the underground man imagines that same technology will be used in the century to follow to more efficiently kill more people than ever before. Little could he envi-sion that the ruins of the Crystal Palace would be used later as a navigational point by the Luftwaffe in its bombing runs over London, nor that morally untethered technology would build concentration camps and nuclear weapons less than eight decades later.

But even more telling, the underground man turns his lens upon himself and describes his own naked emotions and uncensored agendas. "Now then, what does a decent man like to talk about most? Himself, of course. So, I'll talk about myself" (Dostoevsky, 1961, p. 93). His honesty is, to this day, still astounding and justifies the appellation he grants himself: "the anti-hero."

He celebrates his capacity to make others miserable when he moans loudly from a toothache. He acknowledges that he has no self-worth because, of course, he is a man of superior intellect, and anyone of superior intellect will of course know how worthless he really is. He describes his vanities, his petty jealousies, and his elaborate plots to exact revenge for presumptive insults, and he considers torpor superior to the stupidities of those who are activists primarily because they are stupid. The underground man's cumulative catalogue of contumely is over-whelming, but in the end, he turns it around by confronting the superior, judgmen-tal reader by noting that he alone has the honesty to look at himself in the mirror and bear what looks back, while the reader cannot bear to look in the mirror very long at all. Amid his catalogue of shame, the cauterizing virtue of honesty shines with stunning, compelling, and intimidating power on the reader.

In Dostoevsky's trope of "the underground man," we begin to approach the per-spective of depth psychology at last. Perhaps having survived the hell of a Sibe-rian gulag, Dostoevsky could survive the hell of self-knowledge. To what degree can any of us bear to see ourselves through the glass darkly, to use the metaphor of Paul's *Letter to the Corinthians*?[2] The pitiful truth of narcissism is that *the narcissist stares in the mirror and no one stares back*. This is why he or she must use others for reflecting surfaces. If that person is the parent, the child is used to bring positive regard to the parent. One has only to think of the stage mother or the little league father for cultural stereotypes of this pattern. If the narcissist is the employer, the employees do the hard work and the boss takes the credit. If the partner is insecure, he or she depends on the other to make them feel good about themselves. In each of these relational deficits, the heroic task is fled, the task which asks: "what am I asking of that other that I need to address for myself?"

I know a socialite who hired a publicist to ensure that she was seen in the right places, with the right people until she became a "celebrity," that is, somebody "known for being known." Now, propped up with surgeries and pancake makeup, she totters to the same old functions to hold court. How sad, how empty, how alone the child within must feel, even in that big house filled with servants and sycophants. When I once drove a member of a religious order through a particularly affluent neighborhood, my guest, who had devoted her life to the poor, noted with pity the terrible psychospiritual burden that dollar-driven ghetto placed on subsequent generations to produce and sustain such splendiferous facades. And always, she noted, the daily fear of the inhabitants that people like us might not drive through their neighborhood to see them and envy them.

Shakespeare, in *As You Like It*,[3] noted how so many seek "the bubble reputation." The frangible nature of fame as a bubble is not lost on any of us these centuries later in this era of 15 minutes of fame, selfies, and vulgarity paraded as the divertissement of the hour. Beneath all this is our universal desire to be seen and every child's desperate plea to be valued. If we wish to judge the other, we must first recognize that need persists in ourselves. In earlier eras of Western civilization, and in many other parts of the world today, the grinding necessities of survival require a focus on the outer world in service to daily survival. Throughout most of history, one's place in the larger scheme of things has been demonstrably tiny, insignificant. If there is a meaning to one's brief transit through this vale of tears, it is found in an afterlife, a place for a possible transformation through embrace by that transcendent other. Practically speaking, the linkage to that transcendent other is so attenuated today that most people have felt the ground shift beneath their feet, the stirrings of existential angst, and have inflated this moment, this hour, with an urgency far exceeding the *carpe diem* thread of classical Greece and Rome. If, as more and more suspect, the other is not there, or looking elsewhere for a century or two, one must scour one's own image through some transient graffito in the shifting sands of the hourglass.[4]

How often we have heard people say, "I want to know myself," or we have even said it ourselves. But do we, really? Could we bear that? Could we bear the possible revelations that we are "human," *menschliche, alle zu menschliche* (Nietzsche, 1993) after all, with all its anfractuosities, its capacities for brutality and compassion, for selfishness and generosity, for aggression and caregiving? As most of us would like to think of ourselves as improvements on humanity's developmental history, could we bear to be simply the most recent iteration of the whole human project, as Terence in the year 190 BCE suggested: *"Nihil a me humanun alienum puto."*

The ancients recognized our ambivalence before the vision in the pond. Could we afford to stare at our own darkness directly, or that of another, or that of Divinity? We know what happened to those who looked at Medusa directly, and so Athena's bright shield provided a reflective surface, a distancing metaphora perhaps, through which to refract that primal power. As T. S. Eliot (1935) put it in *The Four Quartets*, "Humankind cannot bear too much reality." Jung recognized the role of resistance, the creation of those

> taboo regions which psychology must not touch. But since no war was ever won on the defensive, one must, in order to terminate hostilities, open negotiations with the enemy and see what his terms really are.
>
> (Jung, *CW* 16, para. 374)

For over two centuries now, philosophers, psychologists, phenomenologists, physicists, and others have been telling us that we cannot know things in themselves: Hume, Kant, Heisenberg, Husserl, and so on. All we can "know" is that we do not know, but we do experience, and we experience through various modalities, categories, and mediatorial vehicles. Poets and prophets have always known this. The poet knows he or she cannot speak of love or grief or anything worth it directly, so he or she will find a tangible object, which, because it is more nearly available to the corporeal senses, lends itself to the task of bridging to the essential but illusive other. Thus, "the beloved other" is wholly "other" to Robert Burns, but he says his love is like a red, red rose and we immediately get his angle on her. Thomas Nashe (2016), describing the terror of the approaching Black Death, writes, "Brightness falls from the air;/Queens have died, young and fair;/Dust hath closed Helen's eye." We get the point. If you think you are exempt from the roving eye of Lord Death, think again. If we miss that point, he repeats the refrain, *"timor mortis conturbat me."*[5] So, even if we do not dimly see ourselves in that dark glass, we are, apparently, seen by an eye from which we cannot hide.

Remember when you, the reader, first stared into a mirror, perhaps as a toddler, amused to see another, a simulacrum, a funny other who moved limbs like you, yet not you, for they moved differently. How to explain that? Was it that an alternative world lay within, on the other side of that silvered surface? Could one step through into another world, just like this but not, as through a black hole into an alternative universe? And if so, what did it say about the provisionality of this world, this universe, this I?

Narcissus is judged in our emotionally distanced place because he is captured and possessed by his self-image, but are we not all captives to some extent? Is that not the problem for all of us? Is not the central task of psychotherapy to examine and identify what stories, what concepts, what self-images have captivated us and led us to our current impasse, our suffering, and to bring them to the surface, challenge them, and perhaps replace them with something larger, more capacious? Freud called the process *Nacherziehung*, or re-education, given the need to repair or redeem the original *paideia*, or "education," which instructed us as to who we were and what we were to do with our lives.

When we are young, vulnerable, and utterly at the mercy of the world around us, we desperately "read" the world for clues as to who we are, who the other is, what the world is about, how we are to comport ourselves, and so on. The core perceptions assemble over time into a reticulated, anxiety-driven set of autonomous responses to life's challenges. Were there no psychopathology, namely, the revolt of the *self* (Jung's metaphor for the deep natural wisdom of the whole organism[6]), we would be nothing but a series of reticulated and adaptive mechanisms. The revolt of the self tells us that there is an other within, a transcendent other. As it is transcendent to the ego consciousness, nothing particularly useful or informative can be said about it; thus, a respectful silence is best. As Wittgenstein (2001) put it, "*Wovon man nicht sprechen kann, darueber muss man schweigen.*"[7]

So, when we look in the mirror of the world, do we see ourselves, or do we not see through the distorting lenses of our complexes, those charged clusters of history, those fractal narratives which we assemble, some conscious, some not? Is not most of our life seeing what our history tells us, what our world tells us, or what we thought it told us a long time ago? Is not much of our history a replication of the self-image we have thought reflected to us? I have a client currently whose mother repeatedly told him that he was the cause for her unhappy life. What was he to do with that? As a child, was he to take his own life, get out of the way? He thought of that, but then he thought of his younger brothers and knew he could not leave them unprotected. So, he labored on through the darkness—drove himself through a life of work, overcompensation, and caretaking of others, and only now, in the sixth decade, is he beginning to think of his life reflected in a different pool. As he sends his child off to college, he knows he has made her feel welcome, safe, valued, and empowered to live her own journey. The person she sees in the mirror is quite different that the one her father sees every day. And she has no idea that her father sees himself, or has seen himself, as the unworthy, unwanted impediment in his mother's life all these years. As she heads off on a different journey, I have suggested to him that he share with her something of what his life has been so that she can begin to see him as he is, not as the perhaps overcompensating great guy he has been but as a person who is even more worthy of respect and cherishing than she imagines.

Just as the "self" is a transcendent other, so the encounter with the "other" as God is unknowable. This makes "theology," if one thinks it through carefully, untenable. The transcendent other is that about which one cannot speak for only silence is respectful of the transcendence of the mystery; anything short of that is a construing by ego consciousness and a distortion by complexes. As one wit put it, one may be pretty sure we have made the gods in our own image when they seem to hate the same people we hate (and how much history and contemporary politics does that help explain?). Or, as the ancient Xenophanes observed, if horses and lions could draw, the gods they would draw would look like horses and lions. So, respect for the self as transcendent other means the best we ever get at it is a "sense of self."

In the so-called narcissistic personality disorder which is discussed elsewhere in this volume, the narcissist has essentially lost connection with the corrective ministries of the self. Thus, he or she is consumed by a default program, namely, *self-inflation as compensation for the disconnect from the self.* (This program for living was memorably critiqued by Pearl Bailey, who noted, "Them whats thinks they is, ain't."[8]) Most of us are simply garden variety neurotics, which means that we know we have erred, we suffer our disconnections, we know we are at fault, and we know we have to get back in line with some deeper principle within. This "knowing" represents our attenuated but still living thread to the self.

Today, though we have forgotten much of the wisdom possessed by those who went before us, we also know too much to reconnect. Blake worried about this over two centuries ago and proposed "reorganized innocence," an oxymoron if there ever was one. Wordsworth and Rilke grasped the sad solitude of certainties lost forever, of moments of "wholeness" never to be regained (perhaps fortunately, because most of country music thrives on this dialectic of yearning, loss, and more yearning). And what is it we really long for? Robert Frost (1923), in a poem titled "For Once, Then, Something," reports a moment in his reflection on the matter:

Once, when trying with chin against a well-curb,
I discerned, as I thought, beyond the picture,
Through the picture, a something white, uncertain,
Something more of the depths—and then I lost it.
Water came to rebuke the too clear water.
One drop fell from a fern, and lo, a ripple
Shook whatever it was lay there at bottom,
Blurred it, blotted it out. What was that whiteness?
Truth? A pebble of quartz? For once, then, something.

That canny old Vermonter. He is not writing about a well, and we all know it. He is probing, in his usual way, what there is to probe "beyond the picture, through the picture," the received story, the conventional ego frame, "something white," momentarily visible. Something there. *Da-Sein*? Something from the depths. Visible at last? But no, a drop of water from a branch effaces the surface, and the image crazes in fractured shards. "What was that whiteness? Truth?" Was it that? Was it the promised truth? The Promised One? Or merely a stone shard, another hoax, another distortion through the glass darkly? Frost's perplexity is ours as well.

I imagine that when we stare into the pool we experience what, ultimately, Narcissus experienced to his dismay. He was not just entranced by his beauty; he was stunned by his complexity, his infinite number of selves, his compelling regression into the black hole of the timeless *Unus Mundi*. Like the Quaker on the box of Quaker Puffed Wheat holding a box of Quaker Puffed Wheat holding a box of Quaker Puffed Wheat that so amused, perplexed, and captivated me as a child at the breakfast table, our image in the pool fades in infinite replication and infinite regression into a carnival house of mirrors, a receding puzzle box, a *matryoshka* doll within a doll within a doll, and so on. Narcissus wishes to be seen, and to be seen wholly. And so do we. The religious affirm that only God has that power and that capacity, and perhaps they are right. Perhaps the self is that capacious power within each of us that sees and holds us with care as we tumble through an infinite space into the depths of our own fathomless mysteries. It is a pool of great depth, a pool too deep for human sight to penetrate, but we urgently look and never stop looking.

Notes

1 The author's translation from German.
2 1st Corinthians, 13:12.
3 Act II, Sc. 7, line 142.
4 American soldiers left the phrase "Kilroy was here" everywhere in the world during WWII. Kilroy got around.
5 "The fear of death troubles me."
6 My definition of a Jungian self.
7 "Whereof one cannot speak, thereof one should remain silent," Tractatus Logicus Philosophicus.
8 No date or text reference available. It is attributed to her by oral tradition.

Bibliography

Burns, R. (1794). https://www.poetryfoundation.org/poems/43812/a-red-red-rose
Dostoevsky, F. (1961). *Notes from Underground*. New York: New American Library.
Eliot, T. S. (1935) http://www.davidgorman.com/4quartets/1-norton.htm
Frost, R. (1923). http://www.poetryfoundation.org/poem/173528
Hopkins, G. M. (1916). https://www.poetryfoundation.org/poems/44396/i-wake-and-feel-the-fell-of-dark-not-day
Jung, C. G. (1953–1979). *The Practice of Psychotherapy, CW 16*. Princeton: Princeton University Press
Nashe, T. (2016). A Litany in Time of the Plague. In *English Renaissance Poetry*. New York: NYRB.
Nietzsche, F. (1993). *Menschliche Allzumenschliche*. Stuttgart: Alfred Kroner Verlag.
Shakespeare, W. (*As you like it*, Act. II, Sc. 7, l. 142) http://shakespeare.mit.edu/asyoulikeit/asyoulikeit.2.7.html
Terence (c. 190 BCE). https://www.google.com/search?q=nihil+a+me+human&source=hp&ei= QurRYJi-BpGr5NoP0fyt-AM&iflsig=AINFCbYAAAAAYNH4UvtPpF1FmfmUXQQ9__ XaypAbfOPm&oq=nihil+a+me+human&gs_lcp=Cgdnd3Mtd2l6EAMyBggAEBYQH-jIGCAAQFhAeMgYIABAWEB4yBggAEBYQHjIGCAAQFhAeMgYIABAWEB4yBgg AEBYQHjIICAAQFhAKEB4yCAgAEBYQChAeMgglABAWEAoQHjoFCAAQsQM6C AgAELEDEIMBOggILhCxAxCDAToLCC4QsQMQxwEQowI6AggAOg4ILhCx-AxDHARCjAhCTAjoFCC4QsQM6CAguEMcBEBKMCOggIABCxAxCxCRAjoIC-C4QxwEQrwE6AgguOgsILhCxAxDHARCvAVC2D1jfKmC0MGgAcAB4AIABZIg B6wiSAQQxNS4xmAEAoAEBqgEHZ3dzLXdpeg&sclient=gws-wiz&ved=0ahUKE wiY5_zlsKvxAhWRFVkFHVF-Cz8Q4dUDCAk&uact=5
Wittgenstein, Ludwig. (2001). *Tractatus Logico-Philosophicus*. London: Routledge.

Chapter 4

Verena Kast

As the youngest child in a large family growing up on a farm in the Appenzell foothills of the Alps high above Lake Constance, it was rather unlikely that I would one day become a psychologist and psychotherapist. I was the youngest child—my three older siblings were 7, 8, and 10 years older than me. And on the farm lived my grandfather, who was over 80 when I was born. The two of us—the oldest and the youngest in the family—spent a lot of time together, because we were probably the only ones who had a lot of time. I was a very lively child, and to have some peace and quiet, my grandfather told me fairy tales and horror stories, which I loved more than anything else. The love for stories and for symbolism captured me early.

But I have been out in nature a lot, and I still like to be outdoors. Alone or with neighbour children near our farm, at a pond we watched the frogs, especially in spring; we also plagued them, took them in our hands, wanted to tame them. Around the pond there was loamy soil—and if you walked barefoot over it, it slipped between your toes—a wonderful body feeling.

You could also play in the nearby forest: there were caves to discover and live in, and we could build huts there, in younger years for little "people", as we called certain pieces of wood, and later we built larger huts. In winter, I had built a small stage for a game with logs, to which I gave certain names, and which then "performed" their lives together. I played monodrama, of course, without knowing this name. My imagination was also stimulated by excessive reading—reading is actually a great and wonderful imagination—and through reading, many different ways of life became accessible and interesting to me. Through the imagination, the richness of the world and also the inner world became accessible to me. Even today—especially with increasing age—I appreciate the richness of the imagination and the possibilities that the imagination opens up for me. And I am still very happy when I have an exciting book to read.

At lunchtime, our large family often talked about politics—my father was mayor of our residential community, but he was also politically active beyond the community. My mother was president of the "Landfrauen", the peasant women. Both father and mother had no further school education, which both regretted very much, but they were very clever. It was natural for them to take on responsibility when it was necessary. That may be the reason why I became president of the

DOI: 10.4324/9781003148982-5

SGFAP, then president of the IAAP, and later president of the CGJIZ, Küsnacht, and why I was one of the organizers of the Lindau Psychotherapy Weeks, the largest German-speaking psychotherapy congress. I found, and still find, that one has to do something for the community.

I was a very curious child and loved school more than anything else. I thought it was wonderful what you could know. I didn't like the holidays that much; you had to work on the farm, and it was expected that I would do the same. But I loved to read and used my creativity to find ways to get away from work. None of my siblings had done it like that. Each of my siblings took up a decent profession, but nobody wanted to go to college. I was different from the others—my parents and brothers and sisters were very kind people who didn't let me feel it too much, but they were surprised once in a while as to how they had come to have this child. And I was a little surprised that the others were not interested in what I was interested in—and my grandfather had died in the meantime.

After secondary school, I became a teacher for girls between 14 and 16 years old, which was psychologically very challenging, but I loved to teach, to teach other people, to interest them in something. After that, I decided to study psychology and philosophy. I started this study in 1965—it was a time when psychology, especially everything that had to do with depth psychology and psychotherapy, had great importance and was also connected with the student revolts of 1968. As a student of psychology, it was natural to choose a "school" of depth psychology. So, I visited every institute for psychotherapy in Zürich. The Jung Institute was at that time very little regulated, somehow creative and chaotic, and the lecturers were interesting: I only mention Jacobi, von Franz, Fierz, Riklin. There I stayed and started my education, parallel to my studies at the university in 1965. In the Jung Institute I recovered from the university, while at the university I recovered from the Jung Institute. This double-degree course was very convenient and a time savings for me as a student who had to earn the money for her studies herself. But not only that: the ideas that were discussed at the Jung Institute touched me much more than the mostly cognitive ideas from modern psychology. Jungian psychology also coincided well with my philosophical interests. I became a psychotherapist, a very young psychotherapist at first—and my colleagues thought I was too young for a long time—until I was suddenly too old for some things.

From 1973 to 2008 I worked at the University of Zürich, first as a lecturer and then as a professor. I was very fortunate to also be able to cover depth psychology in my lectures and seminars in the field of anthropological psychology, which meant that I was able to teach on the topics that were closest to my heart and that were also the basis for my books and the lectures that I have given in many countries.

Looking back, I am astonished about what has found a place in my life: teaching, professional involvement, writing books, therapeutic practice, raising the children of a friend who died of cancer at an early age, traveling, swimming in the sea.

And I was always working at the C.G. Jung Institute in Zürich. I still teach today at this institute, which has changed a lot over the years, combining Jungian psychology with modern approaches. For me, Jungian psychology is based on emotions and imagination and, thus, on creativity; that is why it always remains contemporary, for example, when we think about how modern neuroscientific research on imagination is today. Of course, psychology is never complete—many of C.G. Jung's thoughts can be brought into a new form in the confrontation with current streams and thoughts. And it feels good to know that there are colleagues for whom it is important to carry Jung's thinking further.

There have always been people with whom I have lived and worked, with whom I have exchanged ideas, and I have been especially satisfied when the feeling of sharing, the feeling of togetherness, was particularly tangible, together with all of the inspiration and creative ideas that came from it.

Verena Kast
Sant Gallen, July 2020

Complexes and Their Compensation

Impulses From Affective Neuroscience

Originally published in 2019 (German) in *Analytische Psychologie (Zeitschrift)*, 191. Reprinted with permission.

The Basis of Personality Is Affectivity

This is what C.G. Jung wrote around 1906, and it is comparable to what Panksepp said about 100 years later. Jung began his scientific career with the association experiment and thus with complex theory. In other words, he began his career with the study of emotions, which he understood to be the basis of what it means to be a human being. "The essential basis of our personality is affectivity. Thought and action are, as it were, only symptoms of affectivity" (Jung, 1906, §78).

There are two important footnotes to this statement. Footnote 1: Bleuler proposes the term "affectivity" for feeling, sentiment, emotion, affect, "which is to denote not only the affects in the actual sense, but also the light feelings or emotional tones of lust and lustlessness in all possible experiences." Footnote 2: Bleuler says,

> Thus, affectivity is much more than cognition the driving element in all our actions and omissions. Probably we act only under the influence of feelings of lust—and lustlessness; logical reasoning only gets its driving force from the affects associated with it. . . . Affectivity is the broader term of which wanting and striving is only one side.
>
> (Bleuler, 1906, quoted in Jung, 1906, footnote to §78)

An amazing statement by Eugen Bleuler! On the basis of this important statement, Jung established the theory of "emotional complexes", and with it also a link to dreams. In sleep, according to Jung, the complexes appear as dreams (see Jung, 1934, 1967, §202f.).

Now, about 100 years later, Jaak Panksepp, an affective neuroscientist, writes, "It is clear that psychotherapy is in the midst of an emotion revolution. The primal affective aspects of mind are no longer marginalized, but, rather, are recognized as the very engines of the psyche" (Panksepp and Biven, 2012, p. 35).

C.G. Jung and Affective Neuroscience

It seems to me to be the right moment to bring together the ideas of C.G. Jung and Jaak Panksepp, and also those of Antonio Damasio and Frans de Waal and others. These new findings and ideas of affective neuroscience support the theories of C.G. Jung and also show how important they were, both in his time and in the current discussion. Perhaps we can, thereby, appreciate C.G. Jung's more fundamental theories.

The findings of affective neuroscience can also provide input for our work: On the one hand, we will see that C.G. Jung's basic ideas on psychology are in accordance with current findings in affective neuroscience. On the other hand, these findings will teach us to better understand the dynamics of complexes, stimulate us to come up with new ideas for clinical work with complexes and dreams, and also give us new ideas about the roots of the human being.

Basic Emotional Systems

Jaak Panksepp describes seven basic emotional systems in mammals, which he writes in capital letters to make it clear that they refer to neural networks and should not be understood as emotions in the everyday sense. The systems are SEEKING (seeking, rewarding, enthusiasm), sexual LUST (lust), RAGE (anger, rage), FEAR (fear, anxiety) CARE (care, maternal care), PANIC/GRIEF (panic and grief, experience of loss), and PLAY (social play). He calls these systems "primary process psychological experiences (they are among the 'givens' of the Brain-Mind" (Panksepp and Biven, 2012, p. 457). "BrainMind" is written as one word to express the fact that brain and mind are an inseparable unit. Over this biological, emotional basis, he sees various learning and memory processes, which he calls secondary processes of the brain and which he understands as deeply unconscious (Panksepp and Biven, 2012, p. 9). At the top of the brain are various higher mental processes—insights and thoughts that enable us to reflect on our experiences. He calls these processes tertiary processes (Panksepp and Biven, 2012, p. 9). According to Panksepp, therapeutic work takes place on the secondary, and especially on the tertiary level. But at the mammalian level, he sees something fundamental in the power and energy of the primary process-like emotions, something fundamental to our emotional nature, which can be felt by humans but cannot really be researched. But it can be researched in other mammals. And herein lies the importance of studies on animals, such as those by Panksepp and others. Panksepp is convinced that these primary process-like emotional systems can be found in all mammals, including humans. Panksepp adds further comments:

> The raw affects are ancestral memories that are also experienced in animals, we can understand their functions in similar ways. By anticipating survival issues, intrinsic affective states provide immediate guidance for behavior. To the best of our knowledge, we are born with innate neural capacities for the full complement of seven basic emotions that are hardwired into the subcortical networks of all mammalian brains. . . . These pre-propositional emotional energetic states have minds of their own as ancient forms of affective mentation that preceded language and thought by vast spans of evolutionary time.
> (Panksepp and Biven, 2012, p. 453)

Here we have a reference to archetypal processes, archetypes understood as emotional and structural dispositions upon which social and cultural structures with their narratives are built; aspects of our deep emotional systems that are also the basis for unconscious actions. Panksepp sees these basic affects as independent of subsequent environmental experiences (Panksepp and Biven, 2012, p. 21). However, the environmental experiences are based on these primary process-like affective systems: People learn a lot in their ongoing contact with the world in the broadest sense, and so these raw affects become connected with the experiences and images of an individual's life. And so, the primary emotions are connected with and behind our "normal" emotions; in fact, they are the basis and the foundation of our "normal" emotions, such as curiosity, interest, joy, fear, anger, and grief, as well as social emotions such as shame or envy. What we call "primary emotions" in psychology are based on the basic emotional systems, but they are mixed with and enriched by the development of the experiences, thoughts, and fantasies connected with them, thus forming the secondary and tertiary levels of human experience. For Panksepp, art, like spirituality, is based in biology, in our emotions.

Clarification: Emotion, Cognition, and Feelings

Emotions and cognition have a highly interactive effect, and at the tertiary level, according to Panksepp, distinctions are almost impossible. Panksepp suggests a definition, which I am happy to follow here:

> The cognitive aspects are more closely linked to the programming of each individual's higher brain development, while the raw emotions and affects represent the ancestral inherited tools for living. Although the interaction of emotion and cognition is inextricably interwoven in the unique puzzle of each individual's higher mind, we must be able to envision cognition and emotion as different, albeit interconnected, types of mental processing. Anatomically speaking they are as distinct and interacting as our hearts and skeletal muscles.
> (Panksepp and Biven, 2012, p. 468)

Basically, in the view of Panksepp and others, the affects provide the energy and they promote and guide thought (that's what Bleuler thought). The pronounced original emotions of the primarily affective systems are the sources and the roots of our everyday emotions, such as curiosity, interest, joy, fear, anger, and shame, but also of our thinking and behaviour.

We connect feelings with the perception of what is going on in our body and mind when we focus on and reflect on the different emotions. Then we can also roughly name them. Emotions can be understood as the perception of images of what is going on in our body and mind. This view corresponds to the idea that emotional processes are accompanied by ideas, pictures, and thoughts. The experiences that an individual has in everyday life are triggers for emotions, connected with changes in his or her own body (physiologically) and through synchronizations with other bodies, and these also connect again with memory contents and imaginations.

Jung and the Complexes

Complexes are energy centres built around a core of affective meaning, probably caused by a painful collision of the individual with a requirement or event in the environment for which the individual is not ready. Every event in a similar direction is then interpreted in the sense of this complex and further reinforces the complex: the emotional tone (the emotion) that makes up this complex is retained and even reinforced (cf. Jung, 1921, §991). Thus, the complexes denote the crisis-prone areas in the individual. As energy centres, however, they have a certain activity—expressed in the emotion—which makes up a large part of the psychic life.

Complexes hinder the individual in his or her personal development in the area of the complex topic, but in these complexes also lie the germs of new life possibilities (Jung, 1934, 1967, §210). These creative germs appear when we accept the complexes, and when we grasp the narratives, the emotions, and the imagery connected with it. We all have complexes; they are expressions of life topics which have become life problems. They make up our psychological disposition, out of which nobody can jump. So, the symbols and symbolic representations, connected with the corresponding emotions, are both expressions and processing processes of the complexes; dreams and imaginations work on the complexes (Jung, 1934, 1967, §202).

The Complex Episode as Relationship Experience

The term complex episode is derived from a quotation by C.G. Jung. In a lecture in 1928, Jung talks about the emergence of complexes:

> It (the complex) appears to emerge from the clash of a demand for adaptation with the particular and, in terms of demand, unsuitable nature of the individual.
> (Jung, 1921, 1960, §991)

With this definition, the relationship aspect is brought into the centre of the formation of the complex, and the aspect of relationship, also in Jung's theory, has become increasingly important in recent decades. Following this abstract definition, Jung then speaks of the parental complex as the first manifestation of the clash between "reality and the in this respect unsuitable nature of the individual." As a rule, the demand for adaptation probably always emanates from people, which means that our complexes structurally and emotionally reflect the relationship stories of our childhood and later life. Complexes can arise as long as a person lives. However, most complexes, even those that are developed later, associate themselves with earlier complexes. Therefore, in this view of the clash, two people face each other: a child and a significant related person. I call these the two poles of the complex.

Because Jung then speaks of parental complexes, we can conclude that the clashes of which he speaks are those between children and parents or other important caregivers. In connection with the results of the attachment theory, we can safely add the following: an agonizing clash in a situation where a child would have needed an experience of attachment, an experience that someone cares helps, even in a situation parents do not like. Wherever experiences become complex episodes, the point is that the person has been abandoned in a situation of special challenge or in connection with demands, in which the child would have needed caring, supportive relationship persons and in which the child would have felt loved, even if he or she had done something that was not good in the eyes of the relationship persons. Instead, messages such as "you are always a disappointment" and "you never make an effort" are sent with the associated feelings, which in turn trigger special counter-feelings such as despair, anger, or fear, combined with the conviction that things will never be different, and above all never better.

The Past of Complexes: Emotional Contagion as an Early Basis of Complexes

Complex episodes have a past, an emotional basis. Researchers from various disciplines study the phenomenon of empathy and, in this context, the field of emotional contagion: empathy is based on emotional contagion (see Waal, 2011, p. 269, and Hatfield et al., 2009). Emotional contagion means that if someone is angry, we also become angry without any external cause, we are infected. If someone laughs, we laugh too; if someone moves his or her body in a specific way or touches him- or herself, we unconsciously make the same movement or gesture. Currently, it is assumed that emotions are triggered by the synchronisation of the bodies of different people (de Waal, 2011, p. 69). We feel what the other or the other person feels, deeply unconsciously but very effectively. In the analytical process, we try to put emotional contagion into words: We express approximately in images or words what we feel and what may be going on in the analysand—and thus we help the analysand to find words and images for disturbing emotional states. We help to make people aware of emotional and emotional states by perceiving the countertransference, and through processes of mentalising, and at the same time we prevent ourselves from being constantly infected by the analysand's emotions.

Some ideas of developmental psychology: From the beginning of life—also intrauterine—a baby is exposed to the emotions and feelings of the mother and father and other caregivers through movements, voices, and later through facial expressions, and there is no way for the baby to escape this. If children have good attachment bonding, combined with a good release of oxytocin and other hormones, this helps in dealing with stress. But if the bonding is not secure, then stress situations—and these are emotional problems—of the related persons will also influence the baby, and this has an influence on later stress management, as studies have shown (cf. Roth and Stübner, 2014, p. 145ff.), that is, in later life they react more sensitively to conflicts, especially to conflicts in relationships, which are the bases for the formation of complexes.

The baby is infected by the emotions of the caregivers, and this means that the emotions connected with the complex episodes, such as fear, exist long before stories about the complex episodes can be formulated, long before someone can tell about a situation that has caused them so much fear or a situation that is shameful and insulting, and long before the emotions can be expressed verbally or visualized. Panksepp suspects that these early emotional contagions and also overwhelming experiences are all about the fact that the primary process-like basic emotional systems are sensitized or desensitized too much, especially in early childhood, but I also mean later. This is due to "permanent, epigenetically induced high-stress reactivity and excessive primary process negativistic feelings" (Panksepp and Biven, 2012, p. 434).

Panksepp sees these mechanisms at the root of numerous psychological disorders based on a genetic sensitivity background on the one hand and due to stress experienced on the other. Of course, there is a difference in the emotional maturity levels at which the respective emotional stress is experienced. [The decisive difference is probably whether a self (ego complex) already exists and then a trauma was experienced, or whether the child is exposed to a trauma before a self could emerge].

Basically, if we speak of father and mother complexes in a general form, not of individual complex episodes but of the whole of the complex episodes that emerged in relation to the mother and father and to maternal and paternal representatives, then we should not forget that the emotional lives of the parents have a great influence on the emotional bases of the children and thus also on the formation of the complex episodes.

The definition of a complex episode described so far must therefore be supplemented to this effect: Complexes are formed when the individual undergoes a painful clash with an external demand or an event in the environment that is experienced as overwhelming because no caring, or a not caring enough, relationship is available. Through these conflict situations, without sufficient containment, ancestral "family emotions" are also activated, along with the primary emotional systems associated with them.

Constellated Complex Episodes

Complex episodes are expressions of difficult dysfunctional relationship experiences, generated particularly in early childhood and emotionally linked to the emotional heritage of the parents and their history. These relationship experiences constellate again and again in everyday life; similar experiences are occur again and again in relationships or comparable difficulties, or they are interpreted with an emotionally strongly emphasized experience in the sense of the complex episode, and this also occurs in the therapeutic relationship. If these experiences are disturbing in everyday life, such as, "I experience the same rejection again and again, the world threatens me", dysfunctional patterns of relationships are developed out of these convictions, and self-esteem is increasingly weakened. In the therapeutic relationship, we welcome the constellation of the complex episode: an important problem in relationships shows up, and it can be worked on and eventually changed in a situation of attachment bonding—connected with the friendly face of the analyst. Complex episodes become visible in stories of difficult dysfunctional relationship episodes that repeatedly occur in similar ways, consisting of comparable information, particularly about the self-image (Selbstbild) of the child and of the attacking persons. These dysfunctional relationships are accessible in narratives, connected with definite emotions experienced in these difficult relationship situations, and therefore also accessible in emotions. The felt (experienced) emotions bring forth the story lines, more conscious material. The stories concern relationship experiences that have occurred repeatedly and are internalised with episodic memory (Kast, 1998). This means that the whole complex episode (child and aggressor)—usually we can tell a story about it—is internalised and can be active. In the stories there is often an identification with the child part of the complex episode, and the complex bearer (the human being suffering from the complex) is convinced that "all" other people attack them in the way in which the attacking figures of the complex episodes did, but this might be not true. They can also be identified with the attacker—in soliloquies—but also in how they treat other people in everyday life. And this is very important to become conscious about: believing that they are in the position of the victim, unconsciously they are identified with the position of the attacker, treating their fellows as they have approximately felt to be treated in the experiences that created the complex.

Complexes are generated in situations in which bonding would be important. It is a "cutting down" of the need to be with others—to feel attached. If the complex episode is constellated, the patient is psychologically back in this situation of abandonment in a stressful situation. And the stories revolve around the basic needs of human beings: being accepted, being loved even in difficult situations, being seen, being able to be effective and creative, being helpful to others, and experiencing meaning. These stories connected with the complex episodes are linked with the conviction that even new experiences are not possible; they are in the old ruts, the experiences of relationships have always been the same—and will always be the same. Usually psychic life is dynamic—emotions are constantly changing, thoughts and images are changing—but if a complex is constellated, psychic life is frozen. This is the place where we work psychotherapeutically.

Complex Episode Shame: An Example

When we are ashamed, we experience ourselves in the mode of being seen and seeing. We are in the eyes of the others. But, if we are ashamed, we assume that the other person looks at us with an evil, critical eye and denies what we are and what we do. Under this shameful look, our self-esteem crumbles. And then we ask ourselves very precisely: Who am I? The analysis of the gaze of Jean Paul Sartre is, in my opinion, illuminating. In his biography "The Words" ("Les Mots"), Jean Paul Sartre describes an experience that led to shame (Sartre, 1968, p. 48). As a child he experienced adults being very attentive to the actions of the child, keeping a critical eye on the child's behaviour. And then, he adds, even when the adults are no longer in the room, when they are outside, the eyes remain there. His experience: he is always under the eyes, under the evaluating eyes of the adults, either real or imagined. The child has internalized these critical eyes so that he always lives under these critical eyes, under these critical looks. And that is the essence of a complex episode: we have internalised what has happened to us. The relationship episode with the corresponding emotion between the one who is shaming and the one who is being shamed can also be understood as self-talk. Under these critical looks, Sartre says, self-esteem crumbles. This must then be restored. The lowered self-esteem must be defended and compensated: we can try to be extraordinarily perfect so that nobody sees anything wrong with us. Or we can simply hide, hoping not to be discovered by the eyes of others—or we can get angry and fight at best—at worst we become destructive. Jean Paul Sartre solved the problem by saying that the eyes of the others are none of his business, that what the others think of him does not concern him. But this argument devalues the relationship.

In this context, I would like to argue with Levinas' "benevolent eyes." Levinas, also a French philosopher and a contemporary of Sartre, argued that we are often viewed by very friendly eyes—and that we then feel accepted, seen, and valued. But we can also feel ashamed when people look at us in a benevolent way, because we feel that we have gone beyond our limits in the other person's kind look. The shame then shows us our limits, which are often also the limits of the community in which we live. There are not only the critical eyes, there are also friendly eyes—we ourselves can look at each other in an evil critical way, but we can also learn to confront ourselves with very kind critical looks. Of course, the question arises here, too, whether one was looked at in a very kind and critical way as a child, only critically, or only friendly, one will have to learn one or the other (Levinas, 2003, p. 115).

Complex Episode and Narrative

These dysfunctional relationship experiences are also accessible in narratives, linked to the emotions experienced in the difficult episode. The experienced emotions convey the stories, so the emotions are verbalized or illustrated. Usually a "basic narrative" is found, which is given by the analysands as evidence of a complex episode and thus often also of an inhibition, which is a story from the past but that can be enriched more and more. The woman who says of herself that she cannot speak in front of her team, and who therefore cannot or does not want to take a higher position in her professional life, finds a narrative underlying this complex episode based on a dream.

The dream:

> I'm supposed to speak in front of my team. I am in the room in which we meet to talk in reality. But the room is bigger. I have a microphone, and I am not speaking, I am singing. There's a sound coming from somewhere: "Stop that fucking noise". My colleagues look around, come closer to me and ask me to keep singing. The dream fades, but it felt very good and the voices saying "fucking noise" disappeared.

The dreamer is surprised that she sings. She has a very sober job, she says. Singing felt good: terrible when those voices in the background disturbed, wonderful when her team members gathered around her and made her understand that they liked her singing.

The dreamer remembers: she was maybe 13 when her teacher told her that she had a very beautiful voice. So, in the evening she stands at the window of her room and sings loudly and "beautifully", so she thinks. Her father comes by and orders her to stop her "shit noise." Since then, she says, she can no longer "perform" in front of other people. In the dream, however, this complex episode from childhood is not simply repeated, but he has changed it. "Back then" there were apparently no helpers who could have supported the girl against the father's rejection—but now in the dream there are. As a result, the fear that the others might laugh at her has disappeared—and with the imagination a "we-feeling" also arises. Together with the others—not at the mercy of the others—but with those who ask them to sing on. These were important impulses for her. Not the fear of being laughed at, but the good feeling of being together with others and thus being able to stand on her own. No longer the critical look projected onto colleagues, but the friendly look. Not to be pushed into loneliness by criticism, but to stand together in solidarity. Again and again the dreamer imagined the dream: work situations in which she became suspicious, wondering whether her colleagues were really critical now. She also understood her singing as a form of self-exposure—and she dared to address her insecurity in such situations by discussing the topic that worried her and no longer by simply assuming that her employees were questioning her as a person. She learned that in working with others she performed very well as part of a team, but above all that she did not have to be perfect. This dream was one of the dreams that accompanied her for a long time and brought about a change in her social behaviour.

As already mentioned, complexes are generated in situations where the possibility of a bonding experience would have been essential in dealing with the conflict.

This should be kept in mind in the therapeutic process: when the complex episode is constellated, the patient is again in this experience of being abandoned in an emotionally difficult situation and in need of a bonding person, a helper. In this dream, intrapsychic helpers are already appearing, a sign that this complex is in good work, the dreamer has access to helping figures in her own psyche. This is usually the result of experiencing reliable relationships, be it through a good therapeutic relationship but also through trusting relationships with people in everyday life.

The narratives that are told concern experiences that have been experienced repeatedly in a similar emotional tone around the "same" subject and have been internalized with episodic memory. Perhaps the narrated story is a "generalized" story (Kast, 1998, p. 307), which may never have happened in this way, but which psychologically summarizes and depicts the basic experience in a particularly coherent way. Because the whole complex episode has been internalised with episodic memory, this also means that the relationship between the child and the attacker has been internalised and that one can identify with both figures. However, the stories are first told from the perspective of the child, that is, from the perspective of the victim. And those who are marked by a complex episode are initially convinced that "all" people attack them as they were attacked by the characters who set the complex episode. That is not always true. But we can also be identified—usually unconsciously—with the attacker. This becomes clear, for example, in soliloquies, which are often conversations between the "old attacker" and the "old victim. But we can also be identified with the attacker and attack people in everyday life from this position. To perceive these situations, to become aware of them, is very important for the work on the complex episode: sometimes we are convinced to be in the role of a victim, "as always", but unconsciously we are identified with the attacker and treat our fellow human beings in a similar way as we ourselves felt treated in the experiences that caused the complex.

The stories are always about the basic existential needs of humans: they are about being loved and being allowed to love, being seen, being allowed to pursue one's interests, exploring the world, being allowed to be creative, following one's own impulses, being effective, living with relish, being allowed to help and accept help, and being allowed to experience life as meaningful.

These narratives of complex episodes are connected with the conviction that other, new experiences are not possible, that experiences in relationships always move on the old tracks, have always been like this, and will never be different. There appears to be no possibility to have access to creativity on a personal level. Actually, psychic life is dynamic, emotions are constantly changing, and thoughts and images are constantly in motion. But when a complex is constellated, the psychic life is shock frozen. This links to what is understood by ruminating in research on daydreaming (Fox et al., 2018). These are repetitive thoughts that focus on the negative, as is the case with patients with depression and anxiety. These stereotypical negative feelings, thoughts, and fantasies are connected with complexes. That is what we work on for possible change, for possible becoming.

What About Possible Inputs From Newer Theories About Emotions for Working With Complex Episodes?

> Emotional disorders are invariably tied up with one or more of the basic emotional systems.
>
> (Panksepp and Biven, 2012, p. 435)

Panksepp argues that telling the stories and the associated affects that represent the mental disorder over and over again is counterproductive—and I would speak of complex episodes in this context—and that this throws the affect system out of balance. Therefore, he thinks it would be helpful to bring people who are out of balance into a different emotional state, especially by activating the SEEKING system and the PLAY system, which are also the bases for the so-called positive emotions such as curiosity, interest, joy, and inspiration. This idea of Panksepp was already described by Baruch Spinoza (1632–1677) in a comparable way. He was very interested in emotions and described them in detail: Spinoza wrote that when a human being is seized by a deep, difficult emotion, only the opposite emotion—with the same or even more energy—can change the difficult emotion or balance it. When we suffer, we need the affect of joy (cf. Spinoza, 1963, p. 196).

The idea of Panksepp, and of Spinoza previously, to stimulate an emotion opposite to the one that defines the complex is close to Jungian thinking: he also saw complexes as centres of energy (emotion), and in this respect of change as well, as "burning—or nodal points of the psychic life" (Jung, 1921, §990). The idea of compensation, and thus also that of imbalance and balance, is a central theme in Jungian psychology: The psychic life loses its balance again and again and becomes one-sided, and this is connected with emotional problems. In emotional experiences, in dreams and in imagination, one finds indications of aspects that are missing, which allow one to momentarily regain a state of unstable balance. These processes of rebalancing oneself again and again are processes of compensation or creative processes which, as a whole, make up the individuation process. It is not only about overcoming problems or about psychological well-being but, as seen in terms of life as a whole, a process of getting in touch with oneself.

Panksepp also pursues the idea of compensation without using the word. By referring to the SEEKING system and the PLAY system, one moves away from the emotions that determine the complex and into the opposite emotions, that is, primarily into the SEEKING system. For Panksepp, the SEEKING system is involved in all emotional excitement and it initiates the search for resources to survive but also for reward. On the second level, the SEEKING system corresponds to the emotions curiosity, interest, and joy. It is Panksepp's idea that the primary process-based emotional system helps to establish corresponding emotions, as well as thoughts and structures on a higher level. We cannot directly activate the primary process level (dreams can possibly do it). But what we can do is to activate everyday emotions and feelings, which could then affect the primary emotional process level (see Panksepp and Biven, 2012, p. 434).

In practical work it looks like this: Gifted therapists apply this idea without knowing the theoretical background. How often, in a situation of deep sadness of being stuck, does a remark from the analyst cause a smile or even real laughter, and new ideas become possible again, different emotions and feelings are accessible again—not only the one of sadness or anger about being stuck—and this means that imagination, creativity, and joy, are possible again, as are, therefore, fantasies of good experiences. And it goes without saying that therapists are in good contact with the CARE system. This is the basis for the therapeutic relationship that is so important for the success of psychotherapeutic processes.

Affective Balance Therapies

Panksepp suggests making a turn towards more positive emotions in psychotherapy. For this he refers to a form of therapy which he calls "Affective Balance Therapies (ABTs)" (Panksepp and Biven, 2012, p. 434). Above all, he suggests activation of the PLAY system as a counteraction to RAGE, FEAR, and GRIEF. What exactly does he mean by "activating" the PLAY system, which is always connected to the SEEKING system? He means to engage creatively, to take a very kind interest in the mental world of others, a kind of friendly competition. Analysts and analysands play with ideas and content, and both are engaged. It is abstinent in the sense that the analyst does not determine what the analysand has to do, play, or think, but not abstinent in the sense that he or she helps to open a space for creativity, exploration, creative methods, body movements—and all of this is possible through secure bonding in the therapeutic process. Panksepp's conviction: If the SEEKING system gets connected to higher brain functions, this leads to psychological development and to experiences of identity and of meaning. In addition, the activation of emotions is a good way to access repressed cognitive material. In analytical psychology, the SEEKING system is triggered by our deep and lasting interest in the individuation process, connected with our interest in symbols, dreams, images, and imagination, which hopefully will also infect our analysands.

The PLAY System and Dreams

Panksepp plays with the idea that in dreams the PLAY system is at work. The PLAY system prepares us for future challenges, and that, he believes, is also the function of dreams: to test solutions to complex problems. He sees in dreams: "emotion-related cognitive possibilities in the safety of dreaming sleep, thereby perhaps better helping integrate cognitive and affective issues" (Panksepp and Biven, 2012, p. 377). He understands dreams as "a window into our ancient emotional minds" (Panksepp and Biven, 2012, p. 377), In REM sleep especially he sees the activation of original (raw) affects. In this manner, dreams connect cognitive elements in a new way, integrate neglected emotions, and help to find creative solutions for the future.

Complexes and Dreams

There is a connection in C.G. Jung's thinking between the understanding of complexes and dreams and our imaginations. In "The Problems of Modern Psychotherapy", C.G. Jung states,

> The complex forms a small enclosed psyche, so to speak, which . . . develops a peculiar fantasy activity. Imagination is in fact the self-activity of the soul, which breaks through wherever the inhibition by consciousness weakens or even stops altogether, as in sleep. In sleep the imagination appears as a dream. But even when we are awake, we continue to dream below the threshold of consciousness, and this is especially so because of repressed or otherwise unconscious complexes.
>
> (Jung, 1935, §125)

In 1916, C.G. Jung had already pointed out that the emotionally charged aspects of the psyche (the complexes) are the starting point for imagination, for fantasies, for series of pictures: starting points for symbols. This includes the statement that although complexes prevent the individual from developing in the areas of the most important complexes, germs of new life—possibilities for the future—can be found in the complexes (Jung, 1934, 1967, §63). Jung describes the following in his 1916 essay "The transcendental function" (see Jung, 1934, 1967, §131–193): "In the intensity of the emotional disturbance itself lies . . . the energy which he should have at his disposal in order to remedy the state of reduced adaptation" (Jung, 1934, 1967, §166).

These creative germs can be found if we accept the complexes and let them be represented in our imagination or if we experience them in dreams, particularly if we work on them with our imagination (Kast, 2019).

C.G. Jung: "The via regia to the unconscious . . . is the complex which is the architect of dreams and symptoms" (Jung, 1934, 1967, §210). In Jung we find the idea that the emotions connected with the complex episodes trigger the dreams, connected with memories. And these memories can be connected in the dreams in a new way, and with this the emotions change (Kast, 2019). When the emotions in the dreams connect to the primary emotional system, and this is what Panksepp assumes, then the dream has access to the archetypal level and helps to balance the emotional life by connecting to an old evolutionary system in our body.

Panksepp: Thoughts on the PLAY System

According to Panksepp, depressive people have an underdeveloped PLAY system, and therefore it is the task of therapy to activate the SEEKING system and the PLAY system in a situation where the CARE system, as the basis for a therapeutic relationship, unfolds its effectiveness. For Panksepp, therapy means not only to get in contact with emotions but also, and above all, to get in contact with positive emotions "to reframe troublesome memories—to reconsolidate psychic pain within the balm of positive affects" (Panksepp and Biven, 2012, p. 435).

How does it work? Panksepp sees "many ways to use the positive affects of SEEKING and PLAY to counteract the negative affects of depression and anxiety disorders" (Panksepp and Biden, 2012, p. 431). His belief is that "[i]f one modifies affects, cognition will follow, especially with good counsel" (Panksepp and Biden, 2012, p. 432).

A change in thinking only works if emotion is involved, states Panksepp. So the question is, how can we induce emotions and feelings? His answer is through body movement, music, and imagination of experiences that have triggered or will trigger positive emotions. Panksepp is convinced that emotions are triggered by the synchronisation of the human body, and therefore he also sets body reactions to induce positive emotions. In one study, he shows that even when simulating emotional actions, for example, in a situation in which the physical reaction of laughing is imagined without imagining a funny episode, positive emotions are aroused (Panksepp and Biven, 2012, p. 454). I cannot imagine, however, that if we concentrate on the physical expression of laughter, we cannot also imagine a situation in which we once broke out into a big laugh. Panksepp also sees the SEEKING system at work when we allow ourselves fantastic and creative imagination and also in the use of all of our prosocial emotions (such as empathy, joy, love), which are based on the CARE, GRIEF, and PLAY systems. This is a way for him to regulate our emotions in a much deeper sense than we normally do, for example, by mentalising and by becoming aware of emotional contagions. Deeper, because we include these ancestral emotional systems, in our language of the archetypal systems: this creates a better balance, and for him this is the basis for well-being. The idea of balance corresponds to the idea of regulating emotions, and this is also a concern in the work with complexes. But the balance that Panksepp has in mind seems to me to be even more sustainable, more fundamental: he wants to include the energy of the emotions of our ancestors (ancestral emotions) in the form of the wisdom of the body (Panksepp and Biven, 2012, p. 377). And that means inclusion of the energies of the archetypes in the form of emotions—and this is meant quite physically—in order to cope with life in a broad sense but also for the everyday regulation of emotions.

The Importance of the Imagination

Memories are imagination (Schacter et al., 2012) and they are important, but not only memories are associated with complex episodes. In fact, these seem to be rather counterproductive, as they always tell the same stories and describe the same emotions, which does not change the situation but reinforces the emotions involved at the time and the convictions associated with them, leading finally to rumination. When patients ruminate, they speak of difficult situations without being emotionally covered: these descriptions are flat and filled with little emotional content. Therefore, little change can take place. It is not about precise, imaginative, single complex episodes from their life story but about generalized memories, such as everyone was always mean to me, just like my mother. The difficult situations are described from a distance and not really felt emotionally. These patients are too distanced from their problem, which nevertheless, or precisely because of this, does not let go of them. Therapists will sense these feelings, name them, and gradually give them images, making them tangible to the analysand. And therapists will ask about specific situations and about memories of specific experiences—in the form of imagery connected with emotions. Dreams and imagination will be extremely helpful. If the emotions associated with a complex episode are experienced, it is possible to also feel the strength in those emotions, for example, the anger that helps to change life. Or, if one really perceives how one was repeatedly shamed in one's childhood, then one can, with a certain distance, experience sadness about what happened and about the fact that these situations have determined one's life for so long that one could not really live one's own life. And grief also opens the gates to gratitude.

But memories that much more connected with interest, curiosity, joy, and inspiration are also sought. We find this material when we ask for resources at the beginning of therapy or when the analysand complains about not having access to good experiences right now. If these resources are specified, they are at least available as possible experiences that have already been accessible. In the imagination we can bring back into consciousness and feeling the missing joys, interests, and creative ideas that the individual has already experienced in his or her life.

Positive emotions can be awakened by the imaginative visualization of good experiences. For example, one can identify with oneself as a child in a situation in which one was full of joy by putting oneself in the body of the child in that particular situation. In our imagination, we can become infected with joy or situations of interest from the past. In dealing with patients, it is important that each, even fleeting, impression of joy or interest is perceived and named as something significant. These are the treasures that can be brought back to consciousness through imagination. In the process of imagination, we temporarily enter into an emotional contagion with the good experiences and the emotions associated with them. And if Panksepp's theory is correct, we also activate our elementary emotional systems in the process, which should lead to more balance and the possibility of developing new scenarios.

When people are so trapped by complex experiences, it is sometimes difficult to find joy and interest. We find them in regret: people tell us, for example, how much they used to enjoy singing, but now that joy is gone. Joy that no longer exists or seems to exist is remembered, at first with regret, but it is possible to empathize imaginatively with the remembered situations; even through empathic questions from the therapist, the joy can be experienced minimally. But there are also great feelings that can be present in the moment, and by drawing attention to them we can bring about great emotional change. Even people who have a difficult time in life and who are determined by a few complexes or even by one complex alone, and therefore easily get into brooding and ruminating, have touching emotional experiences, as they are presented in the concepts of awe and kama muta.

Awe and Kama Muta

Imagine a wild, roaring sea—a burst of energy, an experience of power—beautiful, full of energy and frightening, yet also fascinating. Overpowering, frightening—and fascinating.

A raging thunderstorm—it flashes and crashes and storms and rains—eerie, yet powerful, impressive.

The first spring flowers, the scent of spring, the first sounds of spring: embraced by becoming in nature.

There are experiences in nature that emotionally grip us, grab us, leave us breathless, and give us the impression of having experienced something wonderful—or even frightening—something that goes beyond our everyday experience and which we cannot grasp at first. It is strange, disconcerting, astonishing, and completely unusual what one experiences: a wonderful or frightened amazement about something overpowering, which we do not really understand at first, seizes us, we are seized by awe.

We feel awe when something big and powerful takes hold of us, something that is far beyond our control, which happens to us, surprises us, exceeds our expectations; it is much more deeply touching than we expected. And this experience suddenly changes our perception of ourselves: we feel small in the face of this fullness of experience, shrinking to a human dimension, and yet, or perhaps precisely because of this, we feel connected to this great, overpowering essence, we feel one with the world around us, and this gives an experience of meaning, of belonging to a great whole. In such moments, one is in a completely different context than the everyday. It is as if a crack has opened up in the clouds and for a certain time we can see ourselves, our lives, and others in a different way.

Most of the time such experiences happen in nature or when we experience culture, like music, but sometimes we are also given them in a dream. These experiences change our self-perception, and this change is well researched. Our mental concepts, according to Keltner and Haidt (2003), must be adapted to this experience. These are moments in which people open themselves to new possibilities, new thinking, new values. In the face of this overwhelming power, people realise their everyday needs and worries are less important and they feel more connected to the world and other people. In Jungian psychology, we speak in this context of an experience of wholeness or a "all-one." (Einheitswirklichkeit) A counter-world to the experience of stuck complex episodes, with many degrees of freedom.

Close to the feeling of awe are the feelings called kama muta—and yet they are also somewhat different, as kama muta is understood as a positive relationship emotion (Zickfeld, Schubert et al., 2019), a feeling that is fed by, but also changes, human relationships. According to various authors, kama muta is a "new feeling", for which these authors use the Sanskrit expression kama muta, most commonly translated as "moved by love," a tender feeling (Fiske et al., 2019).

Kama muta is described as a positive social relationship feeling, which is caused by observing or participating in sudden reinforcements of the communal experience with each other: an experience with others that is moving, touching, and heart-warming. Physically it is accompanied by feelings of warmth in the chest, buoyancy, and cheerfulness, tears, and often goosebumps. It motivates devotion to the community and to community action and stimulates commitment to community service. These feelings can occur when one actually observes other people, but these feelings can also arise when one reads about such situations or remembers them. In all of these cases, it is hardly a matter of self-efficacy: one has not caused these scenarios in a significant way, one is present from an empathic observer and witness perspective (see Menninghaus et al., 2015).

On a practical level, we can ask for a narrative about a situation in which the patient was moved, became tearful, or experienced a feeling of goose bumps—maybe when viewing a sporting event or a celebration. Such an event can be brought back imaginatively; here too, the therapist must encourage the patient to bring the situation back into memory as vividly as possible, visually and emotionally.

Such imaginative situations enliven aspects of the psyche that are not connected with the dominant complex episode, and they enliven experiences that connect us with other people and with nature.

Imagination—The Basis for Various Techniques in Jungian Psychotherapy

Imagination is fundamentally important when it comes to activating these universal basic emotions, to establishing an emotional balance, to playing with images, to perceiving emotions associated with them, and also to perceiving the body's feelings. The perception of a state of being in the body can be an emotional starting point for imagination. We know that Jung valued the imagination highly.

> To the extent that I managed to translate the emotions into images, that is to find the images which were concealed in the emotions, inwardly calmed and reassured. . . . I learned how helpful it can be, from the therapeutic point of view, to find the particular images which lie behind emotions.
>
> (Jung, 1961, p. 201)

The idea that in the affective disorder lies the energy that the suffering human needs for his or her emotional self-regulation, as well as for upcoming developmental steps, is the theoretical basis for the various techniques such as imagination, painting, performing games, and sand play and other techniques that are used in Jungian therapy to make complexes more conscious and to enable creative change. To work with the unconscious and to be attentive to the creative in the psyche, this was Jung's basic idea, and it applies to therapy as well as to everyday life.

For Jung, being in touch with the imagination meant being "alive", becoming more and more alive. "Soul is the living thing in man, that which lives on itself and causes life" (Jung, 1934, 1980, §56). To be in contact with fantasies means to be in contact with the living, but it also means that the everyday things of life become "alive." Imagining always also means playing. The same applies to working with dreams: we play with the themes of the dream, amplify them, collect the feelings connected with them, and connect them with memories and current problems with which we are dealing. We take dreams as a starting point for imagination and then paint them or shape them in a sand game.

If we take Panksepp's ideas even more seriously, we could do even more: we could consciously make contact with the respective counteracting universal basic emotions via imagination, but also via corresponding archetypal stories. We would have to become creative and clearly committed to the PLAY system: can we invent joyful stories? Interesting imagination of future experiences? And, can we share them with others whose imaginations are also involved?

Regulating Emotions: Two Ways

Even though I have now spoken a great deal about the importance of emotions and their associated body perceptions, we should not forget that there are two forms of emotional regulation: biological and sociocultural. In biological regulation, we perceive the corresponding emotions and feelings and also use them for orientation in life (cf. Kast, 2018, p. 97ff.). In sociocultural regulation, we tell stories about these emotions. Films, art, music, and paintings are expressions of emotions, feelings, and thoughts and give us the opportunity to encounter not only our own spirit but also that of others—and thus to be emotionally infected—in a good way, in the awakening of hope. Cultural heritage is a never-ending source to activate positive emotions—if we take the time for it and if we can get in resonance with it. We know the sociocultural way to balance our emotions very well from Jungian psychology; the emotional way, especially the way of emotional compensation, we could use more often. The processes of imagination are connecting the two.

Conclusion

Affective neuroscience provides us with the biological basis for Jungian psychology and psychotherapy. We Jungians could pay more attention to the biological bases of complexes and archetypal stories and make more use of this emotional track, together with the technique of imagination which is inherent in Jungian theory.

Literature

Bleuler, E. (1906). *Affektivität, Suggestibilität, Paranoia*. Carl von Reifitz (Hrsg) Verlag Der Classic Edition. Südwestdeutscher Verlag für Hochschulschriften.

Damasio, A. (2011). *Selbst ist der Mensch. Körper, Geist und die Entstehung des menschlichen Bewusstseins*. München: Siedler.

Fiske, A. P., Seibt, B. und Schubert, T. (2019). The Sudden Devotion Emotion: Kama Muta and the Cultural Practices to Evoke it. *Emotion Review,* 11(1), 74–86.

Fox, K. C. R., Christoff, K. and Dixon, M. L. (2018). Affective Neuroscience of Self-Generated Thought. *Annals of the New York Academy of Sciences* (uploaded October 15, 2018).

Hatfield, E., Rapson, R. L. and Le, Y. L. (2009). Emotional Contagion and Empathy. In J. Decety and W. Ickes (eds.), *The Social Neuroscience of Empathy* (pp. 19–30). Boston, MA: MIT Press.

Jung, C. G. (1906, 1985). Der gefühlsbetonte Komplex und seine allgemeinen Wirkungen auf die Psyche. In *Gesammelte Werke*, Bd 3, § 78. Olten: Walter. In *The Psychology of Dementia Praecox, CW* 3

Jung, C. G. (1921, 1960). Psychologische Typologie. In *Gesammelte Werke*, Bd 6, §991. Olten: Walter.

Jung, C.G. (1934, 1967). Allgemeines zur Komplextheorie. In *Gesammelte Werke*, Bd. 8. Olten: Walter.

Jung, C.G. (1934, 1980). Über die Archetypen des kollektiv en Unbewussten. In *Gesammelte Werke*, Bd. 9/1, § 56. Olten: Walter.

Jung, C. G.(1935, 1971). Die Probleme der modernen Psychotherapie. In *Gesammelte Werke*, Bd. 16, § 125. Olten: Walter. *The Practice of Psychotherapy*. CW 16, § 125

Jung, C. G. (1960, 1969). A Review of the Complex Theory. In *CW* 8, § 202, 203, 210. London: Routledge.

Jung, C. G. (1960, 1969). *The Transcendent Function*. In *CW* 8, § 131–193. London: Routledge.

Jung, C. G. (1962/2011). *Memories, Dreams, Reflections*. Recorded and edited by A. Jaffé. London: Random House.

Kast, V. (1998). Komplextheorie gestern und heute. *Anal Psychology*, 29, 296–316.

Kast, V. (2018). *Immer wieder mit sich selber eins werden*. Ostfildern: Patmos.

Kast, V. (2019). *Träumend imaginieren. Einblicke in die Traumwerkstatt*. Göttingen: Vandenhoeck & Ruprecht.

Keltner, D. and Haidt, J. (2003). Approaching Awe, a Moral, Spiritual and Aesthetic Emotion. *Cognition and Emotion*, 17(2), 297–314.

Levinas, E. (1980, 2003). *Totalität und Unendlichkeit*. Freiburg: Alber.

Menninghaus, W., Wagner, V., Hanich, J., et al. (2015). Towards a Psychological Construct of Being Moved. *PLOS ONE*, 10(6), e0128451. https://doi.org/10.1371/journal.pone.0128451

Panksepp, J. and Biven, L. (2012). *The Archeology of Mind*. New York: Norton.

Roth, G. and Stübner, N. (2014). *Wie das Gehirn die Seele macht*. Stuttgart: Klett-Cotta.

Sartre, J. P. (1968). *Die Wörter*. Reinbek: Rowohlt.

Schacter, D. L., Addis, D. R., et al. (2012). The Future of Memory: Remembering, Imagining, and the Brain. *Neuron*, 76, 677–694.

Spinoza de, B. (1841, 1963). *Die Ethik nach geometrischer Methode dargestellt*. Lehrsatz 7, S. 197, Hamburg: Meiner.

Waal de, F. (2011). *Das Prinzip Empathie. Was wir von der Natur für eine bessere Gesellschaft lernen können*. München: Hanser.

Zickfeld, J. H., Schubert, T. W., Seibt, C. and Blomster, J. (2019). Kama Muta: Conceptualizing and Measuring the Experience of Being Moved Across 19 Nations and 15 Languages. *Emotion*, 19(3), 402–424.

Chapter 5

Stanton Marlan

My passion for Jung and archetypal psychology, for alchemy and its goal, the philosopher's stone, captures an important part of my life and creative efforts. The chapter I have submitted for this book is representative of a transitional moment in my work, a movement from the black sun to the philosopher's stone, from darkness to illumination. It acknowledges the importance of not turning away from darkness, but rather the value of turning toward it, of opening oneself to the unknown and to what the alchemists called the *lumen naturae*, the shine of darkness itself. In so doing, one can discover the complexities of the soul and the interpenetration of life's opposites, its suffering and its amazing gifts.

These concerns have been present in my life since my earliest years, but it is difficult to express one's life in any one frame of reference. Multiple images come to mind; mythic moments and metaphoric expressions rise to the surface. I remember playing with stones as a child, wondering about the organic and inorganic mysteries of life and death, as well as my kinship with stones. When I learned that my name, Stanton, meant "from the stone house," my kinship deepened. The inorganic silence and my love of stones were complemented by my love for organic life, plants, flowers, trees, insects, and animals, things that grow and change, live and die. I loved this introverted time and being close to nature. I remember sitting in the sunroom of our old house. When it rained, I sat by the front window, watching the flow of water rushing along the curb, which gave me a sense of mystery, peace, and well-being.

While I enjoyed my inner life and time alone, my love for family was strong and they appear in many childhood memories. I remember my grandfather holding me up to pick wild cherries from a tree in our backyard and making wine out of them on a handmade press. I recall that my father's nickname was Sonny, and when he entered a room and smiled, it felt as if the whole room lit up. He would often say out loud, "I love my family," and it was a love I felt throughout my life. I have another fond memory of my father from the time when I was in analytic training: I had been searching for, but could not find, a copy of *The Hermetic Museum*, a compilation of alchemical treatises. I mentioned this to my father, who soon surprised me with a copy of the book! I could go on with many such memories, but I will end with one of my most profound joys: the birth of my children and grandchildren, who remain an ongoing delight and carry on my feelings of love into the future.

DOI: 10.4324/9781003148982-6

I realize that in many ways my own life has been protected and privileged, but I have lived long enough to also lament life's tragic shadows. Life can be brutal, cruel, and unfair. We impose these atrocities on each other, from racism and sexism to mass murders and hate crimes. Nature, too, assaults us with natural disasters, from famines and floods to plagues and pandemics—violations some call fate and others the dark side of God. I have seen how we are stripped bare, left feeling anxious and vulnerable—in a dark night of the soul, a *mysterium tremendum*. The dark side of life is never fully abated, and the play between light and dark, good and evil, and life and death appears as a circular and archetypal reality. The powerful truth of such experiences played an important part in my education, in my search for life's meaning, and in answering the question asked by James Hillman, "What does the soul want?" My life experiences led me to the study of philosophy and psychology, both Eastern (Taoism, Zen, Tibetan and Tantric Buddhism) and Western (from Plato to Postmodernism), and ultimately to Jung and archetypal psychology and into alchemy and the search for the philosopher's stone.

These studies were deepened and enhanced in personal analyses, and I am appreciative for my analysts, particularly Edward Edinger, Thomas Kapacinskas, and James Hillman, for their guidance and example. In this process, working with dreams taught me to value images and the imagination as a gateway to the depths of psyche and soul. After a lifetime of searching and education, life remains for me an incredible mystery and a sacred marriage between darkness and light, an illumination for which I am grateful in every moment.

Stanton Marlan, PhD Pittsburgh, PA, May 2020

Hesitation and Slowness
Gateway to Psyche's Depth

Originally published in (2005). *The San Francisco Jung Institute Library Journal*, 24(1), 1–12. Reprinted with permission.

This chapter was first presented at the Congress of the International Association for Analytical Psychology in Barcelona, Spain, on August 30, 2004, and was later printed in *The San Francisco Jung Institute Library Journal*, 2005, Vol. 24, no. 1, 1–12. Reprinted by permission of Taylor & Francis. *He who hesitates is lost*, says an old adage, and such conventional wisdom speaks a truth. There are moments when spontaneous action and quick directness win the day. A moment's hesitation and all is lost. But there are other moments when quickness betrays psyche, when its straight-arrow directness bypasses opportunity—and it is in this absence that psyche resides. Hesitation follows a circuitous, non-Euclidean path; it follows the curve of psyche into empty spaces, into a nothingness where the alterity of the unconscious shows itself and contours are revealed that the direct path ignores or covers over. For the postmodern philosopher Jacques Derrida (1978), it is this "consciousness of nothing, upon which all consciousness of something enriches itself, taking on meaning and shape. And upon whose basis all speech can be brought forth" (p. 8). This recognition is as true for analysis as it is for philosophy. In the context of this reflection, I imagine hesitation as being a fecund opening, a gateway to the unconscious and to the nothingness of which Derrida speaks. It is a nothingness that enriches both the dialectical process of analysis and our theoretical speculation. In this con text, hesitation is also a deepening of interiority and psychological space—which, for James Hillman, increases through slowness. For Hillman (1979),

> This increased interiority means that each new . . . inspiration, each hot idea . . . will first be drawn through the labyrinthine ways of the soul, which wind it and slow it and nourish it from many sides.
>
> (p. 68)

In accord with the alchemists, Hillman refers to "patience as a first quality of soul" (Ibid., p. 94).

The longer I reflect upon and practice analysis, the more it impresses me that hesitation and slowness are a way to psyche's depth. The word *hesitation* generally means to be slow to speak, decide, or act; to hold back, pause, or waver; to vacillate because of doubt or uncertainty about what to do or say. Over the years, my uncertainty has continued to deepen, and with it my sense of curiosity and wonder about analysis. Hesitation can, of course, have many negative meanings; it can refer to inaction such as a fear of beginnings or an obsessional inhibition. As a complex indicator, it points to dynamic conflict and at times to a variety of pathological states. But, at its best, it can show itself in a more conscious and organic reserve of judgment. This places conscious intention in suspension and opens a space for deliberation, repetition, and slow circumambulation. Both Freud and Jung spoke of this reserve. Freud (1958) wrote about an "evenly-suspended attention" (p. 111). His advice to his colleagues was to "withhold all conscious influences. . . [to] simply listen" (Ibid., p. 112). In short, Freud's hesitancy led to an abstinence designed to free the analyst and patient, to respect the other's autonomy, and to create an empty space, a nothingness into which his analysands' projections could unfold.

Likewise, Jung (1954) advised holding in check all "authority and desire to influence" in the name of not doing violence to his patients. While Jung ultimately developed his own dialectical approach, he, like Freud, valued a conscious reserve in his engagement with his analysands. In the work of analysis, I too feel the importance of these gestures of hesitancy and the need to slow down the psychological process, to hear images again and again, and to return to beginnings.

It is strange to be describing these reflections to colleagues because, in one form or another, I believe we all know and practice in this spirit of hesitation. We have learned it from the very beginning of our analytic training, and we teach it to our candidates. Yet, I am *hesitant* to take it for granted. It is a way of being that develops and becomes personalized and assimilated over long years of analytic practice, encounters with psychic reality, and the gravitas of sitting with patients and/or with ideas. For myself, I know I am often still in danger of using shorthand concepts to replace the slow struggle with new understanding. And in working with training candidates in supervision and control analysis, I have often found the need to slow things down, to help them to sit with material, to support its *unfolding*, and to resist the pressure for quick answers, whether motivated by transference demands or by inner compulsions. In *Alchemical Studies* (1953/1968), Jung states that

> deeper insight into the problems of psychic development soon teaches us how much better it is to reserve judgment instead of prematurely announcing to all and sundry what's what. Of course we all have an understandable desire for crystal clarity, but we are apt to forget that in *psychic* matters we are dealing with a process of experience, that is, with transformations which should never be given hard and fast names if their living movement is not to petrify into something static.
>
> (para. 199)

This reserve of judgment is in part a response to an encounter with an other, both inner and outer. When this other is respectfully encountered, it gives us pause. It interrupts our own narrative demand for meaning and solutions, sets us back, and opens the participants for an engagement with psyche—and it requires a relativization of the ego. This sets the stage for a complex dialectical process that is difficult to describe, which varies from patient to patient, and from analyst to analyst.

The living movement about which Jung speaks requires psychic slowness, particularly in the midst of the considerable pressure of a culture that thrives on speed and productivity. Perhaps it is already a cliché to note how medical and psychological treatment have become infected by the rapid growth of technology, producing in its wake an industrialization of psychic reality. Outside the sacred precincts of the analytic consulting room, the press for quicker treatment, drug therapies, and managed care are marks of our time. As analysts, many of us differentiate our practices from these trends. But I believe that the collective demands of our culture have unconsciously slipped into our consulting rooms, and the psyche of both patients and analysts has been infected by what Carl Honoré (2004) has called the "cult of speed" (p. 11). Honoré quotes British psychologist Guy Claxton, who states: "We have developed an inner psychology of speed, of saving time and maximizing efficiency" (Ibid., p. 4). In his book *In Praise of Slowness*, Honoré describes his own life as having "turned into an exercise in hurry," and he notes that American physician Larry Dossey "coined the term 'time-sickness' to describe the obsessive belief that 'time is getting away, that there isn't enough of it, and that you must peddle faster and faster to keep up'" (Ibid., p. 3).

Many years ago, a young Italian man entering analysis complained about his "backward" immigrant parents. They were an old-world Italian family who had a vineyard and grew grapes in their backyard in a contemporary middle-class neighborhood. They embarrassed my patient, and he wanted to distance himself, to fit in and adapt to the modern world. He had a dream about driving a supervehicle at over 200 miles per hour. It was three feet off the ground and everything around him was a blur. The vehicle was called "The Spirit of America." Driven by anxiety and his wish to distance from his family and from their old-world values and attitudes, which he saw as out of step with the times, he experienced life as flying by. There was never enough time to accomplish what he wanted to do, and he had little gratification in his accomplishments. One might imagine his dream to be mirroring the quality of his ungrounded drive and his inability to focus and see things clearly.

The particular quality of manic flight exhibited by this patient can be understood through his personal psychological history, but it also reflects continuing movement in the cultural and archetypal psyche. Such a patient cannot be helped by any analysis that is itself infected by hurry. Jung was already aware of this trend in the 1960s. In *Memories, Dreams, Reflections* (1961/73), he writes about "our up-rootedness, which has given rise to the 'discontents' of civilization and to such a flurry and haste that we live more in the future . . . than in the present" (p. 236). The price paid for "new methods or gadgets . . . are deceptive sweetenings of existence," which "by no means increase the contentment or happiness of people on the whole" Ibid., p. 236). He gives the example of "speedier communications which unpleasantly accelerate the tempo of life and leave us with less time than ever before. *Omnis festinatio ex parte diaboli est*—all haste is of the devil, as the old masters used to say" (Ibid., p. 236).

Likewise, the alchemical text *The Ordinal of Alchemy* notes: "The Devil will do his utmost to frustrate your search by one or the other of three stumbling blocks, namely, haste, despair, or deception" (Norton 1953, p. 22). It goes on:

> For he who is in a hurry will complete his work neither in a month, nor yet in a year; in this Art it will always be true that the man who is in a hurry will never be without matter of complaint.
>
> (Ibid., p. 23)

If all haste is of the devil, then it surely is the case in analysis, which begins with hesitation and pauses, silences that slow, and a holding back that allows psyche's rhythms to come to the fore.

I believe that analysis requires the capacity to endure what Goethe called "infinite nature" or what the painter Ad Reinhardt referred to as "infinite duration." In the arts and philosophy, as in analysis, hesitation and slowness play a prominent role. The philosopher Martin Heidegger, for instance, asked that his thought—and in principle, all thought—be spared the "disaster of an immediate presentation" (quoted in Derrida & Leavey 1989, p. 6), and the projective poet Charles Olsen was once described as "one man who would never be rushed" (Boer 1975, p. 11). Hesitation and slowness would seem to require what the French philosopher Paul Ricoeur (1970) called "a humiliation or wounding of knowledge belonging to *immediate* consciousness" (p. 377). For Ricoeur, as for Jung, this dispossession of the ego requires a shift in "the origin of meaning to another center which is no longer the immediate subject of reflection" (Ibid., p. 54). One might imagine in Jungian terms that the origin of meaning is ultimately shifted to a transpersonal center, an other than the ego. The philosopher Immanuel Levinas amplified this sense of otherness by noting that the "other is not given as a matter for thought or reflection" (Critchley 2002, p. 8). The other is "not a phenomenon but an enigma, something ultimately refractory to intentionality and opaque to the understanding" (Critchley 2002, p. 8). Levinas' work provides perhaps the most radical ethical expression of the concern shared by Freud and Jung not to violate the other person. It is an important reminder for analysts, because it is so easy to become unconscious of the enigma of otherness with our patients as we fall into fast and stereotypical understandings, and the flattening down of a primary encounter, and as we begin to think about them in the hackneyed language of analytic shorthand. Hesitation and slowness—and analytic experience—put us at the threshold of a remedy for this kind of unconsciousness. As analysts, hesitation teaches us that we must learn to wait for psyche and to appreciate the slowness of old man Saturn the Senex, the eternal play of the child, the anima's moodiness, the slowness of gestation and digestion, the organic temporality of the body, the *kairos* of the moment, and the geological time of the self. Up against these clinical realities, the ego's narratives are interrupted and set back. We are forced to wait, to find the indirect way, to resist the temptation of easy technique or quick response. I have always imagined analysis as a bulwark against the black tide of technology, but it is also true that such bulwarks set the stage for an *enantiodromia*. Technology should not simply be disregarded and with it the desire for quickness of insight, to-the-point commentary, and, at times, those spontaneous intuitions that turn out to be more rooted in the objective psyche than in unreflected countertransferences.

Ultimately, the quality of analysis cannot be identified by its literal pauses and temporal hiatus but in a certain richness of engagement. Alongside *omnus festinatio ex parte diaboli est* (all haste is of the devil), it is fitting to recognize the value in the Renaissance maxim taken over by the alchemists, *festina lente*, often translated as "make haste slowly." This adds complexity to the notion of hesitation, which cannot be identified properly in the simple dichotomy of fast and slow. It rather has to do with the *kairos*, the right time, and with *moderatio*, the right degree. The saying *festina lente* has been discussed by Erasmus, who explains the importance of "the right timing and the right degree, governed alike by vigilance and patience, so that nothing regrettable is done through haste, and nothing left undone through sloth" (Erasmus 1991, p. 3; Figure 5.1). At times the adage has been given visual representation, for example, on a "coin issued by Titus

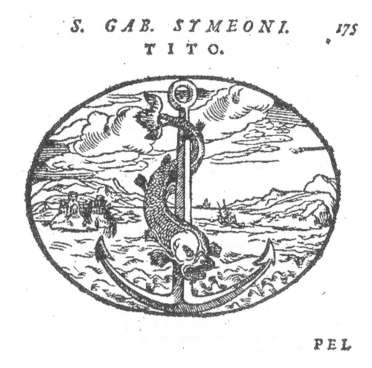

Figure 5.1 Gabriele Simeoni, Imprese Heroiche et Morali, in Paolo Giovio, Dialo-
gio dell'Imprese Militari et Amorose, Lyon, Guillaume Rouville (1574,
p. 175).

Source: Julius S. Held Collection, Clark Art Institute Library, Williamstown, MA. Public
domain.

Vespasianus" (Erasmus 1991, p. 13). On the back side of this coin was an anchor,
the central shaft of which had a dolphin coiled around it. Erasmus noted that:

> the coin itself is a circle and stands for eternity, [which] (has neither begin-
> ning nor end), the anchor (holds back and ties down a ship) [and] stands for
> slowness, and the dolphin expresses speed (as the fastest and in its motions
> the most agile of living creatures).
>
> (Erasmus 1991, p. 13)

The image is a *complexio oppositorum* or a contrast of opposites. Many images
amplify this coincidence of opposites, and alchemy is filled with expressions
of this subtle attitude. The image of the crab and the butterfly is an example
(Figure 5.2).

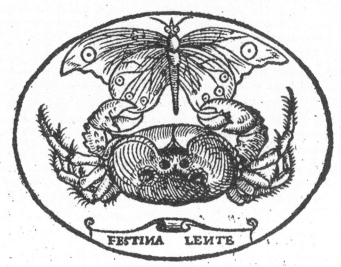

174   *LE IMPRESE DEL*
AVGVSTO.

FESTINA LENTE

Di queſta medeſima natura fu Tito figliuolo di
Veſpaſiano, laquale volendo anch'egli manifeſtare,
in luogo del Granchio e della Farfalla tolſe per im
preſa vn'Anchora con vn Delfino intorno, facendo
vna figura moderata della velocità di que-
ſto, e della grauezza di quell'altra,
nel modo che noi veggia-
mo dinanzi à i libri
d'Aldo.

TITO.

Figure 5.2 Gabriele Simeoni, Imprese Heroiche et Morali, in Paolo Giovio, Dialo-
gio dell'Imprese Militari et Amorose, Lyon, Guillaume Rouville (1574,
p. 174).

I am particularly fond of another expression of this attitude: the well-known image of the Arabian alchemist Avicenna (980–1037 CE) pointing toward a chain that links an eagle to a toad while exclaiming: "The eagle flying through air and the toad crawling on the ground are the magistery" (Fabricius 1976/1989, p. 55). Fabricius suggests that this image reflects "the central idea of the Hermetic procedure: the conjunction of the opposites . . . expressed in the alchemists' arduous attempt to unite the eagle and the toad, spiritus and corpus, intellect and instinct, mind and matter" (Ibid., p. 55). If this is so, for me it also reflects the spirit of *festina lente* (Figure 5.3). I believe that it is in this spirit that we should understand hesitation—not as a one-sided opposition to quickness, but as a sign to express the irrepresentable quality of actions relegated by *Matura,* the wisdom that knows "when things are done neither prematurely nor too late, we call them ripe" (Mnemosyne). This spirit is a grace that beats at the heart of the archetype before it is torn asunder and that is available in a moment's hesitation, intuition, or gesture of integrity. The poet Rumi describes such a moment in a line of a poem: " who comes to the Spring thirsty and finds the moon reflected in it" (Rumi 1997, p. 10). Here the demand of the "instinct" gives way to something more and newly discovered in the pool of psyche. While I am not exactly sure what Rumi

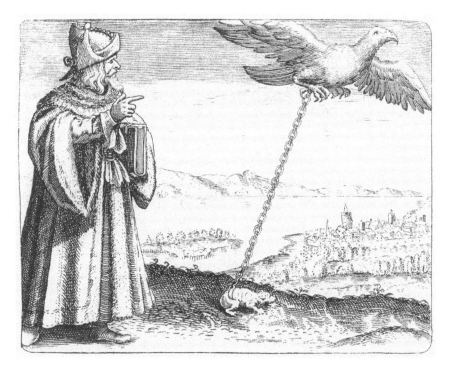

Figure 5.3 Avicenna, in Michael Maier, *Symbola Aureae Mensae* (1617, No. 82).

had in mind here, for me the beauty of the image captures a moment of grace and integrity at the heart of an undivided archetype. It is a moment at the crossroads of time, between heaven and earth, instinct and soul, another example of *enantiosis*, a subtle gesture between the so-called opposites.

This gesture of integrity was also well understood by the practical minds of the Chinese sages in the realm of action and is expressed in the concept *wei wu wei*. It is a saying often translated as " doing-non-doing," and it too is a paradox of contrasting ideas and images. For the Chinese, it is a saying having to do with seamless action and is concerned with the unceasing flow of change. It points to a moment when effort and effortlessness are impossible to describe in any terms seen to be totally independent of one another. The idea is motivated by "a sense of oneself as connected to others and to one's environment" (Hardash, n.d.). It is *not* motivated by a sense of separateness. It is an action that is spontaneous and effortless, but "at the same time it is not to be considered inertia, laziness, or mere passivity" (Hardash, n.d.).

Chung Tzu refers to this way of being as "purposeless Wandering," and I propose that we consider this notion alongside Freud's "evenly suspended attention" and Jung's "holding in check all desire to influence." While the Taoist point of view might be imagined as a romantic *enantiodromia* to our highly technological culture, it may better be seen as another adage signifying a complex notion of hesitation, not unlike *festina lente*. Make haste slowly can now be linked to action-non-action, and in so doing we may be able to see the moon in Rumi's spring, even in the face of instinctual demand. So here I will make haste toward my conclusion.

As we set out to examine our contemporary directions for theory and practice, I am hopeful that we can bring our analytic sensibilities to the work of reflection and that hesitation and slow deliberation can play a role in our considerations. Professional interests are often the site of our most passionate engagements and are subject to the same psychological complexities as all other human endeavors. As we strive to make our contributions, our efforts are embedded in our unconscious "instincts" and our desires—in our needs for recognition, power, self-expression, identity, and relationship to others, both inner and outer.

In addition to the complexes of our personal psychology, archetypal contents can press us toward speedy and premature clarity and ontological closure. Our theories often resemble the gods and goddesses in whose thrall we labor to work out our visions and in whose service we become warriors for their truths. We become purveyors of particular points of view—classical, developmental, archetypal, modern, or postmodern. Our truths lie rooted in psyche or biology, in philosophy, physics, or poetry, or even in the deconstruction of any point of view. We cannot escape the gods; they are necessary. They offer us sanctuary, not only in our inner but also in our outer worlds—our professional organizations, universities, consulting rooms, and private studies.

Still, as analysts, we strive to free ourselves from the grip of such personal or archetypal demons. When in their grip, our feeling function remains primitive.

But hesitation may allow us to reserve judgment and to resist one-sided formulations. It may allow us to stand firm against the pressure for clear and distinct ideas that devitalize our work and foreclose an openness to psyche on the threshold of meaning and of that nothingness upon which psyche enriches itself. When that open space collapses, we fall into unconsciousness, our theories became stultified, and we lose something essentially human.

I would like to end with a passage from the poet Rainer Maria Rilke. In his *Letters to a Young Poet*, he writes,

> Allow your judgments their own silent, undisturbed development, which, like all progress, must come from deep within and cannot be forced or hastened. *Everything* is gestation and then birthing. To let each impression and each embryo of a feeling come to completion, entirely in itself, in the dark, in the unsayable, the unconscious, beyond the reach of one's own understanding, and with deep humility and patience to wait for the hour when a new clarity is born: this alone is what it means to live as an artist: in understanding as in creating.
>
> In this there is no measuring with time, a year doesn't matter, and ten years are nothing. Being an artist means: not numbering and counting, but ripening like a tree, which doesn't force its sap, and stands confidently in the storms of spring, not afraid that afterward summer may not come. It does come. But it comes only to those who are patient, who are there as if eternity lay before them, so unconcernedly silent and vast. I learn it every day of my life, learn it with pain I am grateful for: *patience* is everything!
>
> (1984, pp. 23–24)

To reclaim the art of analysis, analysts would do well to remember our complexes, to recall and to release our gods, and, in my mind, it does not hurt to consider Rilke.

Reference List

Boer, C. (1975). *Charles Olsen in Connecticut*. Chicago, IL: The Swallow Press Inc.

Critchley, S. (2002). Introduction. In S. Critchley & R. Bernasconi, Eds., *The Cambridge companion to Levinas* (pp. 1–30). Cambridge, UK: Cambridge University Press.

Derrida, J. (1978). *Writing and difference* (A. Bass, Trans.). Chicago, IL: Chicago University Press.

Derrida, J. and Leavey, J. P., Jr. (1989). *Comment donner raison:* 'How to concede, with reasons?' *Diacritics: A Review of Contemporary Criticism* (Heidegger: Art of Politics), 19 (3/4), 3–9. doi.org/10.2307/465384

Erasmus, D. (1991). *The collected works of Erasmus, vol. 33* (R.A.B. Mynors, Trans.). Toronto, CA: University of Toronto.

Fabricius, J. (1976/1989). *Alchemy: The medieval alchemists and their royal art*. London, UK: Diamond Books.

Freud, S. (1958). Recommendations to physicians practicing psychoanalysis. In *The collected works, vol. XII*. The Hogarth Press.

Hardash, T. (n.d.) Taoism—The Wu-Wei Principle, Part 4. Taoism—The Wu-Wei Principle—Part 4. https://jadedragon.com/archives/june98/tao.html

Hillman, J. (1975). *Revisioning psychology*. New York, NY: Harper and Row.

Hillman, J. (1979). Peaks and vales. In *Puer papers* (pp. 54–74). Irving, TX: Spring Publications.

Honoré, C. (2004). *In praise of slowness*. San Francisco, CA: HarperSanFrancisco.

Jung, C. G. (1954). Principles of practical psychotherapy. In G. Adler, Ed., & R.F.C. Hull, Trans., *The practice of psychotherapy: The collected works of C.G. Jung, Vol. 16.* (pp. 3–20). Princeton, NJ: Princeton University Press.

Jung, C. G. (1953/1968). Paracelsus as a spiritual phenomenon. In G. Adler, Ed., & R.F.C. Hull, Trans., *Alchemical studies: The collected works of C.G. Jung, Vol. 13* (pp. 109–189). Princeton, NJ: Princeton University Press.

Jung, C. G. (1961/73). *Memories, dreams, reflections* (A. Jaffe, Ed., & R. & C. Winston, Trans.). New York, NY: Pantheon Books.

Norton, T. (1953). The ordinal of alchemy. In *The hermetic museum, Vol. 2*, (pp. 3–67). London, UK: John M. Watkins. (Originally published in 1678).

Ricoeur, P. (1970). *Freud and philosophy* (D. Savage, Trans.). New Haven, CT: Yale University Press.

Rilke, R. M. (1984). *Letters to a Young Poet* (S. Mitchell, Trans.). New York: Random House.

Rumi. (1997). *The illuminated Rumi* (C. Barks, Trans.). New York, NY: Broadway Books.

Chapter 6

Renos K. Papadopoulos

It was a warm afternoon in 1957. I was waiting for my turn to have my piano examination at the music conservatory, housed in an ancient two-storey building on the main commercial road of the old quarter of Nicosia, surrounded by the bulky Venetian walls. Whilst waiting, I went out onto the balcony overlooking the narrow busy road and watched people walking up and down, shopping and chatting. The pupil being examined at the time was playing Mozart's "Rondo Alla Turca," and I was humming along to the piece, impressed by how well she was playing without making any mistakes. All of a sudden, deafeningly loud, I heard several gunshots and saw some men falling on the ground, hardly 50 yards away from me, and a couple of young men running away, whilst placing their handguns hastily inside their jackets.

It was one of the years that Greek Cypriots were involved in an armed liberation struggle against the British colonialists, and what I had witnessed was the execution of British soldiers in civilian clothes by members of our liberation organisation. I was stunned. I was 10 years old. On the one hand, I was excited to be privileged to see our heroes in action, inflicting a deadly blow against our oppressors, and, on the other hand, I was upset to see people dying in front of me. In the evening, at home, as usual, we were angry when the news bulletin on the colonial radio station characterised our freedom fighters as "terrorists."

That incident shook me. I was confronted by two sets of fundamentally and diametrically opposed perspectives. Killing people was not good, and yet fighting for your freedom was noble. The very same event could be understood completely differently from two contrary perspectives, both equally valid. A very difficult and unsolvable conundrum, indeed. The naming of the same people as freedom fighters or terrorists was a similar conundrum, but it was less incomprehensibly troublesome because it was not taking place "within" me; unlike the first, it was enacted by two different groups of people who viewed the same phenomenon from two opposite positions.

Following the independence of Cyprus (in 1960), the intercommunal strife between the Greeks and Turks on the island exposed me to many more, similarly perplexing challenges, so that I painfully came to realise the deadly effects of polarised convictions. In the midst of all the violence, during that same period, as a pupil of a classical gymnasium, I was reading philosophical and psychological

DOI: 10.4324/9781003148982-7

books, including Freud, Jung, Kierkegaard, and Nietzsche, and Jung appealed to me, particularly because of his intentional avoidance of blind dogmatism. I was also enchanted by Rabindranath Tagore's poetry and fascinated by Mahatma Gandhi, even giving a lecture on his philosophy of non-violence. Then, my years in South Africa (1970–1980, lecturing in psychology at the University of Cape Town) during the height of apartheid, the ultimate regime of inhuman racial discrimination, were another agonising reminder of the fatal consequences of the inflexibility of those in power, who are unable to appreciate the realities of the oppressed.

When I was asked by my university to start the first course on psychotherapy for clinical psychology trainees, I faced a dilemma as to how to structure the course. Earlier, during my own university education (with a UNESCO scholarship, I had studied in Yugoslavia), our psychotherapy professor, Dr Matic, was a Freudian, who had actually studied in Vienna and attended some of Freud's famous Wednesday meetings. Although I learned a great deal from him and respected him enormously, I was uneasy being inducted in one approach and made to understand the relevant phenomena from within one closed system. Inevitably, I reached out, exploring the budding world of behaviour therapy and, in fact, wrote my graduate dissertation on comparing and contrasting the two schools.

In Cape Town, some colleagues and I became involved in the emerging human potential movement of humanistic psychology, which was also in tune with our anti-apartheid positions, working with multiracial groups (which was, then, illegal). Moreover, following the visit of Donald Bloch (then director of the Ackerman Institute, New York), I became enthusiastic about systemic approaches that were more amenable to working in community settings. My deep engagement with these four different schools made me realise that, although they used different languages and emphasised selectively different aspects of the work, essentially, all of them had their strengths and weaknesses.

It was in the context of this awareness that my interest in Jung, "my first love," was reignited, acquiring new meaning and relevance. His non-dogmatic and "non-denominational" messages that "we miss the meaning of the individual psyche if we interpret it on the basis of any fixed theory, however fond of it we may be" (Jung 1926: 93) and "I have set up neither a system nor a general theory, but have merely formulated auxiliary concepts to serve me as tools, as is customary in every branch of science" (Jung 1952: 666) made perfect sense and were immensely appealing to me, avoiding narrow dogmatic entrenchment and bigotry. And it was this understanding that became the basis of the psychotherapy course that I finally formulated.

Whilst lecturing in Cape Town, I also completed my PhD. Not surprisingly, it was on Jung and the phenomenon of otherness, titled "The dialectic of the other in the psychology of C.G. Jung: a metatheoretical investigation," which was the first PhD on Jung completed on the continent of Africa and the first time that the concept of the other was used in relation to Jung.

After moving to the UK and working at the Tavistock Clinic, where I was the first clinical psychologist who was also a systemic family therapist and Jungian analyst, it was satisfyingly surprising that, on one occasion, when I intervened in a heated argument of polarised positions during a clinical team meeting, by identifying positive elements in each position, a Freudian colleague remarked with genuine admiration, "Of course, only a Jungian analyst could have possibly achieved this."

During the wars that resulted in the break-up of Yugoslavia, I was the only clinical psychologist in the UK who spoke the languages of that part of the world and also had personal connections with mental health professionals there (without originating from those lands). Accordingly, I was invited to assist on the ground with psychosocial projects, which, unintentionally, solidified my additional specialisation in this field. Ever since then, I have been working in many countries with refugees, tortured persons and other survivors of political violence and disasters. Although my approach is never explicitly "Jungian," nevertheless, the framework that I developed over the years is based on many Jungian insights, even if they are not phrased in the traditional Jungian language, for example, his non-pathologisation of human suffering, the growthful potentiality of adversity and his epistemological agility.

Tragically, I have been disappointed to witness that many Jungian colleagues adopt the very opposite stance that Jung espoused, treating his concepts and positions very much as a closed system, indeed as a "fixed" and "general theory," waving jingoistically their Jungian banners against all the "infidels."

But I cannot, possibly, forget the "Rondo Alla Turca."

The Other Other
When the Exotic Other
Subjugates the Familiar Other

This is a shortened version of the paper published in the *Journal of Analytical Psychology*, 2002, 47, 163–188. Published with permission.

The problem of otherness is both enormous and complex, and it has implications for several disciplines and approaches to the study of human nature (De Certeau, 1986; Derrida, 1985). Therefore, it would be imprudent to try to address it within the limitations of this chapter, unless an appropriately limited perspective were to be developed, and this is what I shall endeavour to undertake here: to construct such a perspective on the other that would enable us to grasp some crucial features of this theme and then to propose a new differentiation between two kinds of other.

The Other Other

So, what is the other? To begin with, colloquially, the "other" is not the "this," whatever the "this" may be. In all of its grammatical forms, as an adjective, noun, conjunction, pronoun and adverb, the other is dependent on something that has been referred to already. If the reference is to a "me" or "we," then the other refers to anything or anybody that is not "me" or "we." However, the relationship between the "this" and the "other" is not always that of opposition or conflict. After an etymological and linguistic analysis of the other, Papadopoulos (1984) observed that there is a range of meanings, including "some seemingly contradictory" (p. 56) ones. Logically, this relationship could cover a wide range of possibilities, from opposition to complementary, from difference, separation or distinction to alternative, remaining or supplementary. Yet, this wide range of potential relationships is not always kept in mind; the main associations to the other tend to refer to the antagonistic, oppositional, hostile and conflictual meanings of the other.

In Greek, the two words that refer to the other are "heteros" and "allos," and there is no substantial difference between them, the first being the Attic form of the second (Papadopoulos 1984, p. 55). However, derivatives of these words have slanted the meaning in terms of specific emphases. The meaning of words such as heterodoxy, heterogeneous and heterosexuality as well as allopathic, allochthonous and allomorphic offers an indication of the shades of connotations and denotations that these two forms of the other can take.

Concluding his observations, Papadopoulos (1984) used a phrase from Plato to develop a working understanding of the other. In *Meno* (88d), Plato refers to "alle psyche" ("other soul"), which in English (Barber 1968) is rendered as "the *rest* of the soul."

> This neutral translation implies that there is still some *other* part of the psyche which constitutes the rest of the one already mentioned. Therefore, the inherent duality of meaning in the 'other' may be comprehended as follows: if the rest is added to the existing part, a wholeness, a totality may be achieved; but if the rest is left apart, then a separation, a division will result.
>
> (Papadopoulos 1984, p. 56)

This means that the other could be understood as something that, regardless of its inherent oppositionality, marginality or complementarity to a this, somehow belongs together with the this and together they are part of a larger entity, a bigger whole. Logically, even opposites share something in common (Jarrett 1979; Ogden 1967); unrelated entities cannot be oppositional to each other. We refer to something as being opposite if, in relation to a certain dimension, it lies at the opposite pole. However, often entities belong to several dimensions, and it is possible that in relation to one dimension they may be opposite to each other while in relation to another dimension they may be complementary. What matters is where the emphasis lies in the context about which we speak—their similarities or their differences. For example, men and women are both human beings and at times what matters most is their membership in the human race, whereas at other times, depending on the context, we may emphasize their differences; then, the one becomes the other's other. When referring to the otherness of other human beings or ethnic groups, the focus is on their characteristics and/or the circumstances which highlight their strangeness and their differences rather than their commonality with the referent group. In the case of inner otherness, the emphasis is on the experience that parts of a person (under certain circumstances) appear to him/her as not belonging to the self-image he/she has of him/herself.

Paul Ricoeur has contributed substantially to this debate by arguing (in his seminal book *Oneself as Another*) that "the selfhood of oneself implies otherness to such an intimate degree that one cannot be thought of without the other" (1994, p. 3). This means that there can be no self without the other and no other without a self. Logically, philosophically and psychologically, the one is a constituent element of the definition of the other.

Otherness is an area that has received much attention in recent years across the social sciences in various forms (e.g., Fowler & Hardsley 1994; O'Barr 1994; Said 1978, 1994; Sampson 1993). With reference to otherness in social groups, what is usually referred to is the tension between two groups of people, regardless of whether the one group aspires to imitate the other group or despises and wants to distance itself from the other group. Concluding a review on "Theorizing representing the Other," Wilkinson and Kitzinger caution that,

> Unless we actively engage with the process of Othering as *topic*, we run the risk of uncritically reproducing it in our own research and writing. Only by making Other*ing* (rather than Other*ness*) the focus of our attention, and by exploring the ways in which it is done and undone, reinforced and undermined, can we open up the possibility, finally, of interrupting its oppressive discourse.
>
> (1996, pp. 27–28)

Thus, in effect, Wilkinson and Kitzinger make the relevant distinction between the act of othering and the accepted result of othering—a perceived given otherness. Their plea is for paying attention to the actual process which produces otherness, and their emphasis is on the active process of othering others rather than identifying the other in terms of its various "other" characteristics.

In philosophy, the other has been treated directly or indirectly by virtually every philosopher. The relationship between the subject, the being, the me, the selfhood and the other human being or the otherness in culture and/or within oneself has always occupied a central position in our understanding of personal identity and of the human condition in general.

Paul Ricoeur introduced a helpful distinction between two types of identity which has instructive implications for our understanding of the other. To begin with, it is important to be reminded that identity is closely connected with the definition of the other (Papadopoulos 1997), because a person understands his or her identity in relation to what he/she is not. Following the Latin origins of "identity" ("idem" and "ipse"), Ricoeur argued that identity can be understood in terms of sameness (permanence in time: idem) and selfhood (identity of character: ipse). He clarified that, "By 'character' I understand the set of distinctive marks which permit the re-identification of a human individual as being the same" (Ibid., 1994, p. 118). Ricoeur argued that although the ipse and idem perspectives on identity are different, they inevitably overlap:

> [P]recisely, as second nature, my character is me, myself, *ipse*; but this *ipse* announces itself as *idem*. Each habit formed in this way, acquired and become a lasting disposition, constitutes a *trait*—a character trait, a distinctive sign by which a person is recognized, reidentified as the same—character being nothing other than the set of these distinctive signs.
>
> (1994, p. 121)

What is of relevance to our investigation here is that Ricoeur sees that these two sides of identity overlap through what he calls a "narrative identity." For him, we have "another model of permanence in time besides that of character." It is that of keeping one's word in faithfulness to the word that has been given.

> Keeping one's word expresses a *self-constancy* which cannot be inscribed, as character was, within the dimension of something in general but solely within the dimension of "who". . . . The perseverance of character is one thing, the perseverance of faithfulness to a word that has been given is something else again. The continuity of character is one thing, the constancy of friendship is quite another.
>
> (Ibid., p. 123)

In identifying the "narrative identity," Ricoeur introduces another important realm (within the context of language interactions) which can accommodate sameness despite the occurrence of differences across time.

Thus, the narrative identity that Ricoeur introduces, which is the identity that one develops in the context of interactions in language, is an important element that bridges the two sides of identity, that is, the sameness over time (idem) and uniqueness of character (ipse). This is an important type of identity in terms of our everyday life. Consequently, it could be argued that this identity suggests another formulation of the other, an other that is not in line with the narrative identity that an individual has developed about him/herself. This could take the form of competing or supplementary narratives that can create an otherness of oneself, with considerable consequences. A simpler form of this would be reflected in the various roles we play in life and the different groups to which we belong and within which we interact and define ourselves in connection with them. These roles can be competing, and we can therefore have several narrative identities and, hence, several others to ourselves.

The psychoanalyst who has been responsible for the greatest contribution to the introduction of the other in analytical vocabulary is Jacques Lacan (1968,

1977a, 1977b, 2000). Summarizing the various concepts Lacan covers by the term "other," Anika Lemaire outlined the following:

> The Other is (i) language . . . the symbolic. . . . (ii) the site of the intersubjectivity of patient and analyst, and hence the analytic dialogue. . . (iii) the unconscious. . . (iv) the third party witness invoked in analysis as soon as it is a question of formulating a truth . . . (v) the Father or the Mother.
>
> (1977, p. 157)

These meanings of the other connect in some way with Ricoeur's narrative identity insofar as they involve the order of language and the symbolic as well as the interaction between two persons in an intimate context (analyst and analysand, child and parent). Stephen Frosh offers a comprehensive discussion of Lacan's use of the other and clarifies that for Lacan, "the self . . . is actually constructed by means of identification with something external, fundamentally other than the subject itself" (1999, p. 143). However, he further notes that,

> in Lacan's theory . . . there is no complete unity or Otherness that inhabits the universe; there is only the search for this Other that reflects and constructs the absences each individual feels inside and which are fantasized as fulfilling the desires that have had to be repressed . . . the desire to be the object of the other's desire.
>
> (Frosh 1999, pp. 222–223)

Thus, one of Lacan's contributions has been the elucidation of the psychoanalytic contingencies of the other, emphasising both the integral nature of the other in the constitution of the subject and the elusive nature of completeness with the other.

In her book *Shadow of the Other* (1998), Jessica Benjamin argues for the usefulness of distinguishing two kinds of "other" or other individuals. The first considers the other as an independent being capable of entering into a reciprocal relationship of knowing one another, whereas the second uses the other as a repository of unwanted characteristics cast from the self. Although she mainly focuses on the implications of this dual relationship for the male-female hierarchy, her approach is of relevance to the wider debate on identity, intersubjectivity and the definitions and relationships between the self and the other. Benjamin's approach concentrates on the dynamics of the interrelationship between the self and the other, and her main contribution lies in the discussion of how we turn others into our other, that is, our rejected selves. In addition to these formulations of the other, there are, of course, also extreme and pathological positions. More specifically, with reference to internal otherness within an individual, in the extreme, we have pathological conditions such as schizophrenia or double personality or even multiple personality syndrome. One interesting, recently identified syndrome is that of the "the anarchic hand," which is the condition when a person, at times, cannot control the movements of his/her own hand. This syndrome is caused by a lesion in the motor area of the brain and results in the hand occasionally acting against the will of the person (Della Sala 2000; Kritikos et al. 2001; Marchetti & Della Sala 1998). However, apart from these extreme pathological and neurological conditions, otherness and the other are much more common phenomena.

The general theme of the other, in its various forms and permutations, has been used extensively in novels and in poetry. Classics such as Robert Louis Stevenson's *The Strange Case of Dr Jekyll and Mr Hyde* (1886) emphasised the extreme forms of the good and evil sides of human nature, whereas more modern novels such as Alberto Moravia's *The Two of Us* (1972) have treated the other in lighthearted, but telling ways; in this case, the hero (Federico) is tyrannised by his penis, which assumes an independent personality and even is given a name (Federicus Rex—a parody on Oedipus Rex). The story is about the constant comic exchanges between these two "heroes" (Federico and Federicus Rex).

In short, for general orientation purposes, it would be useful to distinguish between "internal" and "external" others, although the difference between them is not always as obvious as it initially appears. Moreover, the relationship between internal and external others (if we accept them as distinct and separate) is not so simple. For example, the evil within Dr Jekyll or Federico's sexuality are not unrelated to external evil and the wider sexual discourse in society.

Thus, a working summary of the other could outline the relationship between the "self" and his/her "other" (be it internal or external) within the broad scheme of the following possibilities:

1   the self encounters the other in a conscious way, and this could lead to either positive or negative consequences, or
2   the self does not encounter the other in a conscious way, and their contact remains only as an unconscious impact which, of course, could lead to various forms of acting out.

Jung and the Other

Jung made repeated explicit references to the other in his autobiography (*Memories, Dreams, Reflections*). He observed that in his childhood his personality was composed of two distinct parts, whom he named Number 1 and Number 2 personalities. Number 1 was the ordinary personality that obeyed his parents, went to school and attended to his everyday commitments, whereas Number 2 was his "other" or "second" personality, which was a "grown up—old, in fact . . . remote from the world of men but close to nature . . . above all close to the night, to dreams" (Jung 1961, p. 62). Jung referred to his Number 2 personality as his other and discussed in detail the dynamic interactions between his two personalities. However, this was not the only reference Jung made to the other.

Papadopoulos (1980) undertook the first systematic study of the other in relation to Jung. Beginning with an overview of the problematic of the other, he attempted to discern a specific theory of the other in the works of Heraclitus, Plato and Hegel, despite the fact that none of these philosophers addressed this problem directly or explicitly. The dialectic emerged as a shared approach that these three great thinkers employed to tackle this problematic, and he discussed the similarities and differences in their treatment of their dialectic of the other. Then, he focused on Jung, his life and his work and offered a new reading of his theoretical opus from the perspective of the other. Finally, he revisited the three philosophers, comparing and contrasting them with the Jungian approach to the dialectic of the other.

One of the arguments Papadopoulos (1980, 1984) advanced was that Jung's preoccupation with the other predated his relationship with Freud, and it was to this concern that Jung returned after his professional relationship and personal friendship with Freud came to an end. Moreover, Papadopoulos claimed (with documentary evidence) that Jung's engagement with the other played a central role in his initial attraction to Freud's ideas, as well as in his final break-up with his great master. According to Papadopoulos (1980, 1984), Jung had the initial impression that Freud had a similar involvement with the other, and he hoped that Freud would assist him with advancing further his understanding of the other. Jung parted company with Freud when he gradually realized that his Viennese master could not, in fact, assist him with his original quest for the other.

Papadopoulos' study proposed a new reading of Jung that was based on the hypothesis that the Jungian opus could be appreciated more fully if it were to be seen as a series of progressive reformulations of his understanding of the other. Throughout, Jung was deeply concerned with the nature, composition and dissociability of the psyche and keenly observed the meaning of the various others which he encountered; these ranged from the objects of his imaginary games as a child ("his" fire, "his" carved manikin and "his" pebble from the Rhine) with which he had a special relationship and were, in a sense, part of him to the Number 2 personality within himself. Later, during his professional life, he understood the other in terms of complexes, which were intrapsychic structures that had a semi-independent and autonomous existence within one's personality. The other-as-complex was followed by Jung's reformulation of the other-as-symbol; symbols were similar to complexes, but they were not restricted within an individual's intrapsychic world and had a wider, collective applicability. Finally, Jung's reformulation of the other-as-archetype was characterized by the intricate combinations between intrapsychic and collective dimensions. Overall, Jung's reformulations of his preoccupation with the other followed the movement from animistic, external other objects to a rather unsophisticated, global internal other (Number 2 personality), and then from intrapsychic individual functions (complexes) to more collective forms of structuring principles (symbols). The other-as-archetype represents the pinnacle of Jung's theoretical endeavours as it offers a structuring principle which is also connected with broader cultural and societal perspectives. This reformulation represented a dialectic between the internal and external, specific/individual and general/collective, and personal/intrapsychic and societal/symbolic. Appreciated in this way, Jung emerges as an important theorist of the other who was able to combine many of the facets of the other that others addressed (before and after him).

Jung's theory of opposites offered the backdrop to his explorations of the other and enabled him to develop a fairly elaborate approach to understanding the other. One of Jung's main principles was that the tension between opposites was the very source of psychic energy itself [e.g., "there is no energy unless there is a tension of opposites" (1943, p. 53)]. Characteristically, Jung also claimed that, "Where there is no 'other,' or it does not yet exist, all possibility of consciousness ceases" (1951, p. 193). So, the very source of life (energy) and consciousness itself was the product of the interaction between an entity and its other or its opposite. That is why Jung often felt close to Heraclitus, who had proclaimed that conflict is the father of all.

After Papadopoulos (1980, 1984), others have explored facets of Jung's treatment of the other, adding important insights. For example, Adams (1996) examined the otherness in Jung in connection with race and culture, Giegerich (1998) used the other to interpret myths, and Hauke (2000) discussed the other in Jung in relation to ego consciousness, gender and the shadow. David L. Miller (1990) argued for the return of Jung's other, his Number 2 personality, in relation to his adult theories. More specifically, Miller attacked the increasing "Jungian fundamentalism" (which he implied was connected with Jung's Number 1 personality) and made a plea for the return of the "other Jung" who was not preoccupied with the concerns of everydayness but was fascinated by the openness of the unpredictability of the self. Miller privileged Jung's Number 2 personality ('Jung's other'), to whom he attributed the excitement of the unknown and of discord as, for example, expressed in the following:

> The concept of the unconscious *posits nothing*; it designates only my *unknowing* . . . the united personality will never quite lose the painful sense of innate discord. Complete redemption from the sufferings of this world is and must remain an illusion.
>
> (Miller 1990, p. 325)

However, in addition to these understandings of the other in connection with Jung, it will be argued here that there is still another perspective that has not yet been explored. This perspective will be developed on the basis of an investigation of Jung's own position with regard to the social and cultural contexts of his approach.

Jung's Other Others

To begin with, it is important to be reminded of Jung's argument that our psychology, in effect, is Eurocentric. He demonstrated this by the repeated reference to the differences in the approach to various issues between European and non-European perspectives. Characteristically, he pointed out that

> the predominantly rationalistic European finds much that is human alien to him, and he prides himself on this without realising that this rationality is

> won at the expense of his vitality, and that the primitive part of his personality
> is consequently condemned to a more or less underground existence.
>
> (Jung 1961, p. 273)

This quote encapsulates Jung's position, as (1) it distinguishes between two different approaches—the European and the "primitive"—and (2) it privileges the "primitive" (which is more "vital") over the European (which is more "rationalistic"). Regardless of the accuracy of his specific observations (Papadopoulos 1998), and regardless of the fact that this stance led him to slip occasionally into inappropriate political gaffes (to put it mildly), what is important is that Jung was a pioneer in acknowledging the fact that "our" psychology is indeed limited due to its Eurocentric nature. Consequently, Jung articulated the need to expand our Western psychological epistemology into wider parameters in order to avoid its inherent limitations.

The second point that is important to keep in mind in developing our argument here is that Jung repeatedly emphasised that he did not have a psychotherapeutic system of his own, and he claimed that he based his approach on clinical and empirical evidence: "I have set up neither a system nor a general theory, but have merely formulated auxiliary concepts to serve me as tools, as is customary in every branch of science" (Jung 1952, p. 666). Moreover, he maintained that the set of principles he employed in his work did not follow blindly the contemporary European tenets (of rational and causal-reductive science) but he was also drawing on insights gained by other approaches that were practised in previous historical times in Europe (alchemy) and are still used now by different cultures (in Africa, India, etc.). In effect, what Jung claimed was that his therapeutic approach was not time or place specific, but instead it was a formalized version of the distilled wisdom derived from the timeless general therapeutic principles from ancient as well as from contemporary traditional practices.

Taking these two claims together (his observation that our psychology is Eurocentric and that his therapeutic approach was based on well-proven practices over time), we see that Jung discerned two interrelated realms—the one upon which European psychology (and psychotherapy) was based and another, which he claimed was more balanced and more wholesome, which he identified with traditional wisdom as expressed in alchemy and other ancient healing rituals and which, he claimed, still existed in more traditional cultures outside of Europe, in our times.

It would not be far-fetched if we could name this second realm the other because Jung himself connected it with his own internal other, his Number 2 personality. Thus, in addition to the reformulations of the problematic of the other, which we could distinguish in Jung's explicit theoretical work (as sketched previously), we may now identify another kind of other that occupied an equally important place in the Jungian opus. This is the other realm, which is different and indeed foreign to our European mentality and epistemology. However, Jung claimed that this other realm was not totally foreign to us, as it was part of our forgotten European heritage which was neglected and suppressed by the development of our rationality and technological advances. Thus, Jung saw it as his mission to reconnect us with this forgotten vital other realm. In not very ambiguous terms, Jung declared that the healing potential in our culture and communities, in our beliefs and rituals has disappeared, and his psychology was one way of reactivating this potential in us as individuals. He believed that all agencies that promoted this healing potential (mythologies, religious rituals, community narratives, etc.) had lost their potency to do so, and it was left to modern analytical psychologists to carry out this function. Jung was particularly critical of what he called "institutional religion" which, according to him, was now impotent to provide modern humans with much needed effective meaning. Hence, Jung accepted that his own therapeutic approach represented a serious attempt to reinstate this healing function in reformulated structures that fit with modern psychotherapeutic contexts.

Characteristically, in his essay on "The spiritual problem of modern man," Jung wrote,

> The psychological interest of the present time is an indication that modern man expects something from the psyche which the outer world has not given him: doubtless something which our religion ought to contain, but no longer does contain, at least for modern man. For him, the various forms of religion no longer appear to come from within, from the psyche. . . [modern man] tries on a variety of religions and beliefs as if they were Sunday attire, only to lay them aside again like worn-out clothes.
>
> (1931, p. 83)

Such an undertaking, of course, can be quite a grandiose project, and it amounts to an actual mission. No wonder that glimpses of messianic and redemptive imagery have been closely associated with Jung the person and his work. Undoubtedly, this seductive element in the overall Jungian package still attracts a considerable number of people to Jung as followers and as trainees, analysts or patients.

Be that as it may, the main point here is that, by distinguishing these two discourses, Jung in effect created another important other—a cultural and epistemological other that he kept as a constant and an ideal, and against which he compared and contrasted the European approach. Moreover, he did not hide his preference for that other discourse (that of traditional wisdom and healing rituals) and his criticism of the European perspective. With great reverence, Jung marvelled at the thaumaturgical effects of the primitive cultures in which, he believed, people are closer to their unconscious and are thus more natural and less spoiled by our corrupt civilization. Finally, he construed his own therapeutic theory and practice as an attempt to bridge the gap between these two discourses, and his aim was to invent appropriate and creative ways of recreating the lost potential of the other discourse in our contemporary European contexts.

Placed in its historical and sociopolitical context, this was not an atypical move. It fits within the tradition of a colonialist approach and the modernist project in which the other cultures are "explored" and "discovered." The aim is to safeguard and increase our own domination and power either by conquering the other and thus eliminating all dangers it may pose for us or by exploiting and appropriating from it whatever can be of use to us. In the realm of knowledge, to conquer the other in a modernist context means further expansion of our own concepts, doctrines and ideologies by incorporating parts of the other in ways that do not threaten our own dominance. Insofar as the modernist project is to create grand theories (and, in this context, grand theories of human nature and of suffering), the inclusion of the other becomes an essential part of this pursuit.

Many authors consider that the Freudian project falls within the same parameters, insofar as Freud tried to discover the otherness of human beings, their unconscious realms, and then make the unconscious conscious. Jung's formulation of the same project appears to be different from the Freudian one as Jung's encounter with the other discourse mostly took the form of idealisation rather than that of a rationalist appropriation.

Regardless of its similarities to and differences from the Freudian project, the Jungian venture was heavily biased towards the other discourse, the discourse of the other, the discourse of the Number 2 personality. However, the way in which Jung went about it could be characterized, at worst, as a subtle form of patronising the "primitive," idealising the native and adoring the "noble savage" and, at best, as an attempt to critique the limitations of European rationalism; the latter, of course, has similarities with the main thrust of the Freudian project—to puncture a hole in Western rationality. However, by idealizing the "primitive," regardless of the genuine good intentions behind it, Jung ignored the sociopolitical and economic plight of the disadvantaged and created a romantic tendency for a return to the lost paradise of simplicity and pure and uncontaminated wisdom—"intuitional activity can be observed most easily among primitives," Jung wrote epigrammatically (1948, p. 137). Undoubtedly, there are valuable elements in this approach, but unless the negative consequences are appreciated, it is likely that this kind of uncritical adoration of the other would produce unfortunate results.

The Exotic Other and the Familiar Other

Emmanuel Levinas (1906–1995), the Lithuanian-born French philosopher who was one of the main modern thinkers who concentrated on a human's relation to the other, wrote characteristically:

> Transcendence is only possible with the Other (Autrui), with respect to whom we are absolutely different . . . transcendence is only possible when the Other is not initially the fellow human being or the neighbour; but when it is very distant . . . when it is the one with whom initially I have nothing in common. . . . Transcendence seemed to me to be the point of departure for our concrete relations with the Other; all the rest is grafted on top of it.
>
> (Peperzak et al. 1996, p. 27)

With these words, Levinas implies a distinction between a distant other and another other which could be called a familiar other. That passage was, in fact, in response to Minkowski's suggestion that, "in everyday life we have three terms for the Other: other, fellow human being and neighbour (autrui, semblable, et prochain)" (Peperzak et al. 1996, p. 26). Levinas insists on the distance between the me and the other (Peperzak, 1993). Although his notion of transcendence will not be considered here, it may suffice to explain that by this term he refers to what could be called a transformative encounter.

Using this prompt from Levinas, it would be useful to propose a distinction between two kinds of others—a distant or exotic other, with whom one feels very different, and a familiar other who is closer to one or even part of one. According to Levinas, the point of departure, the very first step in our pursuit of the other, is the encounter with what could now be termed the exotic and distant other. It is in that encounter that a felt transformation can take place, and then many other processes can be grafted "on top" of that.

Viewed from this perspective, it is understandable that Jung first had to identify the distant other realm of the exotic "primitive." However, what was the familiar other in his case? Why did Jung not identify and comment on the familiar other? What dynamics are involved in the neglectful treatment of the familiar other and his overemphasis and adoration of the distant and exotic other?

Jung compared and contrasted the West (North America and Western Europe) with the distant and exotic others of the Middle and Far East, Africa and native North America; he also included in the distant others the past traditions of European culture (mainly alchemy). However, in doing so, he ignored other others that are not so distant culturally, geographically or temporally—not only the Near East (which covers mainly the territories of the former Ottoman Empire) but a territory much closer to home: all of Eastern Europe and Russia. It is astonishing that, with all of his erudition and widespread research, Jung totally ignored these territories not only in terms of their historical realities but mainly in terms of their cultural and religious traditions. In his *Collected Works* there is scant reference to this world, and wherever we do find mention of it, it reflects an almost shameful ignorance and an inexcusable prejudice against it.

Jung constantly commented on the limitations of Christianity, but the Christianity he considered was the reality of Western Christian denominations. It is incredible that he ignored the entire tradition of the Christian East and the Eastern Orthodox Church. Following the Great Schism in 1054, there was a separation between the Roman Catholic Church and the Orthodox Church; subsequently, the Protestants broke off from the Catholic Church and, gradually, the hundreds of various denominations resulted. Throughout, the Orthodox Church remained the same, continuing with its long tradition. It is astonishing that Jung virtually blocked out the entire Byzantine culture and legacy which form the foundation of Eastern Orthodox Christianity. Similarly, although Jung drew a great deal from the richness of the Greek classical pagan civilization, he made no reference to the modern Greek Orthodox heritage and reality.

It is interesting to note that it was Jung's own daughter (who was definitely not his "best son," as Freud referred to his own daughter, Anna) who expressed a keen interest in the Russian Orthodox tradition. Throughout, Hélène Hoerni-Jung remained outside the analytical movement and resisted joining her father's pursuits. Mrs Hoerni-Jung, Jung's own other as a woman and a non-analyst, seemed to redress her father's negligence and inattention. More specifically, Mrs Hoerni-Jung seriously studied the Eastern Orthodox Church and in particular Russian icons, about which she wrote (e.g., Hoerni-Jung 1991, 1997) and lectured. Her writings express a deep and sincere appreciation of these forms of religious art, which are not abstract artefacts but have always been central to the actual devotional rituals and lives of Orthodox Christians. Anybody who has spent any time in Russia or Greece will have witnessed that rituals there are by no means dead; it would, therefore, become apparent to any observer that what Jung was contrasting with the exotic East and "primitive" communities was not the totality of modern Christianity but the increasing rationalism of Western Christian institutions and practices.

The point here is not to extol the virtues of Eastern Orthodox Christianity at the expense of Western Christianity. What is of importance is to observe how Jung overlooked precisely that for which he was looking: the Orthodox Church has retained alive rituals and resisted the rationalist Enlightenment; its institutions have not been dominated by secularist concerns; its emphasis has remained on holistic approaches; and the individual has not been allowed to become alienated from the community (cf. Ware 1973). If anything, the Orthodox Church has been criticized for this stance, which is considered by some as anachronistic and at times asphyxiating for the individual. However, these are the very elements for which Jung was looking in the exotic other traditions, and yet these were available to him in an alive and functioning tradition (the Orthodox Church) right at his doorstep. It is important to reiterate that the Orthodox Church is not idealized here, and it is not, by any means, introduced as the image of perfection. The paradox is that although Eastern Orthodox Christianity embodies many qualities that Jung was seeking in other cultures, he failed to acknowledge its existence and he also missed the opportunity to engage in serious debate with Orthodox issues. This is more surprising because he was not unaware of Orthodoxy. Gilles Quispel (2001) introduced Orthodox themes at the Eranos Conferences (e.g., Quispel 1951), and he had discussions with Jung on these matters. Quispel felt that Jung was, by then, an old man with already well-established interests, and it was difficult for him to accommodate a new paradigm. Quispel was of the impression that, at that time, Jung did not have the stamina to take on board new projects and, therefore, he was not in a position to consider the serious impact of Orthodoxy. However, what is equally astonishing is that the same neglectful stance on Orthodoxy was continued, by and large, by Jung's followers.

Quispel's view cannot be accepted as the definitive explanation as to why Jung failed to engage with a closer and familiar other, instead of searching for the virtues of the distant and exotic other. Despite the fact that the literature on Orthodoxy that was available to his daughter Hélène was also available to Jung, and there is evidence of that in his *Collected Works*, what is astounding is, in fact, his hostility towards it. For example, in commenting on the Russian Church, paradoxically he ignores his usual argument about living rituals, and in a scathing tone he writes,

> We need feel no surprise that in Russia the colourful splendours of the Eastern Orthodox Church have been superseded by the Movement of the Godless—indeed, one breathed a sigh of relief oneself when one emerged from the haze of an Orthodox church with its multitude of lamps and entered an honest mosque, where the sublime and invisible omnipresence of God was not crowded out by a superfluity of sacred paraphernalia.
>
> (Jung 1936, p. 180)

When are "sacred paraphernalia" elements of living religious rituals and when are they just superfluous "colourful splendours"? Which mosque was Jung comparing to which church? It is all the more interesting to observe Jung's prejudicial comments when we know that he never even went to Russia.

One may claim that Jung, a typical Swiss conservative, writing during the height of the Cold War, saw Russia only in terms of its communist ideology (of which he was uncritically dismissive) and failed to appreciate the cultural wealth and spirituality of that world. Although there is a lot of truth in this claim, in the passage just quoted, Jung seems to almost justify the emergence of "Godless" communism as a reaction to what he saw as the meaningless "sacred paraphernalia" of Orthodoxy. Not only does he fail to grasp any positive potential in these rituals but he also finds it difficult to hide his contempt of Orthodoxy.

Thus, we see that Jung had a genuine adoration of the distant and exotic other, whilst he had nothing but contempt for the close and familiar other. This stance cannot be explained away in terms of either Jung's ignorance or his political conservativism and, therefore, it requires further investigation.

Shadow, "Minor Differences," "Narcissism-Socialism" and "Nameless Dread"

The distinction between two others (the exotic other and the familiar other) enables us to appreciate that the psyche may be involved in a selection of different material to project onto each one of the others. Evidently, in the example given previously, Jung projected all idealisations onto the exotic and distant other (of the non-Christian, Oriental, African, and other "primitive" realms), whilst he ignored or scorned the familiar other (Eastern Christianity). This is not an uncommon phenomenon and it is encountered frequently in clinical work, when analysands idealise one other and denigrate another other. There is a great variation of positive and negative responses, of course, to these two others, for example, fearing one and admiring the other, being repulsed by the one other and being attracted by the other other, noticing and valuing the one other whilst ignoring the other other, etc.

The usual way in which Jungian psychology understands our relation to others is either in terms of projections of our own material (positive or negative) onto them or in terms of the way in which these others activate in us certain images which may then exert their power on our psyche and evoke our response. With regard to the first possibility, the focus is on the contents and processes within our own psyche which are then projected onto the others, whereas in the second possibility what is emphasized is the archetypal nature of the others themselves, which then get a grip on us in specific ways that make us react accordingly. More specifically, analytical psychology often approaches these issues (without, of course, naming them as "the other") in terms of projecting the shadow and scapegoating (e.g., Henderson 1990; Perera 1986) or in terms of idealisation and projection of images of lost paradise (e.g., Bishop 1989, 1995; Hillman et al. 1997; Jacoby 1985). These are useful and appropriate ways of understanding these processes, but they lack the precision that can be introduced when there is an appreciation of the differentiation of the two others and, consequently, the relationship between the two others. The fact that the two others themselves are in some relationship with each other brings a new level of complexity to our understanding.

One of the main ways in which Freud attempted to understand these phenomena was by means of his ideas on *Narzissmus der kleinen Unterschiede*, usually translated as the "narcissism of minor differences." He claimed that,

> It is always possible to bind together a considerable number of people in love, so long as there are other people left over to receive the manifestations of their aggressiveness. . . . It is precisely communities with adjoining territories, and related to each other in other ways as well, who are engaged in constant feuds and in ridiculing each other.
>
> (1930, p. 114)

In this passage, we see both the relationship between the two others and the hostility towards the familiar other. However, we observe that the others are related in terms of the intrapsychic dimension of the individual rather than due to any of their own characteristics. According to this passage, our aggression towards an other is determined mainly by our own impulses—depending on whether we have an other group that we hate, we can afford to also have a group of people to love. Moreover, Freud's understanding of "minor differences" implies that the differences can be either minor or major, and it certainly matters whether they are major or minor. If they are minor, then one is closer to the other, and the proximity creates not only a certain familiarity but also the possibility of a closer identification with predictable consequences.

However, the differences between us and the other are not fixed as minor or major. Differences that are minor under certain conditions may change to become major and vice versa (cf. also the preceding discussion). These changes can be socially constructed, and often there is nothing static or inherent in some differences being small or big, minor or major. To return to Ricoeur, narrative identities may alter this balance; political alliances, changes in the balance of power and other conditions can incur the most dramatic changes in terms of determining the type of differences between the various others. Michael Ignatieff (1999) used this mechanism to account for the ferocity of contemporary war, especially in the Balkans, in his book *The Warrior's Honor*. Following Freud, he argued, for example, that the close similarities between Serbs and Croats could be responsible for the viciousness of their conflict. One of Ignatieff's arguments is that nationalism is not an expression of "some primordial essence, formed by history and tradition" but essentially a "relational" construct: "A Serb is someone who is not a Croat. A Croat is someone who is not a Serb" (1999, p. 37). This, essentially, constructivist approach to nationalism is important, and it demonstrates some of the dynamics involved in the othering process. Under certain circumstances and conditions (e.g., fear, oppression, violence), the relational identities change, the minor differences become major, and the positioning of the one against the other alters radically, often with calamitous consequences (Papadopoulos 2000a). However, these circumstances and conditions do not appear *ex machina*; they are not unrelated to the societal structures and sociopolitical and economic realities. Often they follow or develop wider societal discourses which can be expressed in terms of articulate ideologies or specific propaganda campaigns. Often these discourses emerge as dominant, subjugating all other minor discourses. Thus, in Yugoslavia, the dominant discourse of "brotherhood-unity" among the constituent ethnic groups of that country under Tito was subjugated by the new emergence of a dominant discourse which exalted nationalism. The process of othering an ordinary citizen at the individual level is strongly influenced by the dominant discourse at the time, and it is also a product of complex interactions in the collective and personal realms.

Narcissus represents the epitome of the impossible state of "otherlessness." Narcissus has no other but himself to relate to and to admire, or rather, more precisely, his only other is his own image of himself. However, by excluding external others, Narcissus creates another powerful otherness—his external and public image, the part of himself that relates to others. Bion referred to an internal conflict that can be used here to throw more light on this facet of narcissism. Bion argued that there is a constant conflict between the bipolarity of instincts which "refers to their operation as elements in the fulfilment of the individual's life as an individual, and as elements in his life as a social, or as Aristotle would describe it, as a political animal" (Bion 1992, p. 105). Bion further proposed the existence of a central conflict between what he termed a person's "narcissism" and "socialism":

> experience shows that there is in fact such a conflict—not between sexuality and ego instincts, but rather between [a person's] . . . narcissism and his socialism, and this conflict may manifest itself no matter what the instincts are that are dominant at the time.
>
> (1992, p. 106)

In other words, even if one were to be enwrapped within a narcissistic state ignoring the other, ultimately that would still ignite the conflict between one's own "narcissism" and "socialism," between the impossibility of solipsistic narcissism and its narrative identity.

Bion's helpful insight furthers the investigation into the distinction between the two others and the conditions under which they are fixed and unfixed. The internal conflict between one's "narcissism" and "socialism" can contribute to the perception of minor or major differences in the other, in addition to the dominant societal discourse.

The Trauma Discourse as a Dominant Other

There is an increasing demand for psychology and psychotherapy to provide coherent responses to the painful questions about the nature and meaning of conflicts and violence in our world today. Despite the variety of theories about these issues, it seems that there is a consensus in considering almost everybody affected by these events as being "traumatized." The word "trauma" has been appropriated by every commentator on these conflicts regardless of their psychological sophistication. The word "trauma" has become synonymous with any form of painful experience. Trauma has been

> appropriated by journalists, politicians, social commentators, and demagogues and used indiscriminately to render respectability to their claims. . . . The power of the word 'trauma' lies in its widespread (and seeming) intelligibility which, of course, is deceptive because if pressed, those who use it would find it difficult to define what they mean by 'trauma'.
>
> (Papadopoulos 2001a, p. 5)

Therefore, it is justified to accept that "there is a prevalent and indeed dominant discourse in society which makes people hold the conviction that when a person is exposed to adversity automatically he or she is traumatized" (Papadopoulos 2001a, p. 5). A particularly powerful form of this dominant trauma discourse applies to refugees. However, although the "refugee trauma" discourse dominates our understanding of the refugee experience, in fact it addresses (if it is at all valid) only one segment of the wide spectrum of the refugee experience. Papadopoulos (2000a, 2000b, 2001a, 2001b) has identified four major phases of this experience, which he named "anticipation" (when people sense the impending danger and try to decide how best to avoid it), "devastating events" (this is the phase of actual violence, when the enemy attacks and destroys and the refugees flee), "survival" (when refugees are safe from danger but live in temporary accommodation and uncertainty) and "adjustment" (when refugees try to adjust to a new life in the receiving country). "Unmistakably, the 'refugee trauma' discourse privileges the phase of 'devastating events' and blatantly downplays or even ignores the consequences of the adverse nature of the other phases" (Papadopoulos 2001a, p. 5). In actuality, the refugee trauma discourse exerts a tyrannical effect on both refugees and workers, insofar as it subjugates the pain and suffering involved in all of the other phases of the refugee experience.

Why is the trauma discourse so dominant and how does it relate to the problematic of the other?

According to this dominant discourse, refugee trauma is understood in a monocausal way and as referring to the phase of devastating events. In this way, it offers a simple, convenient and discrete way of conceptualising human suffering under otherwise difficult circumstances. Such a simplified formula can be most consoling in addressing highly complex situations which are not only difficult to grasp intellectually but also painful emotionally as well as confusing epistemologically. The idea of a trauma defined in terms of that specific devastating event which happened in a country far away from the therapists, and which clearly did not form part of our own experiences, creates a safe distance which shields us as therapists from the "nameless dread" which is in danger of engulfing us.

In other words, the power of the trauma discourse is largely based on the exotic and distant otherness, which has the function of protecting us from overwhelming feelings of despair, helplessness and destructiveness.

However, the simplification that the refugee trauma discourse offers can do violence to an already multifaceted and multidimensional field such as the refugee situation. Despite the misleading "self-evident" situation, as we have seen, the source or the cause of refugee trauma is not just one single and identifiable event. Moreover, our justified abhorrence of the atrocities that are considered the cause of refugee trauma may force us into creating a simplistic causal relation between the atrocities and the trauma, thus ignoring the possibility of a non-pathological response to the condemnable atrocities. In other words, the epistemological confusion between morality and pathology may lead to uniform pathologisation of the refugee situation.

Other interrelated implications of accepting this widespread and predominant version of the refugee trauma discourse include the distance that is created between therapists and the suffering refugees, the fostering of dependence, the diminishment of psychological complexities, the setting up of polarised situations, the creation of victim-saviour dyads and the denial of resilience and other positive outcomes.

The denial of complexity (which the refugee trauma promotes) may also deprive therapeutic work in these contexts from accessing the totality of psychological functions and abilities of refugees. Ultimately, human beings have the capacity to process internally and within their families and communities painful events and experiences and to transform them into potential growth situations. Therapeutic work that is focused too closely on the refugee trauma as a monocausal pathological phenomenon will fail to capitalise on this potential; the positive use of the roles of imagination and symbolization as well as the whole transference-countertransference matrix may be underestimated or completely ignored.

Thus, the example of refugee trauma discourse as an exotic other demonstrates how the lack of vigilance regarding the nature, function and impact of the othering processes can perpetrate further violence in these tragic situations.

Heart of Darkness

A mature South American woman of European extraction came to see me with intense feelings of depression, complaining that she feared she would be overwhelmed by her own passivity. She was a successful professional who presented an immaculate external image of an efficient, gregarious and likeable person. Shortly after we began working together, it emerged that she was petrified of "going mad," and she associated this fear with her compulsive practice of native religious rituals from her home country. Although she had lived in England for a long time, she had continued to practise these rituals in secret. She lived alone but had a wide social circle and led a lively social life. In the past she believed in those rituals, but gradually she lost any real faith in them yet was unable to stop practising them. In many ways, she led a double life, continuing to go regularly to the Catholic Church and, at the same time, practising her secret rituals at home. Prior to coming to see me, her sense of meaning lessness and pain had increased to an unbearable degree, and she often contemplated suicide. Neither the Church nor her rituals offered any substantial solace.

To begin with, she blamed her Catholic, intellectual and bohemian parents for introducing her to these rituals early in her life, and she was able to get in touch with her enormous anger towards them. She felt that they did not prepare her for real life and that their idealisation of the pagan practices had damaged and trapped her. Moreover, she now considered them responsible for leading her further into "madness."

The work was difficult and full of pain, especially as more psychotic-like features of her personality began to emerge. She was plagued by images of "Catholic purity" as well as of "pagan darkness." Not unexpectedly, her transference to me was equally powerful and split; interchangeably, she saw me as a Christian saviour and as a pagan initiator, idealising and admiring me as well as fearing me and attacking me. She was struggling with the meaning of the duality of others—the familiar other of the Catholic Church and the exotic other of the native rituals. She felt a strong connection both with her Catholic identity and with her native rituals, but she was completely enwrapped in their confusion and anguish.

One significant step in our work was her "accidental" (!) discovery of Joseph Conrad's novel *The Heart of Darkness* (1898). She identified with Kurz, and then with great excitement she realised the connection between this novel and Coppola's film *Apocalypse Now*. Many sessions were dominated by her discussion of images and themes from both of these masterpieces. My concern was to not allow her to fly into abstract intellectualisations, but, at the same time, I was aware that this intense interest had a therapeutic function and acted as a form of active imagination for her and in the way we used it. The safety of this other medium enabled her to delve into her own dynamics, and the formalized images of these works acted as vehicles for her to both develop a much needed reflective stance and connect with her own material in a deeper way.

The last words that both Mr Kurtz and Colonel Walter E. Kurtz utter before their deaths—'the horror, the horror'—received particular attention from her.

Gradually, she came to feel that they conveyed not only the horror that these two tragic heroes witnessed in their encounters of the other in the depths of the heart of darkness but also the heroes' own horror about how they themselves had ended up identifying with that darkness.

The novel and the film enabled us to approach the complexities of her own predicament from a safe distance both in terms of her intrapsychic turmoil and in terms of her external circumstances. The idealisation of the exotic other was grasped in terms of both her inner need for a mystery and a yearning for a connection with her shadow and her liberal politics of wanting to identify with the oppressed. In time, the compulsiveness of her ritualistic practices weakened, and then she stopped them completely. A new energy began to spring to life in her which was not so formalised and contrived. The quality of her human connections changed, and she felt that she was able to relate to people with freshness.

This brief vignette of a success story cannot possible convey all of the elements of the others discussed in this chapter, but it offers one illustration (admittedly, of an exotic nature) in which the identification of the others and their dynamics approached via stylised artistic images enabled a person to free herself from a most crippling condition. Needless to say, none of these issues was addressed in our sessions with this terminology; instead we used ordinary language referring to the intricate nuances of the othering processes. My analysand was enabled to appreciate the complex effects of her assimilation into foreign cultures, the function of her liberal politics, the dynamics of her family predicament and her own inner forms of otherness.

References

Adams, M. V. (1996). *Multicultural imagination. Race, colour and the unconscious*. London: Routledge.

Barber, E. A. (ed.) (1968). *Lidell, Scott and Jones' Greek—English Lexicon: A Supplement*. Oxford: Clarendon Press.

Benjamin, J. (1998). *Shadow of the Other*. London: Routledge.

Bion, W. R. (1992). *Cogitations*. London: Karnac, 1994.

Bishop, P. (1989). *The Myth of Shangri-La: Tibet, Travel Writing and the Western Creation of Sacred Landscape*. London: Athlone.

Bishop, P. (1995). *An Archetypal Constable. National Identity and the Geography of Nostalgia*. London: Athlone.

Conrad, J. (1898). *The Heart of Darkness*. London: Dent, 1974.

De Certeau, M. (1986). *Heterologies. Discourses on the Other*. Manchester: Manchester University Press.

Della Sala, S. (2000). 'Anarchic hand: The syndrome of disowned actions'. *Creating Sparks, The BA Festival of Science*. www.creatingsparks.co.uk.

Derrida, J. (1985). *The Ear of the Other. Texts and Discussions*. Lincoln: University of Nebraska Press.

Fowler, D. D. & Hardsley, D. L. (eds.) (1994). *Others Knowing Others: Perspectives on Ethnographic Careers*. Washington, DC: Smithsonian Institution Press.

Freud, S. (1930). 'Civilization and its Discontents'. *SE* 21.

Frosh, S. (1999). *The Politics of Psychoanalysis*. London: Macmillan, 2nd edition.

Giegerich, W. (1998). *The Soul's Logical Life*. Frankfurt am Main: Peter Lang.

Hauke, C. (2000). *Jung and the Postmodern. The Interpretation of Realities*. London: Routledge.

Henderson, J. (1990). *Shadow and Self*. Wilmette, Il: Chiron.

Hillman, J., et al. (1997). *Haiti or the Psychology of Black*. Thompson, CT: Spring.

Hoerni-Jung, H. (1991). *Maria. Bild des Weiblichen. Ikonen der Gottesgebaererin*. München: Koesel-Verlag.

Hoerni-Jung, H. (1997). *Unbekannter Petrus. Schlüssel zum Menschsein*. München: Koesel- Verlag.

Ignatieff, M. (1999). *The Warrior's Honor. Ethnic War and the Modern Conscience*. London: Vintage.

Jacoby, M. A. (1985). *The Longing for Paradise*. Boston: Sigo Press

Jarrett, J. L. (1979). 'The logic of psychological opposition'. *The Journal of Analytical Psychology*, 24, 4, 318–325.

Jung, C. G. (1931). 'The spiritual problem of modern man'. *CW* 10.

Jung, C. G. (1936). 'Wotan'. *CW* 10.

Jung, C. G. (1943). 'The psychology of the unconscious'. *CW* 7.

Jung, C. G. (1948). 'Instinct and the unconscious'. *CW* 8.

Jung, C. G. (1951). 'Aion'. *CW* 9ii.

Jung, C. G. (1952). 'Religion and psychology: A reply to Martin Buber'. In *CW* 18.

Jung, C. G. (1961). *Memories, Dreams, Reflections*. London: Fontana, 1995.

Kritikos, A., Mattingley, J. B. & Breen, N. (2001, April). Anarchic Hand Syndrome: Bimanual coordination and sensitivity to irrelevant information in unimanual reaches. *Inaugural Australian Conference for Cognitive Neuropsychology and Cognitive Neuropsychiatry*. (Abstract published in *Australian Journal of Psychology*, 53 (Suppl.).)

Lacan, J. (1968). *The Language of the Self. The Function of Language in Psycho- analysis*. Baltimore: Johns Hopkins University Press.

Lacan, J. (1977a). *Ecrits. A Selection*. London: Tavistock.

Lacan, J. (1977b). *The Four Fundamental Concepts of Psychoanalysis*. London: The Hogarth Press.

Lacan, J. (2000). *The Seminar of Jacques Lacan*. New York: W. W. Norton.

Lemaire, A. (1977). *Jacques Lacan*. London: Routledge & Kegan Paul.

Marchetti, C. & Della Sala, S. (1998). 'Disentangling the alien and anarchic hand'. *Cognitive Neuropsychiatry*, 3, 191–207.

Miller, D. L. (1990). 'An Other Jung and an Other . . .'. In *C. G. Jung and the Humanities. Toward a Hermeneutics of Culture*, ed. K. Barnaby & P. D'Acierno. London: Routledge.

Moravia, A. (1972). *The Two of Us*. London: Secker & Warburg.

O'Barr, W. M. (1994). *Culture and the Ad. Exploring Otherness in the World of Advertising*. Boulder: Westview Press.

Ogden, C. K. (1967). *Opposition. A Linguistic and Psychological Analysis*. Bloomington: Indiana University Press.

Papadopoulos, R. K. (1980). *The Dialectic of the Other in the Psychology of C. G. Jung. A Metatheoretical Investigation*. PhD Thesis, University of Cape Town.

Papadopoulos, R. K. (1984). 'Jung and the concept of the Other'. In *Jung in Modern Perspective*, ed. Renos K. Papadopoulos & Graham Saayman. London: Wildwood House.

Papadopoulos, R. K. (1997). 'Individual identity and collective narratives of conflict'. *Harvest: Journal for Jungian Studies*, 43, 2, 7–26.

Papadopoulos, R. K. (1998). 'Jungian perspectives in new contexts'. In *The Post-Jungians Today*, ed. Ann Casement. London & New York: Routledge.

Papadopoulos, R. K. (2000a). 'Factionalism and interethnic conflict: Narratives in myth and politics'. In *The Vision Thing. Myth, Politics and Psyche in the World*, ed. Thomas Singer. London & New York: Routledge.

Papadopoulos, R. K. (2000b). 'A matter of shades: Trauma and psychosocial work in Kosovo'. In *Psychosocial and Trauma Response in War-Torn Societies; the Case of Kosovo*, ed. N. Losi. Geneva: International Organization for Migration.

Papadopoulos, R. K. (2001a). 'Refugees, therapists and trauma: Systemic reflections'. *Context; the magazine of the Association for Family Therapy*, No. 54, April, 5–8. Special Edition on REFUGEES; eds. Gill Gorell Barnes & Renos Papadopoulos.

Papadopoulos, R. K. (2001b). 'Refugee families: Issues of systemic supervision'. *Journal of Family Therapy*, 23, 4, 405–422.

Peperzak, A. (1993). *To the Other. An Introduction to the Philosophy of Emmanuel Levinas*. West Lafayette: Purdue University Press.

Peperzak, A. K., Critchley, S. & Bernasconi, R. (eds.) (1996). *Emmanuel Levinas. Basic philosophical Writings*. Bloomington: Indianapolis University Press.

Perera, S. B. (1986). *Scapegoat Complex: Toward a Mythology of Shadow and Guilt*. Toronto: Inner City Books.

Quispel, G. (1951). 'Time and history in patristic Christianity'. In *Man and Time*, ed. Joseph Campbell. Collected Papers from the Eranos Yearbooks. New York: Princeton University Press, 1957.

Quispel, G. (2001). Personal communication.

Ricoeur, P. (1994). *Oneself as Another*. Chicago: Chicago University Press.

Said, E. (1978). *Orientalism*. New York: Pantheon.

Said, E. (1994). *Culture and Imperialism*. London: Vintage (1993).

Sampson, E. E. (1993). *Celebrating the Other: A Dialogic Account of Human Nature*. London: Harvester.

Stevenson, R. L. (1886). *The Strange Case of Dr Jekyll and Mr Hyde*. London: Dent, 1925.

Ware, K. T. (1973). 'Orthodoxy and the West'. In *Orthodoxy: Life and Freedom*, ed. A. J. Philippou. Oxford: Studion Publications.

Wilkinson, S. & Kitzinger, C. (eds.) (1996). *Representing the Other*. London: Sage.

Chapter 7

Denise G. Ramos

The checkered wool skirt had to be 30 cm from the floor. Our blouses were white and long-sleeved, and this in a heat close to 100 degrees Fahrenheit. Even so, in the suffocating humid air, I loved walking in the white marble courtyards of the school in which I studied, a copy of an Italian palace. There everything was silent. In the interval between classes, while a colleague read aloud the life of the saints, we cross-stitched flowers on towels.

The college, run by Italian nuns, was a refuge in the noisy city. There I learned to have compassion and love for others. It took me a while to learn what prejudice was. At home, people of any origin and color were very well treated; it never occurred to me that black people might be suffering from the projected inferiority stamped in the color of their skin.

Many, many years later, when I taught in the city of Salvador, my eyes were opened. I was doing an exercise with word association, when I noticed a tearful look from a black student. Eighty percent of Salvador's population is of African descent, and it was in this city that most ships from Africa docked. The word that triggered so much emotion was "ship", which the student associated with "*negreiro*" – the name given to the ships that brought the slaves. I woke up to a reality that had gone unnoticed.

At the historic center of this city, I studied the great variety of paintings and interviewed street vendors and the owners of old canteens. I was clearly discriminated against – whatever was a "white bitch" doing here, nosing around like a scientist? One of the main figures in the neighborhood agreed to be interviewed. I sat there waiting for 2 hours. I felt that I was being tested; he was not going to serve me just because I wanted. This made me feel how he himself felt. When he finally noticed that I was there, he opened the door and served me a delicious cup of coffee. We could not be more different and more equal. He was black and poorly educated, and I was white and had a graduate degree. We ended with a hug that went beyond all differences.

I presented this research at the IAAP International Congress and opened a research group at my university about intergenerational trauma due to slavery.

But before going into psychology, my passion was ballet. The strict discipline and the severe Russian teacher went hand in hand with the education I had received. Dancing, I wanted to fly. The power to control my body and the pain following the

DOI: 10.4324/9781003148982-8

pulsating rhythm of Chopin's waltzes were all a dream. But being a dancer was a short career. It did not satisfy my need to be independent, and so dance became a mere hobby. I moved on to science. My curiosity about how the mind worked led me to read everything that fell into my hands. Even more mysterious than the mind was the mystery of our origin and destiny. I had to expand my horizons.

While studying psychology, I spent a period at the Esalen Institute (Big Sur, CA). This period was rich in various forms of therapy, including drugs, nudity, Gestalt therapy, massages and Rolfing, and it awakened the question: how do body and mind connect? My vacations were spent seeking out new experiences, which included going with the Arica group (USA) to practice different techniques of awareness development. In New York, I attended workshops with Alexander Lowen, the father of bioenergetics. I already admired W. Reich's work, especially his character analysis associated with body tension rings. The psyche was there, in the body. With A. Lowen, I felt the neurosis present in my body and how to transform it. No longer was it possible to study a dissociated psychology.

My university was essentially humanistic, and C.G. Jung's theory was being introduced into the curriculum. Jung talked about me; how could he possibly know me so well? When I won a Fulbright scholarship, I decided to study in New York to be able to attend the Jungian Institute and do my analysis. My analyst was Estelle Weinrib. Upon entering her office and seeing a bookcase full of tiny toys, I asked if she attended children. Smiling, Estelle introduced me to the world of sandplay. As a teacher member of the International Society of Sandplay Therapy, I have acted as vice president and chair of the academic committee, as well as supervising theses on the effectiveness of the technique, one of which won the award for best thesis in Brazil.

But, in an interconnected circle, my trip to New York resulted in a conflict between love and professional training. In a sexist country like Brazil, it is clear that a woman is expected to serve her husband. I lost in this argument – and this drama came at a price: depression added to cancer. The pain crystallized in my body showed me the essential ingredients of my doctoral thesis: psychosomatics, which later transformed into books and lectures. Another circle closed in Moscow, where I dedicated my psychosomatic lecture to my Russian ballet teacher Madam Olenewa, the first to teach me how to enjoy the body I was given.

Meeting colleagues from around the world has always been extremely rewarding at IAAP. I have made some great friends. Invited to run for an administrative position, I spent 12 years on the executive committee and 3 of them as vice president. This period taught me a lot about national identity differences and equality.

At my university, I have always enjoyed total freedom to develop my research, sharing ideas and projects with students and colleagues at the Center for Jungian Studies, created after my doctorate.

Another circle opened with an invitation from T. Singer to contribute to the book *Cultural Complex*. Here I had the motivation to research a phenomenon that has disturbed me for as long as I can remember, namely, the endemic corruption that plagues my country. I was very pleased with the result, for it had and continues to have repercussions in the social sphere.

The circle already referred to that involved the breakup of a relationship was transformed into the Center for Assistance to Victims of Violence and Abuse and in a large survey entitled. And here I close yet another circle – and free myself from feeling any "guilt" for a decision made in the past.

These, then, are the various circles of my life that open up and connect with one another. They keep on spiraling round, and I am curious – looking forward to – the next step that appears on the horizon.

Jungian Theory and Contemporary Psychosomatics

Unpublished.

One of the most intriguing questions in science is how the psyche and the body relate to one another. This matter, which has been studied since the early philosophers down to the most advanced of today's scientists, still remains at some distance from a solution. Many attempts have been made, including by S. Freud in 1895, to construct a neuroscientific model of the mind. In his project to develop a scientific psychology, the master set out to define "the nature of the relationship between the brain and the mind." He was finally obliged to give up when he realized that most of the fundamental concepts upon which he based his ideas amounted to mere speculation. Freud argued that biology had not advanced enough to be helpful to psychoanalysis (Freud, S., 1950/1895; Solms, 1998).

More than a century later, in spite of the remarkable progress in the biological sciences, a good number of psychoanalysts still continue to maintain Freud's view, and at times in an even more radical manner. Some affirm, for example, that "the science of the mind and the science of the body utilize different languages, different concepts, different sets of tools and techniques." According to this view, "there is no way to unify the two by translation into a common language, or by reference to a shared conceptual framework" (Reiser, 1975, p. 479).

On the other hand, as early as the 19th century, those involved with the practice and study of psychology observed the influence of the emotions on illness and adopted the term "psychosomatic" to define an area of study and practical application. Introduced to science in 1808 by the German doctor J.C. Heinroth, "somatopsychic" or "psychosomatic" medicine reached its peak in the middle of the 20th century, only to be abolished later by the academic milieu, who felt that it lacked a scientific basis. The failure of Franz Alexander's theory (Chicago Institute for Psychoanalysis), among others that tried to establish a correlation between profiles of personality and certain illnesses, together with the rapid development of biomedical medicine with its precise, determinist measurements led to this area of knowledge being viewed as invalid, presenting results that were not very practical and more dependent on faith than on science (Alexander, 1965; Ramos, 2005).

Reductionist and organicist reasoning easily laid low the argument that emotions or stress could be related to organic diseases. Biological proof of organic disturbances that became increasingly easier to detect by means of sophisticated apparatuses and biological measurements led to a rapid weakening of psychological theses. So, the word "psychosomatic" was eventually execrated from the scientific world.

It is ironic that today these same sophisticated measurements are what enable us to observe with greater technical precision how stress, anguish and other psychic disorders affect the functioning of the organism and vice versa, such that a new approach to the relation between psychology and biology is now beginning to appear.

Although contemporary approaches to biomedical research exalt the roles of genetics and molecular biology, social and psychological research shows that the components of health, genetic factors and environmental exposures interact with social and economic factors. Despite the emphasis on the need for behavioral technologies that could promote a sound way of living, the literature in health psychology clearly documents that behavioral change is complex and difficult to achieve. Patient advice or simple patient education rarely achieves its goal, and health programs tend to produce only short-term benefits (Kaplan, 2009). More research is needed to learn how to improve these behavioral approaches. In reality, we need a sound theory and a set of validated methodologies to address these issues.

Jungian Psychosomatics

As early as 1936, C.G. Jung stated, in a lecture given at Harvard University, that "although psychology claims for its own rights in its special field of research, it has to admit that there is a close correspondence between its data and the data presented by biology" (C.G. Jung, 1972, *CW* 8, para. 232).

Nonetheless, difficulties of observation, added to the lack of a holistic theory to allow for a unified reasoning between the various levels of our being, have been the major obstacle in this area. The hope that neurology and the cognitive sciences would resolve the situation was unquestionably a new reductionist way of facing the problem. Without disregarding the importance of new discoveries in the area, it must be admitted that reduction of the psyche to a chain of physiological reactions is quite unsatisfactory. This would be like saying that music and the piano are of the same order of grandeur. To continue this metaphor, music depends on an instrument, but it is not reducible to the material of which it is made. Just as the piano does not make the music, the matter of the brain does not make the psyche, although one does not exist without the other. As with music, we could say that all human production comes from a factor that transcends the matter and consciousness itself, that is to say, the symbol which is the fundamental factor in constructing human beings and culture.

A brief reflection is sufficient to observe that analytical psychology presents us with a full description of the bases for the new paradigm. Although C.G. Jung did not contribute in a direct manner to this controversy, the principles of the holistic model may be found in the psychotherapeutic theory and method that he proposed.

Today, Felix Deutsch is considered to be the first author to introduce the term "psychosomatic medicine" in 1922, although it was Helen Dunbar with her book *Emotions and Biology Changes. A Survey of Literature on Psychosomatic Interrelationships: 1910–1933* who provided the principal bases for the formation of this area with systematic observations and the application of scientific methodology. A little before writing her book, Dunbar visited Jung in Zürich (Kornfeld, 1990) and later, influenced by him and Deutsch, founded the American Psychosomatic Society and journal (*Psychosomatic Medicine*) in 1939.

At this time, Jung was involved with studies to test psychophysiological reactions resulting from the activation of complexes and with the study of typology and physical manifestations. He states the following:

> The distinction between mind and body is an artificial dichotomy, an act of discrimination based far more on the peculiarity of intellectual cognition than on the nature of things. In fact, so intimate is the intermingling of bodily and psyche traits that not only can we draw far-reaching inferences as to the constitution of the psyche from the constitution of the body, but we can infer from psychic peculiarities the corresponding bodily characteristics.
>
> (Jung, 1971, p. 916)

The earliest tests of word association, developed by C.G. Jung in 1902, proved that the emotions and psychic phenomena have physiological correlates and that the constellation of a complex provokes a simultaneous alteration on both the physiological and psychological levels, irrespective of whether the individual notices these alterations.

Complexes are mostly responsible for the formation of symptoms. C.G. Jung defined them in the following manner:

> [A] collection of imaginings, which, in consequence of this autonomy, is relatively independent of the central control of the consciousness and at any moment liable to bend or cross the intentions of the individual.
>
> (C.G. Jung, 1973, *CW* 2, para. 1352).

The core of the complex is a painful or traumatic conflict that upsets the nervous system and disturbs the systems that are not under the control of the superior brain structures. According to Kolk, "traumatic experiences are initially imprinted as sensations or feeling states, and are not collated and transcribed into personal narrative . . . traumatic memories come back as emotional and sensory states with little verbal representations" (van der Kolk et al., 2007, p. 296).

It is noticeable that profound existential or traumatic situations can provoke unconscious emotional and organic excitability that cannot be expressed on the verbal, abstract level. This excitation, a reaction of either freeze or fight or flight from some threatening stimulus or strong emotional charge, stays fixed in the organism as a muscular contraction, provoking a hormonal alteration or lowering the efficacy of the immunological system, for example, which makes it all the more vulnerable and prone to illness.

The different individual reactions to adverse stimuli, however, are important and depend partly on the structure and dynamic of the personality. External or internal events can stir incoherent reactions when they stimulate or touch a complex, that is to say, they can trigger intense physiological reactions when they "reproduce" the central dynamics of the complex. Accordingly, a seemingly harmless stimulus can be transduced by the organism as adverse and menacing, thereby producing a disruption of the organism's homeostasis.

By transduction we mean the conversion or transformation of information from one form to another. We know that the basic function of the sensorial systems is to perform the transduction of the information contained in the external or internal environment to the language of the nervous system to enable the individual to use this codified information in the perceptual or functional-control operations called for at each and every moment. Different mechanisms of synaptic integration engage in action throughout this chain of transmission to enable an analysis of the various attributes of the stimuli and their subsequent use them in other physiological processes or to mentally reconstruct the objects (Albertz, 1994; Rossi, 1986).

If we envisage the human body as a network of informative, genetic, immunological, hormonal and other systems, we shall see that each one of them has its own code. The transmission of information among the various systems requires some type of transducer to allow the code of a system to be transposed to the code of another system. The capacity to symbolize in linguistic or extralinguistic fashion can also be considered as a way to codify, process and transmit information related to the organism from the psyche to the *soma* and vice versa (Rossi, 1986).

The sight or smell of some positive stimulus, for instance, will set off a chain reaction of transductions that will possibly lead to a sensation of pleasure and homeostasis, whereas an aversive stimulus is transduced into physiological alterations that are responded to with alarm and stress. Once the danger is over, the organism normally returns to its homeostatic state.

Often this psychophysiological excitation, which is initially protective, is not registered in consciousness; it can occur dissociated from any perceiving subject, who may feel, for example, a certain discomfort or a vague physiological sensation of pain without relating this to the triggering event. In the case in which there is an overexcited or aggressive reaction incompatible with reality, it is likely that the dynamism of a complex is at play.

The dilemma for us as psychotherapists is how to reach these organic, unconscious levels where words have no effect because the excitation is registered in primitive regions of the cerebral structure.

If the disorder is psychophysiological, the language is that of sensation and motricity, which obliges us to work on the physiological and corporal levels, as well as with nonverbal expressive symbology. Once the lesion is fixed in preverbal structures, we will hardly be able to provoke alterations using psychoanalytical techniques. Pierre Marty himself, founder of the Psychosomatic School of Paris, proposes a therapeutic non-psychoanalytical form of work, because according to him somatization does not have a symbolic significance and is but a signal of a dysfunction (Ramos, 2005).

However, unlike the psychoanalytical school, Jungian understanding of the symbol allows for a new approach to the psychosomatic phenomenon. Here the word "symbol" is understood in its etymological sense, derived from the Greek *synballein* (*syn*, together + *ballein*, throw), meaning a joining of opposites, throwing together the known and the unknown (the unconscious). Insofar as symbol implies the union of something conscious with something unconscious, it always provokes emotion, that is to say, a "movement outward" (*e* + *motion*), a movement of the vegetative, sympathetic and parasympathetic nervous systems. Working on the nonverbal symbolic level, we can transduce the organic polarity of the symptom to the verbal, conscious level.

However, we need to remember that, around the complexes, defense mechanisms "protect" the nucleus of the traumatic conflict, and, to avoid pain, the patient resist any therapeutic measure or conscious advice that could change his/her pathological behavior. Some physicians do not realize that although patients would like to follow his/her medical advice, they cannot because a symptom may work as a defense mechanism against unbearable suffering and a change of habit will be just temporary. This problem becomes clear in studies such as that by D. Holman, R. Lynch and A. Reeves (2018), who observed that although, in recent years, health behavior interventions have received a great deal of attention in both research and policy as a means of encouraging people to lead healthier lives, the results are not satisfactory. Their conclusion is that it is necessary to focus on individualized approaches drawn from behavioral psychology and behavioral economics, suggesting more interdisciplinary collaboration to advance the field.

Only an approach that deals with the unconscious mechanisms that protect the traumatic nucleus may promote a permanent change of habits.

Clinical Practice

In clinical practice, the application of Jungian psychosomatics has effectively produced psychosomatic transformations and promoted a permanent change of habits, as we are going to see in the following examples.

An "Angry" Gastritis

A 46-year-old patient suffering from gastritis, who had already been operated on for a duodenal ulcer, sought out an analyst due to uncontrolled anxiety. He underwent fits of rage that he justified by the improper behavior of others. His difficulty in tolerating anything that caused him annoyance involved him in many conflicts, which at times ended up with him in hospital with stomach pains. His extremely violent parents had abandoned him, which caused constant psychological abuse that led to defensive mechanisms being built around a complex. This traumatic complex made apparently inoffensive episodes take on enormous dimensions because they touched on an unconscious conflict, which provoked an excitation that could not be verbalized and a generalized commotion that was transduced by the autonomous nervous system as a threat to life. In this case, verbal arguments or interpretations were innocuous, failing to reach the lower layers of his organism, which reacted with alarm. While working with the sand-play technique, the patient broke into tears upon sinking his hands into the sand. Regressive behavior made him want to "get inside" the sand, because in his childhood the beach was a warm place where he could hide from the family squabbles. The patient also liked to use a straw to drink chocolate milk from a little bottle: a clear allusion to the lack of maternal milk. He said that this calmed him down, despite his doctor's recommendation that milk could worsen his symptoms. He drew his stomach as a place that bled and hurt. In one exercise of imagination he asked it why it hurt, and the answer was fear, anger and impotence. It bled because he was afraid of his violent father and then he remembered the beating that his little sister took. Watching this scene without moving while thinking that he would be next made him freeze. He could neither flee nor fight. Drinking milk was an unconscious way for him to "calm down with his good mother" the rage and terror he felt. In therapy, the psychophysiological excitation had to be transduced from the organic to the conscious level, from the right hemisphere to the left, using nonverbal techniques. Little by little the patient managed first of all to identify in his body the excitation and the triggering stimuli and subsequently to transduce his suffering into images and then into words so as to hold it in his consciousness. The excitation that had remained stagnant in one of his somatic systems, being repeated compulsively, gradually subsided. The gastritis was a symbol that expressed his consternation: he could not "swallow" the offenses and rejections, and his digestive system reacted angrily to the "intruders who wanted to destroy him."

Here we hold the key to psychosomatics: by observing the symptom as the best expression that his organism produced to defend itself from suffering—a nonverbal symbol—we reached the profound organic layers that were inaccessible to consciousness. Sick or healthy creative productions are symbolic productions, for they bring to the surface unknown material that provokes emotions not controlled by consciousness. Although we lack the space here to delve further into the psychoneurological bases of this approach, it is crucial to observe that "therapeutic interventions that enhance neural integration and collaborative interhemisphere function may be especially helpful in moving unresolved traumatic states toward resolution" (Solomon & Siegel, 2003, p. 15).

Neurological Correlates

The neuroscientist A. Schore (2003, 2010) provided a substantial amount of evidence that supports the proposition that the early developing right brain generates the unconscious and that the left and right hemispheres process information in different ways. According to contemporary neuroscience, he points out that the right side of the brain is dominant for an "emotional" and "corporeal" sense of self and operates a distributed network for rapidly responding to danger or any challenge, stress or pain. This hemisphere is deeply nonverbal, nonconscious, holistic, corporeal and more dominant for emotional communication. It operates in a primary process manner typically observed in states such as dreaming or reverie. The emotional, affective or traumatic presymbolic and preverbal experiences are encoded in this hemisphere.

It is possible that, when a complex is activated, the individual will feel that an apparently neutral situation is extremely dangerous. This illusion will activate the right hemisphere and trigger, in a synchronous manner, physiological reactions— reactions of defense, flight or fight. As there is no real danger, the patient's symptomology seems incomprehensible. However, his body was expressing, without words, a rich symbolism. In this case, interpretation is limited and does not reach implicit memories embodied as physiological disturbances and uneasy feelings. As these sensations related to defensive reactions to trauma are stored with images and metaphors, the work with them (trough transduction) facilitates reaching the physiological levels of the organism. Another case illustrates this point.

A Constant Diarrhea

The patient was a senior CEO of a multinational company. He had very humble origins, and his father severely punished him whenever he got anything but all A's. This father's expectations were that his son would be rich and support him. His success and leadership position were achieved with great effort. He would have diarrhea whenever he was nervous; however, in the last 10 years this symptom became more frequent, occurring about every day. All clinical exams were normal. He complained that he suffered embarrassing situations in his job, especially when traveling, because he always needed to have a bathroom close by due to sudden and severe diarrhea. His physician sent him for analysis, but the patient was very resistant and uninterested in this process. He just "wanted to get rid of the symptom", which greatly reduced his quality of life. He enjoyed his job very much, working 12 hours a day, and he seemed very upset with his problem, which prevented him from traveling in small airplanes without a bathroom. So, he preferred to spend long hours traveling by car so he could stop to go to the bathroom wherever he felt discomfort. He did not remember his dreams and reported no family or social problems. He could be described as an alexithymic. Looking for a thread that could take us to his unconscious, I asked if he had any hobbies besides reading reports and newspapers. He said that he enjoyed looking for pictures of imminent disasters on the internet and brought some of them. We watched videos of tsunamis and September 11 several times. I could see the anguish and pleasure he felt while imagining the terror of the people involved in these tragedies. The pictures showed exactly what he felt when he had to make a difficult decision or when he was stressed in a meeting: as if an uncontrollable disaster was imminent—an excitation that made him run to the bathroom. The stress of a relatively common situation in his daily life was felt as a near death experience. In therapeutically working with these images, it became clear that the dynamic of a business meeting was touching a negative father complex, and his response was about the same as the people he had seen in the videos: fight, flight or freeze.

Conclusion

By promoting holistic reasoning, compatible with theories from other fields of knowledge, Jungian psychosomatics enables deep psychodynamic reflection on the phenomena related to the healthy functioning of human beings. So we may say that all illnesses are psychosomatic, regardless of their physical, organic or emotional causality. When poorly adapted psychophysiological mechanisms cause an individual to suffer, he/she can fall ill and in this way express his/her suffering more emphatically, either in organic or in psychic polarity. Techniques that facilitate transduction between the different systems can intervene in the process of sickness and health, even when the cause is explicitly external. Skin cancer as a result of exposure to the sun, for example, lies inside an organism with a psyche that reacts to it.

Among the techniques that have been most useful in the process of transduction are nonverbal expressive modalities such as painting and pottery, active imagination and sandplay therapy.

In conclusion, understanding the psyche-body phenomenon and the use of expressive and imaginative techniques are the bases of efficacious clinical work, because they promote and permit the work of interdisciplinary teams that develop holistic health practices derived from different spheres of scientific knowledge.

References

Albertz, B. (1994). *Molecular Biology of the Cell*. New York: Garland Science.

Alexander, F. (1965). *Psychosomatic Medicine*. New York: W.W. Norton Incorporated.

Freud, S. (1950/1895). A project for a scientific psychology. *SE1*, 295–387

Holman, D., Lynch, R. & Reeves, A. (2018). How do health behaviour interventions take account of social context? A literature trend and co-citation analysis. *Health*, 22(4): 389–410.

Jung, C.G. (1971). *Psychology Types. CW*:6.

Jung, C.G. (1972). *The Structure and Dynamics of the Psyche. CW*:8.

Jung, C.G. (1973). *Experimental Researches. CW*:2.

Kaplan, Robert (2009). Health psychology: Where are we and where do we go from here? *Mens Sana Monogr*, January–December, 7(1): 3–9. Doi:10.4103/0973-1229.43584

Kornfeld, D.S. (1990). The American Psychosomatic Society: Why? *Psychosomatic Medicine*, 52(4): 481–495.

Ramos, D.G. (2005). *The Psyche of the Body*. Hover: Brunner-Routledge.

Reiser, M. (1975). Changing theoretical concepts in psychosomatic medicine. In *American Handbook of Psychiatry*, 2nd ed., vol. IV. Ed. Reiser, M. & Arieti, S. New York: Basic Books.

Rossi, E.L. (1986). *The Psychobiology of Mind-Body Relationship*. New York: W.W. Norton.

Schore, Allan (2003). *Affect regulation and the repair of the Self*. New York: W.W. Norton & Company.

Schore, Allan (2010). The right brain implicit self: A central mechanism of the psychotherapy change process. In *Knowing, Not-Knowing and Sort-of-Knowing: Psychoanalysis and the Experience of Uncertainty*. Ed. Petrucelli, J. New York: Karnac Book.

Solms, M (1998). Before and after Freud's Project. *Annals of the New York Academy of Sciences*, 843: 1–10.

Solomon, M. & Siegel, D. (2003). *Healing Trauma*. New York: W.W. Norton Company.

van der Kolk, B., McFarlane, A. & Weisaeth, L. (2007). *Traumatic Stress: The Effects of Overwhelming Experience on Mind, Body, and Society*. New York: The Guilford Press.

Chapter 8

Susan Rowland

One advantage of being trained as a literary scholar is to read in the mode of a quest: reading is an asking of what writing is or could be. Of course, any form of training involves exploring different models of writing and the history of literary representation. We all read with presuppositions of what a particular kind of writing should contain or offer. On the other hand, an education in literary studies encourages a questioning, an opening up, of conventions of writing. Fiction is not wholly separable from factual literature if both use many of the same techniques. Imaginative writing and scientific prose are not as distinct as parts of our culture assume.

When reading Jung for the first time, I found myself experiencing some of the pleasures of poetry, mythical tropes, speculation and humour and saw these not to be ornamental or even detractions from the "psychology", but rather as fundamental to its expression. Jung was intrinsically literary, I concluded. I began to recognize that not only was this writing especially suited to literary analysis but also it belonged to literary categories. Above all, Jung's writing is responsive to reading as quest because it is writing as quest. Jung's work belongs to post-Romantic literature, when writing stopped being valued for strict adherence to past models. Romantic works do not obey rules. They are rather in search of rules and theories by which they might be comprehended.

To me, Jung's writing is a quest for meaning; a quest that embraces fictional, poetic, mythic, rhetorical and logical, empirical strategies. Part of its questing nature is to address and unravel distinctions between science and art. Reading Jung is to engage the whole psyche because much of the so-called literary qualities invoke the "other," parts of ourselves that our developmental path in modernity has sited/cited beyond the ego. For Jung's writing is historically acute. Not only does it reveal the hardened ego of post-Enlightenment definitions of reason, but his writing also seeks to overcome ego boundaries. Jung's writing is literature that incorporates the reader's psyche, remaking its map of the soul in modernity.

Here is writing that fulfils the radical program of Romanticism—a psychic revolution to undo aged conventions that have calcified psyche and society. It remains a revolutionary literature by embracing the search for knowledge as a quest for its rules rather than an enactment of them.

DOI: 10.4324/9781003148982-9

It is for these reasons that my reading of Jung has never been concerned with issues of translation. While the study of "original" manuscripts is a fine and legitimate act of scholarship, it is nevertheless built upon an ideal of knowledge as something that is ultimately fixed, pure and knowable. If the essays that make up *Collected Works* Volume 12 were originally written in German, then study of the translation and the related search for Jung's original manuscript will produce a truer text than the English version. Such scholarly research is undeniably valuable as a contribution to a bigger picture. However, it presupposes that writing is hermetically sealed and possessed of full and rational meaning and that is all that can be construed as knowledge.

So, I suggest that if we read Jung as a challenge to the divisions between literature and science, the search for the "original" version or pure and knowable intentions of Jung as author is a mistake. It misreads the radical revolutionary possibilities of his writing. I do not want to read Jung for what the rationalized ego of the once living man might have meant (itself not a realizable goal given the complexity of authorship and revisions), but for what the non-ego qualities of the writing might offer us now. I want to read Jung as a quest to find fertility in the contemporary imagination. I want his words to be seeds to grow and flower in readers today and in the unimaginable future. My work is an attempt to explore and develop the fecundity of Jung as a writer.

Feminism, Jung and Transdisciplinarity

A Novel Approach

Originally published in Gardner, L. & Gray, F. (2017) *Feminist views from somewhere: Post-Jungian themes in feminist theory*. UK: Routledge. Reprinted with permission.

Introduction

In "The Carrier Bag Theory of Fiction," Ursula K. Le Guin offers what amounts to an archetypal theory of Western culture in Jungian terms (Le Guin 1986). Moreover, it is one distinguished by a primal division of gender, not in sexual or somatic structures but rather based on formal distinctions arising from labour. While prehistoric hunters, not slowed down by suckling infants, had exciting adventures shooting spears at nimble prey, the gatherers were forced to multitask. Typically, they were searching for berries while taking care of children. Given that the earliest cultural artefact surviving from these times is a spear point, it seems organically linked to the earliest extant literature of heroic adventures. The spear point stories of combat suggest the primacy of "epic," a genre characterized by male heroes and splendid weapons fashioning a sense of linearity and phallic potency.

Epic's high cultural status propels it into modernity where its heroic quest for supremacy over the "other," be that other a monster, an opposing city, nature or the other gender in its binary logic, becomes a *forming* influence on modern science and its propensity to develop pointed missiles as weapons of war. So far so patriarchal in the historical imagination of a Western modernity that privileges the durable quality of flint arrowheads as indicative of where we come from. But what if the spear point is not the first cultural artefact?

> A leaf a gourd a shell a net a bag a sling a sack a bottle a pot a box a container. A holder. A recipient.
>
> (Le Guin 1986: 150)

If we measure a significant development of the human psyche by the first "thing" groups of humans probably used to enable their communal lives, then the first cultural object must have been a container, something used to drink from, cook with, or carry water or food. The first cultural artefact was probably the proto-carrier bag! In this sense, the "container" is at least equally significant as a founding structure of human consciousness. Here Le Guin proposes another crucial descendant of the primal gourd in the art form that is the well-populated novel, as opposed to the epic's focus on a single, testosterone-fuelled hero. The novel *contains* heterogeneous elements forced into a relationship.

Recognition of this probability enables a shift of perspective from a sense of inevitability about masculine or epic dominance of cultural structures. Taking the lead from Le Guin here, such a shift is where I would position feminism. Whatever feminism is in the twenty-first century, it can be posited as a carrier bag that contains the radical shift of perspective *engendered* by perceiving such archetypal structures operating over the centuries. This is not to suggest that these are the only two archetypal dynamics nor to imply that C.G. Jung—not mentioned by Le Guin—identified them in this way. Rather, I want to suggest in this chapter that extending Le Guin's identification of the founding carrier bag with the novel form into Jungian and archetypal psychology opens up a feminist space for making and critiquing knowledge. In particular, such a *novel* environment can be grounded in adherence to feminist principles of respecting difference and, partly for that reason, be offered to multiple disciplinary locations via the new paradigm of transdisciplinarity.

First of all, it is worth looking at Jung's own turn from epic transcendence into novelistic immanence, for his writing in *The Collected Works* provides two contributions to this chapter's feminist transdisciplinarity: the embodied presence of archetypes and his textual capaciousness to other voices. He is provoked, of course, by the feminine.

C.G. Jung as Feminist Novelist

> The anima has an erotic, emotional character, the animus a rationalising one. Hence most of what men say about feminine eroticism, and particularly about the emotional life of women, is derived from their own anima projections and distorted accordingly. On the other hand, the astonishing assumptions and fantasies that women make about men come from the activity of the animus, who produces an inexhaustible supply of illogical arguments and false explanations.
>
> (Jung 1925/1954, *CW* 17: para. 338)

In this quotation we see the delightful slippage between Jung the epic pioneer of psychological concepts and Jung the novelist whose carrier bag writing contains "other" voices. For these three succeeding sentences begin by offering a binary notion of psychic gender only to have this humorously grounded in an obviously partial perspective. First of all, "anima" and "animus," those properties of the other gender in the unconscious, are polarized between "emotion" and "irrationality" in a sentence positing an objective, detached view. Then the voice switches to a masculine position affirming the impossibility of detaching anima-generated emotionality from an understanding of women. The third sentence is charged with just such anima distortions that were indicted in the second. Is Jung falling into a trap he has just announced, or might this be a net for the unwary reader? If it is the anima and not the ego who speaks of the "inexhaustible" irrationality of women, has this writer noticed it and does he expect his reader to?

The assumption we might make about Jung's authorial position here is indeterminable. We cannot know whether this is a conscious or unconscious trickster at work. Is he deliberately setting a trap for the reader, or unthinkingly falling into it himself? What is apparent are the dual voices at play in this so-called theoretical writing. In fact, we have both a lofty assertion of opposing concepts of anima and animus and a very *situated* demonstration that both reinforces and simultaneously challenges such transcendent epistemology. A feminist approach here can take a hint from the title of this volume and see this proposal of gender theory as *from somewhere* as well as purporting to be from nowhere and everywhere.

My suggestion is that Jung's writing needs to be read as just such an intervention into a feminine epistemology as critical, multiple and grounded, whether deliberate or not on his part. For I argue that his whole *Collected Works* amounts to an attempt to rebalance the gendered psyche of modernity in a way that can be further illuminated by at first a structuralist and then a transdisciplinary paradigm; moves that themselves are mythically described by James Hillman on Jung as Dionysian. Jung, too, turns out to prefer people to heroes.

Jung's Turn to the Feminine

Three moves in Jung's overall project characteristically enact Jung's attempt to reorient consciousness to end exclusion of the feminine. They are his adoption of

Eros and Logos as gendered styles of consciousness, the ambivalent figure of the gender fluid trickster and his far-reaching idea of synchronicity. All three bear the marks of his own psychic resistance to a portrayal of female equality. In effect, Jung summons a powerful feminine, the "mater" of the goddess, in order to shore up the fragile signifying of the masculine in modernity. His innate conservatism nevertheless has truly revolutionary properties.

First of all, Eros and Logos appear as essentialist designations of a male's consciousness determined more by discrimination and the disembodied spirit, Logos. This is mirrored by a female's intrinsic orientation to feeling and relatedness or Eros (Jung 1951, *CW* 9ii: para. 29). So far so binary. However, Jungian individuation, the process of becoming more individual and more whole by an ever-growing relationship with the unconscious, counters essentialism. It is not only desirable but inevitable that Eros, associated with a male's unconscious anima, be integrated through individuation. So too a woman's animus will bring Logos alive in her psyche, even if Jung was at times sceptical of its success (Ibid.).

What is suggestive here is how Eros and Logos, as inhabitants of the human psyche that *require* mutual accommodation, evoke a structuralist notion of myths of consciousness proposed by Jungians, such as Ann Baring and Jules Cashford in *The Myth of the Goddess* (1991). They describe the building of the modern Western psyche as resulting from the unequal relationship of monotheism's Sky Father who succeeded an animistic Earth Mother. Prior to the arrival of the three great monotheisms of Judaism, Christianity and Islam, religions centered on the reverence of the Earth as alive, sacred, generative and the source of all being. This Earth *Mother* was not a woman as opposed to a man because she existed prior to gender division. She gave birth to women, men, animals, rocks and plants equally. For her, matter and spirit are one being. Most often she was figured through animistic cultures, which saw nature as animated, full of individual and articulate spirits.

Monotheism drove animism to the margins and installed a dominant dualism because its Sky Father god created nature as separate from himself, and so non-divine, non-embodied. Separation and disembodiment characterized Sky Father religions in structuring a dualism between God and nature/matter that became mapped into human culture as hierarchical divisions between spirit or mind and body, human and nature, men and women. Here Jung's Eros and Logos consciousness can be seen as a stark attempt to reorient the founding creation myths of the Western psyche. For Earth Mother never disappeared of course. She became marginalized to reappear in the animated matter of art in painting and sculpture, as well as the multiple inspirited characters of the non-hero-driven novel, as Le Guin showed.

Earth Mother also lived on, I suggest, in the figure of the trickster, and as such found a place in Jungian psychology.

> Even [the trickster's] sex is optional despite its phallic qualities: he can turn himself into a woman and bear children. . . . This is a reference to his original nature as a Creator, for the world is made from the body of a god.
>
> (Jung 1954/1959, *CW* 9i: para. 472)

Capable of either gender or multiple variations of the same, the trickster is the embodied, amoral, protean psyche itself. In "his" infinite variety we see the seed-bed of an animistic vision of matter as sacred. Trickster is all feeling and no logical or rational separation from what *matters*. Of course, he demonstrates the core principle of *The Myth of the Goddess*, the need for both types of consciousness without one dominating over the other.

Later in his career, Jung found the goddess again in a perspective upon creation itself that is Earth Mother. For in his notion of synchronicity is an alternative to the narrative of Genesis in which God creates and then steps back from His creation. Union with the creator can come only with death or the end of this created world. By contrast, synchronicity is described by Jung as "*acts of creation in time*" (Jung 1952/1960, *CW* 8: para. 965).

Synchronicity is meaningful coincidence, such as when the psyche and material reality come together in a way that forges meaning rather than a causal connection. It is a vision of reality from within his depiction of the psychic quality of Eros, the "feminine" function of relationship, as opposed to (inevitably) the "masculine" Logos principle of conscious discrimination. So nature is to be investigated because and *by means of* the human psyche that is part of it. True knowledge here is that which takes account of the psyche. By contrast, rational ego-led enquiry is a form of "knowing" that is constructed out of the repression of relating to unconsciousness; it is knowledge as separate and transcendent of the matter to be investigated. Logos knowledge relies upon the hero myth as the sole arbiter of what is to be valued as "science."

> For [experimental science] there is created in the laboratory a situation which is artificially restricted to the question and which compels Nature to give an unequivocal answer. The workings of Nature in her unrestricted wholeness are completely excluded. . . . [W]e need a method of enquiry which . . . leaves Nature to answer out of her fullness.
>
> (Jung 1952/1960, *CW* 8: para. 864)

Perhaps here is Jung's Earth Mother at "her" most complete because "she" is Nature as wholly creative and divine. This is the animistic universe in which dreams inform about momentous events otherwise unknown, and feeling and somatic archetypal images prove prophetic and meaningful beyond the rational understanding of a mechanistic or causal approach to reality.

Synchronicity forced Jung to reassess the fundamental Logos orientation of modernity that separated psyche from non-human nature. He proposed an animistic universe in which archetypes extend beyond the human psyche to its union with matter in the psychoid. In so doing, his entire project fulfils what James Hillman described as his treatment of the myth of Dionysus. Moreover, it indicates that Jung the feminist novelist may have Dionysus as his archetypal foundation!

Hillman on Jung and Dionysus

In "Dionysus in Jung's Writings," archetypal psychologist James Hillman points out that C.G. Jung stresses "dismemberment" as his key narrative in the many myths of the god Dionysus (Hillman 1972/2007). In Jung's treatment of the dismemberment of the divine being, Hillman discerns the possibility of psychic rejuvenation in the corporeal breaking apart of an aging god. He calls Christian modernity too Apollonian, seeing in Apollo the emphases of Sky Father dualism taken to excess. So in Hillman's analysis, an era dominated by one god, defined by distance and disembodiment, is to be followed by dismemberment and multiple stories of being in Hillman's preferred polytheistic approach to psyche. However, I shall show that Jung's dismemberment of Dionysus has possibilities unexplored by Hillman.

According to Hillman, Jung sees a two-stage dismemberment process: first comes a separation into opposites, such as the very notion of Apollo and Dionysus itself. This separation satisfies Jung the lover of polarities, who is reluctant to truly integrate the feminine. Yet, Jung the rebalancing psychologist of the modern Western psyche needs Earth Mother animism in the form of bisexual, embodied, ecstatic Dionysus. In the second stage of Dionysian dismemberment, the god is scattered in pieces.

Opposition is then transformed into multiplicity, with a wider dispersal of the divine in matter, which both Jung and Hillman call archetypal. To Jung, archetypes are inherited potentials in the human psyche for certain sorts of images and meaning (Jung, *CW* 8: para. 352–353). They represent the possibility of many different modes of psychic functioning or, as Hillman later puts it, a polytheistic psyche in which the gods are diverse ways of being in the world (Hillman 2007). Hillman also points out that this second stage of Dionysian dismemberment entails an entry into a different type of consciousness. We enter a new cosmos with the dispersed fragments of the body of the god (Hillman 2007: 26). Distance from the divine becomes interiority and animistic multiplicity within the domain of the god.

> The movement between the first and second view of dismemberment compares with crossing a psychic border between seeing the god from outside or from within his cosmos.
>
> (Ibid.)

Here we find ourselves in Jung's realm of synchronicity, of "*acts of creation in time*", or as Eros knowing, connected, feeling, relational and embodied. Second-stage Dionysian dismemberment is the synchronous universe, Eros, trickster and the feminine mode of knowing and being. Symptomatically, Hillman notes that *zoe*, the life force of the body in Eros, is awakened by this process of divine dismemberment (Ibid.: 29). This new consciousness or zoe is an intimation of wholeness that does not erode differences. The new enlivening zoe is animistic in a particular way of awareness of its own *partial* consciousness, aware of itself as *parts*.

> Rather the crucial experience would be the awareness of the parts *as parts* distinct from each other, dismembered, each with its own light, a state in which the body becomes conscious of itself as a composite of differences. The scintillae and fishes eyes of which Jung speaks . . . may be experienced as embedded in physical expressions. The distribution of Dionysus through matter may be compared with the distribution of consciousness through members, organs, and zones.
>
> (Hillman 2007: 28)

So I suggest that, in this way, Earth Mother consciousness returns again in Jung's work as dismembered Dionysus, the fragmented divine body seeding the universe with its archetypes. It is time to look at other returns of the Earth Mother in order to see how her offspring, the literary form that is the novel, may be an *informing* participant in feminist knowing and being.

Earth Mother Evolution: Complexity and Transdisciplinarity

Frequently hidden in plain sight is the return of the Earth Mother as the mythical narrative of the theory of evolution first proposed by Charles Darwin in *On the Origin of Species* (1859). Fundamental to Darwin's thought was that the world came into being of itself without an exterior divine creator. He, therefore, needed to portray nature as supremely generative and found himself forced to personify "her" as the primal source and maternal matrix of everything. In effect, Darwin reanimates the Earth Mother mythical narrative as the story of creation that is whole (posited to encompass all) but not complete (because Darwin knew his scientific approach and language resources could not rationally account for all). Earth Mother in *On the Origin of Species* is profoundly alive as myth in a Jungian sense as a narrative creating and finding the border between the knowable and the unknowable.

Darwin's divinely created earth is succeeded in evolutionary science by another theory of generation that is well aware of its limitations in producing a complete and rational account of the fabrication of our world. Tacit knowledge and complexity evolution are also Earth Mother and potentially "Jungian" notions through his feminine practices such as synchronicity.

Jung's synchronicity is the notion of an ordering in nature that is accessible to the human psyche. A parallel perspective is to be found in the work of Michael Polyani, in *The Tacit Dimension* (1967), and that of Wendy Wheeler, in *The Whole Creature* (2006). Wheeler brings Polyani's depiction of "tacit knowledge" into her imaginative construction of new work in the evolutionary science of complexity. She finds in his work an understanding of nature that is significantly oriented around the body as a knowing organ, not unlike Hillman on Jung's consciousness of the dismembered Dionysian body.

Polyani's tacit knowledge is the kind of embodied, partly unconscious knowing that we acquire by the body and psyche working together at levels not accessible to ego (separation) consciousness. Effectively, tacit knowledge is knowledge based on body and connection where consciousness of the parts as dismembered parts can be mutually activated. So tacit knowledge cannot be captured in words abstracted from embodied acts. Mythically, tacit knowledge is constellated in the *zoe* or body life force of the Earth Mother.

> Tacit knowledge is creaturely skillful phenomenological knowledge. Human creatures *know* they have it . . . which cannot be put into words, but which is experienced in all creative artisanship and art, and in creative and skillful living generally. This is language as semiosis which is not reducible to words, but which is embodied in acts.
>
> (Wheeler 2006: 47)

Tacit knowledge is potentially meaningful because it is ordered and communicated. What makes it tacit is that it is always part of an intimated order that is far greater than can be articulated, just as a dismembered body cannot simply be stuck back together as one physical being (Polyani 1967: 50). In effect, tacit knowledge bridges humans and nature in the new complexity science, as Wheeler clarifies. Furthermore, tacit knowledge, with its deep rootedness in nature through the human body, is the feminine origin of newness in art and culture.

Whereas the West's adherence to the dominance of Sky Father values emphasized disembodied abstraction as the proper basis for knowing (Logos), tacit knowledge is the psyche and the body working together at their psychoid interface or Eros.

> When we make a thing function as the proximal term of tacit knowing, we incorporate it in our body—or extend our body to include it—so that we come to dwell in it.
>
> It is not by looking at things that we understand them, but by dwelling in them.
>
> (Wheeler 2006: 63)

I suggest that Wheeler's "dwelling in them" as the better form of knowing is both Earth Mother and Dionysian, invoking consciousness as zoe. Wheeler uses Polyani's tacit knowledge to re-situate the body in nature as an organ of knowing indivisible from the psyche. Both exhibit the profound desire to reanimate and *re-embody* Earth Mother consciousness in her dispersed yet carnal mode. Art and culture flourish through tacit knowledge, Wheeler argues. It is through the incarnated creative and multiple psyche that the "new" happens. Moreover, what is crucial is that tacit knowing infers a complexity greater than can be measured by rational methods. Such complexity is not confined to cultural change. Rather, complexity is now regarded as key to evolution Herself.

The recognition of a definitive role for unmappable complexity marks a significant development in the theory of evolution after Darwin. Evolved nature is not so much a competition between wholly separate species, as Darwin originally envisaged, but is more like successive, ever more complexly interpenetrating environments.

> Complex systems evolve via the emergence of strata of increasing complexity. Biological evolution proceeds in this fashion, as, we have now seen, does human culture and human knowledge. Human discovery and invention— human creativity—proceeds via tacit knowledge and our sense that we are in contact with a complex reality of which there is more to be known.
>
> (Wheeler 2006: 67/8)

Culture is therefore nature *creating through the tacit, unarticulated knowledge of human beings*. Tacit knowledge is *realizing* (making it "real" by articulation into human language) the synchronous nature of nature! Tacit knowledge invokes zoe and thereby has implications for the whole project of our traditional disciplines of knowledge, as I shall demonstrate.

Similar to complexity evolution, Jung calls synchronicity "*acts of creation in time*," specifically associating these meaningful coincidences with "nature" as mother (Jung 1952/1960, *CW* 8: para. 965). Jung's unconscious psyche, like Wheeler's and Polyani's, is also embodied. His "synchronous events" are apprehended through and as tacit knowledge in the body as somatic intuition. Effectively, he too embraces the creativity of nature through tacit *significance* into culture.

To sum up: What is being argued here is that nature has an underlying rationality that is too complexly entangled for objective human measurement or for the abstracted ego to grasp. This intricate rationality is part of a constantly evolving complexity of totalities. Such complexity is arguably another way of describing the consciousness engendered by the Earth Mother or dismembered Dionysus; it is tricksterish, archetypal and synchronous. Fascinatingly, complexity theory is also effective in accounting for how *culture* evolves in the sense of how societies and groups creatively interact and mutate beyond the capacity of rational analysis. In this sense, animistic Earth Mother is alive and her zoe is the life force wherever creativity is generated in ways too complex to calculate, predict, control or consciously measure.

Nature's "complex" totalities include human cultures, which are where the signifying potential of nature flowers into human language. Semiotics becomes what Wheeler calls "biosemiotics," the signifying of animated life (Wheeler 2006: 139). Although Wheeler does not make use of Jung's archetypal sense of animism, nor myths of Dionysus, nor Earth Mother, this consciousness, what Jung called "synchronicities," includes moments where tacit, embodied, Earth Mother knowledge grasps just a little more of nature's creativity as she portrays it.

> Creativity is in many ways a word for describing autopoiesis as biosemiotic life: all nature and culture is creative becoming and change. In human complex systems, creativity is semiotic liveliness: liveliness in language and

liveliness in the processes via which tacit knowledge can emerge in concepts which can be articulated or, rather more accurately, *are* articulated as the process of such emergence.

(Wheeler 2006: 139)

Everything said here about nature is also appropriate to Jung's view of the unconscious. Jung's unconscious is embodied and so embedded in our nature as continuous with the non-human. Synchronicity is one aspect of Jung's theory where he *grounds* his unconscious as being in meaningful semiotic *interconnectedness* with nature as Nature.

The psyche is not only inside our corporeal being. To be more precise, the psyche shows "inside" *and* "outside" to be powerful cultural metaphors. Language shapes our relation to the world; it is not a neutral medium. So it is time to look at a way of dealing with the "animistic" multiplicity of academic disciplines with their different languages. How can such a dismemberment of knowledge find its zoe, its Dionysian animation? For we seek disciplines that manifest *realization*, the making real of their plurality *as parts*.

Transdisciplinarity and Dionysus

First appearing in 1970, from Jean Piaget in the sense of "a total system," "transdisciplinarity" has been most helpfully theorized by Basarab Nicolescu (2002). He gave a valuable overview in his talk at the Congress of Transdisciplinarity in Brazil in 2005, which was later published as "Transdisciplinarity—Past, Present and Future" (Nicolescu 2005). Nicolescu rejects the totalizing project inherent in Piaget's definition and dismisses any possibility of a hyperdiscipline, one capable of subsuming all disciplines of human knowledge into a system of perfect knowledge or ultimate truth. Rather, Nicolescu prefers to stress what he calls "beyond disciplines" in his transdisciplinarity, which appears to mean beyond the pretensions of any one epistemological construct to encompass all meaning.

Where Nicolescu is particularly persuasive is in his building of transdisciplinarity on the post-quantum human subject and in his move to embrace the implications of complexity theory for human knowing. Arguing that quantum discoveries end the primacy of the traditional scientific method of repeatable experiments, Nicolescu posits a new human subject for *all* research. Quantum physics discovered that some reality cannot be judged by the criteria of objectivity or absolute separation between the observer and the observed, because the way in which phenomena are measured changes the results radically.

Transdisciplinarity aims for a sense of human knowledge as a unity but an "open" unity, by which Nicolescu means accepting that humans live on several levels of reality at the same time and it will never be possible to rationally know all of them. These realities cannot be eroded or simplified (Ibid.: 4). Such a recognition of irreducible differences indicates that transdisciplinarity must be considered as theoretical, phenomenological and experimental. Nicolescu proposes three axioms of transdisciplinarity to replace those of traditional science, which go back to Galileo.

Hitherto, many scientific disciplines adhered to the following axioms or fundamental principles:

1   The universe is governed by mathematical law.
2   These laws can be discovered by scientific experiment.
3   Such experiments, if valid, can be perfectly replicated (Ibid.: 5).

As Nicolescu points out, such privileging of "objectivity" has the unfortunate effect of turning the human subject into an object by stripping out feelings and values (Ibid.). The problem lies in the positing of *one* level of reality as foundational to all others. This single way of structuring knowledge then subsumes realities like the social or psychological to their objectivizing paradigm.

By contrast, Nicolescu's transdisciplinarity explicitly disavows mathematical formalism because of the human subject's complexity in both simple and theoretical senses, as we will see. Nicolescu's fundamental principles, or three axioms, for the methodology of transdisciplinarity are as follows.

1   The ontological axiom: *There are, in Nature and in our knowledge of Nature, different levels of Reality and, correspondingly, different levels of perception.*
2   The logical axiom: *The passage from one level of Reality to another is insured by the logic of the included middle.*
3   The complexity axiom: *The Structure of the totality of levels of Reality or perception is a complex structure: every level is what it is because all levels exist at the same time* (Ibid.: 6).

This approach to what we know and how we know it amounts to a transformation of the approach to the universe as multidimensional. Reality is now complex. So are human beings. Nicolescu insists that no one level of reality, such as sight perception, for instance, can constitute a dominant position for knowing. No sense organ or academic discipline is capable of understanding all of the other levels of reality in total. Knowledge in any of its forms is necessarily incomplete or "open" (Ibid.: 7). Academic disciplines cannot pretend to a hierarchy in which one is privileged above all of the others. Moreover, such an approach does away with the interior-exterior boundary of knowing.

> Knowledge is neither exterior nor interior: it is simultaneously exterior and interior. The studies of the universe and of the human being sustain one another.
> (Ibid.: 8)

As Nicolescu reiterates, his transdisciplinarity crucially undoes the classical subject-object division in favour of the ternary: subject, object and hidden third that is both subject and object (Ibid.). This "included middle," explicitly prohibited by the previous rational paradigm where A could not also be non-A, does not, he notes, eradicate those types of logical knowing that do insist that A cannot be non-A. Rather, it shows them to be incomplete: they are one level of reality, not a primal truth framing all of them. Traditional objective science has its place as one *part* of the dismembered body of academic knowledge that we call "disciplines."

"Complexity" too needs a context for its inclusion in Nicolescu's transdisciplinarity. Some theorists are looking for a mathematical rendering of complexity, which would, in this notion of transdisciplinarity, limit the levels of reality that it could encompass. So Nicolescu offers the structure of horizontal and vertical axes.

> It is therefore useful to distinguish between the horizontal complexity, which refers to a single level of reality and vertical complexity, which refers to several levels of Reality.
>
> (Ibid.: 13)

Symptomatically, Nicolescu notices the ancient lineage of complexity theory as interdependence: everything really is connected to everything else (Ibid.: 13). He sees his three axioms as innately value generating. The hidden third or included middle emphasizes the interdependence of the model. Where humans and the universe are regarded as interdependent, then we have either values or chaos.

For this reason, higher education needs to convert to transdisciplinarity so that it can develop the three main types of intelligence: rational analytical, feeling and of the body (Ibid.: 15). These intelligences demand complexity on the question of meaning. So here, "horizontal meaning" is what most traditional academic disciplines do; they situate meaning at one level of reality. By contrast, a transdisciplinary education would provide meaning vertically, at several levels of reality with none privileged over the others. Nicolescu suggests poetry, art or quantum physics as providing vertical or multiple levels of meaning (Ibid.: 17).

Interestingly for Jungian studies, Nicolescu rejects attacks on psychoanalysis from those preferring chemical interventions for the mind. Scientists and medics who reject taking the cure are guilty of simplifying different levels of reality into one, the biochemical (Ibid.). To illustrate his revolutionary vision of knowledge, Nicolescu contrasts traditional academic disciplines providing fragments of one level of reality with cultures and religions which anticipate transdisciplinarity by spanning multiple realities. What he calls "technoscience," the alliance of instrumental technology with the traditional science of repeatable experiments, is confined to the zone of the "object" in his tripartite vision of subject, object and hidden third (Ibid.: 17). He calls for technoscience to become a "culture" by entering into dialogue with religion that would expand its zone of reality to all three (Ibid.).

For the world of education in disciplines, I will argue that Nicolescu's vision is remarkably similar to the ethos of Earth Mother consciousness and its *articulation* into dispersed Dionysus.

> The transdisciplinary education, founded on the transdisciplinary methodology, allows us to establish links between persons, facts, images, representations, fields of knowledge and action and to discover the Eros of learning

during our entire life. The creativity of the human being is conditioned by permanent questioning and permanent integration.

(Nicolescu 2005: 14)

Here is education in the framework of complexity theory that positions the human *within and part of* the creativity of non-human nature. Nicolescu's Eros is Earth Mother in knowing and synchronous in epistemology. Symptomatically, Nicolescu betrays his core concern with traditional science in his persistent, yet helpful motif of subject, object and the hidden third that is both. However, his insistence that knowledge is both interior and exterior unites complexity theory with transdisciplinarity's challenge to the atomization of education in discrete disciplines. Because far from acknowledging dismembered Dionysus, separate academic disciplines are all too used to rejecting any consciousness of each other as viable, yet different levels of reality. In the modern university, our mutually indifferent, or even antagonistic, disciplines have no consciousness of themselves as dismembered parts. They therefore have no zoe, no dynamic life force in their separate incompleteness.

It is transdisciplinarity, I suggest, united with complexity theory that embraces Jung's and Hillman's vision of dismembered Dionysus. Moreover, this transdisciplinary ecstatic god had followers well before the hysterics of early psychoanalysis identified by Hillman (Hillman 2007: 17). I propose that those early wild women of Dionysian rites include the sedate Jane Austen in the female-dominated rise of the novel. For example, her *Sense and Sensibility* (1811) demonstrates the clash of values over contrary relations to nature that are also different realities coming into contact.

> Edward: "I like a fine prospect, but not on picturesque principles. I do not like crooked, twisted, blasted trees. I admire them much more if they are tall, straight and flourishing. . . . I have more pleasure in a snug farmhouse than a watch-tower—and a troop of tidy, happy villagers please me better than the finest banditti in the world."
>
> Marianne looked with amazement at Edward, with compassion at her sister. Elinor only laughed.
>
> (Austen 1811: 122–123)

Edward and Marianne reveal their very different adoption of Eros in knowing the countryside where Marianne's once privileged family is living in comparative poverty. She is "Romantic" in espousing the ideals and excited sensibility of cultural Romanticism in regarding nature as a source of ecstatic feeling. Totally at odds here is Edward, whose disposition draws back from the implications of Romantic philosophy. His temperament finds a home in religious beliefs (he wants to be a clergyman) that to him entail pastoral care for the poor. He therefore celebrates the prosperous farming landscape as an extension of religious and social principles.

The novel brings both highly complex constructions of reality into a relationship without negating either, nor suggesting that either is complete: the conditions of transdisciplinarity. Marianne has vertical axes of psyche, poetry and the freedom-loving culture of Romanticism. Edward possesses the vertical axes of religion, its extension into the social with pastoral care and even a protoscientific vision of successful farming and interest in trees as "flourishing." Taking a cue from Le Guin's novel as carrier bag, the novel genre is, I propose, Earth Mother in its animism and also specifically Dionysian in its zoe of life force generated in its *complex*, skilful articulation of different parts of reality in conversation. The novel fosters such conversation that promotes, as here, awareness of these perspectives as *partial*, or as *parts*.

Perhaps Nicolescu's included middle should be seen as feminist and novelistic, as well as importing as non-marginal the intelligences of feeling and the body?

Feminism and the Included Middle: Jung's Symbols, Archetypes and Novels

As argued earlier, Jung's *Collected Works* are closer to novels than to conventional scientific writing. They are feminist novels in the sense that their animistic nature serves his project by turning to what has been marginalized in modernity as feminine. Such a feminine includes what he calls feeling and connection as Eros, as opposed to discrimination and separation as Logos, the trickster androgynous plurality of Earth Mother and "her" complex creativity that he named synchronicity.

Jung the feminist novelist is also Dionysian, as Hillman diagnosed in his two-stage dismemberment. First of all there is dualism, the rending into oppositions that pepper Jung's terminology. More profound and more feminist-friendly is Jung's second-stage of Dionysian dismemberment into parts that are aware of themselves as parts with an emphasis on the Earth mother, or embodied consciousness. Jung's trickster and animistic writing here is the dispersed corporeality of the ecstatic god.

Taking this unlikely push of Jung into feminism even further, we may consider his writing as proto-transdisciplinary. Crucially, Jung's stress on the impossibility of complete knowledge given the indigenous mystery of the psyche is one factor that his work shares with that of Nicolescu. Jung has the potential to be a significant stabilizing force in Nicolescu's transdisciplinarity, where the latter repeatedly warns against the trap of erecting some hyperdiscipline as a pretension to control all meaning.

This is one instance of how Jung might contribute to the transdisciplinary project. There are many more as we start to perceive psychoanalysis and Jungian studies as intrinsically transdisciplinary in their acceptance of multiple levels of reality. Dreams, for example, are real. They are also necessarily of a different order of reality than social engagement, historical events (no longer present to the senses), bodily perception or cultural representations. Depth psychology of the Freudian and Jungian persuasions has a particular expertise in working with multiple levels of reality as simultaneous and *complex* forms of knowing.

As an example of taking Jung's Dionysian feminism a stage further into trans-disciplinarity, I want to consider the Jungian symbol as an instance of the hidden third, to be brought into knowing here as the included middle. Jung writes about the symbol as a specific type of image, which is itself a manifestation of the unconscious as "imag[e]-ination" and the psyche as intrinsically image-making. Looking primarily at images in words, Jung called "signs" those images standing for a relatively known or stable meaning, while "symbols" are pointers to something relatively unknown or not yet known (*CW* 15: para. 105).

Symbols connect the conscious ego to the archetypal collective unconscious. They therefore are prime examples of Nicolescu's "vertical" or multiple levels of reality, being on one level perceptual, on another intuitive and on yet another "spiritual" in the sense of pertaining to the immaterial unknown. Here I want to emphasize that Jungian symbols are far from icons of disconnection to the embodied world. Given that Jungian archetypes are inherited potentials, they have a bodily as well as spiritual pole (Jung, *CW* 8: para. 367). In transdisciplinary terms, symbols derived from archetypes operate vertically to manifest realities of body, feeling and spirit.

In this way, symbols can activate all of Nicolescu's intelligences of body, feeling and analytical intellect. They are the *third* term between the different levels of reality evoked. The symbol of a rose in a love poem can be felt somatically and erotically as well as analytically as an idea about love in ways that are profoundly human and connecting as well as divine and transcendent. A Jungian symbol connects the psyche to what matters. It does so because it is the third that is both matter and psyche in the Sky Father binary logic that there is the human psyche *inside* us and matter *outside*. The symbol is the included middle.

Finally, we must notice that this symbol as included middle is an engine of complexity in the sense that it is a portal between human and non-human nature. Jungian symbols are scraps of the dismembered Dionysian body. They materialize zoe; they are the animated sparks that embody the Earth Mother, the creatures that make the feminine texture of the novel. A symbol for Jung is an image of the deep psyche that stitches us into the cosmos as an act of feminine knowing. Such symbols are necessarily fragments that are aware of themselves as parts. To end this chapter, I want to give an example of a Jungian symbol in and as a literary form. Modern detective fiction, I suggest, provide a healing integration of the wilder aspects of Dionysian dismemberment.

From Dionysian Trickster to Athena Containing the Furies in Detective Fiction

Earth Mother is not a "woman" for she is prior to gender division into dualism. Much of her divine abilities occur in bisexual Dionysus, a complex trickster. In *The Ecocritical Psyche* (2012), I argued that the ancient trickster myth sponsors the modern detective narrative, a form distinguished by its deceptive qualities vis-à-vis the reader. However, there are other archetypal energies in detective fiction that become visible once we see this trickster novel through a Dionysian lens.

Dionysian dismemberment, as Hillman intuits in Jung, has to move beyond oppositions that would posit the Apollonian Sky Father as all rational, matched by Dionysus as total unreason. Maenads tearing men to pieces inspired by the ecstatic god is not the ideal, nor indeed necessary, consequence of divine dismemberment. The literal rending of bodies may be one possible consequence of replacing one dominant archetypal structure (Sky Father, Apollo) with its opposite (Earth Mother, Dionysus), but it is not the desired aim of animistic and transdisciplinary creative multiplicity. Put another way, multiple archetypes require polytheistic solutions. So the possibility of trickster detective fiction going too literally Dionysian invokes a very different type of god(dess): Athena.

Athena is the goddess not only of the city but of what makes communal life possible. We see her at work in Aeschylus's play *The Eumenides*, persuading the Furies not to tear apart guilty Orestes who has murdered his mother to avenge the slaughter of his father (Aeschylus 458 BCE). Athena stops the cycle of revenge. The Furies are incorporated into the city as aliens but as great sources of its fertility. They become zoe, *contained* by Athena as the city goddess who is also the divine bringer of weaving and pottery.

Athena *contains*. She exists in detective fiction in tension with Dionysus and mitigates his more literal bodily qualities of tearing apart. Detective novels are Athena containing and integrating the Furies in us that threaten chaos at the crime of murder, the crime that makes human community impossible if it is not solved. In this sense, detective fiction as a literary form is a symbol in the Jungian sense. It is a temple of Dionysus and Athena (and other gods too). Detective fiction is the included middle between psyche and matter, not least because it deals with what *matters*.

I began with the feminine nature of the novel and so end with its variously gendered gods. The novel is a powerful location for marginalized and feminine energies, a model for multiple and transdisciplinary knowledge, and a trickster stealing her way into Jung's *Collected Works*. She is novel, news from somewhere within the fragmented body of the goddess.

References

Aeschylus. (458 BCE) "The Eumenides," in *The Oresteia*, trans. Robert Fagles, New York: Penguin Books, 1966, pp. 227–277.

Austen, J. (1811/1990) *Sense and Sensibility*, Oxford and New York: Oxford University Press.

Baring, A. and J. Cashford (1991) *The Myth of the Goddess: Evolution of an Image*, New York and London: Vintage.

Darwin, C. (1859/2006) *On the Origin of Species; By Means of Natural Selection*, New York: Dover Thrift Editions.

Glotfelty, C. and H. Fromm. (eds) (1996) *The Ecocriticism Reader: Landmarks in Literary Ecology*, Athens and London: The University of Georgia Press.

Hillman, J. (1972/2007) "Dionysus in Jung's Writings," first published in *Spring: A Journal of Archetype and Culture*, 1972, in *Mythic Figures: Uniform Edition of the Writings of James Hillman, volume 6.1*, Putnam, CT: Spring Publications Inc., pp. 15–30.

Jung, C. G. (1925/1954) "Marriage as a Psychological Relationship," in *Collected Works, Volume 17: The Development of Personality*, Princeton: Princeton University Press, pp. 187–204.

Jung, C. G. (1951) "The Syzygy: Anima and Animus," in *Collected Works, Volume 9ii: Aion: Researches into the Phenomenology of the Self*, Princeton: Princeton University Press, pp. 11–22.

Jung, C. G. (1952/1960) "Synchronicity: An Acausal Connecting Principle," in *Collected Works, Volume 8: The Structure and Dynamics of the Psyche*, Princeton: Princeton University Press, pp. 417–532.

Jung, C. G. (1954/1959) "On the Psychology of the Trickster Figure," in *The Archetypes and the Collective Unconscious, CW9i, The Collected Works of C. G. Jung*, pp. 255–274.

Le Guin, U. (1986/1996) "The Carrier Bag Theory of Fiction," in C. Glotfelty and H. Fromm (eds) *The Ecocriticism Reader: Landmarks in Literary Ecology*, pp. 149–154.

Nicolescu, B. (2002) *Manifesto of Transdisciplinarity*, Albany, NY: State University of New York Press.

Nicolescu, B. (2005) "Transdisciplinarity—Past, Present and Future," paper presented at second congress of world transdisciplinarity, Brasil 6–12 September 2005, published in *Cetrans: Centro Educacao Transdisciplinar*, pp. 1–24; www.cetrans.com.br accessed February 7th 2015.

Polyani, M. (1967) *The Tacit Dimension*, London: Routledge & Kegan Paul.

Rowland, S. (2012) *The Ecocritical Psyche: Literature, Evolutionary Complexity and Jung*, Hove and New York: Routledge.

Wheeler, W. (2006) *The Whole Creature: Complexity, Biosemiotics and the Evolution of Culture*, London: Lawrence & Wishart.

Chapter 9

Sonu Shamdasani

My work has pursued three main intersecting strands: the reconstruction of the formation of modern psychology, psychotherapy and the work of C.G. Jung. The following summarizes the main lines of my work on Jung.

1988: Through meeting Michael Fordham, I discovered that, contrary to what was held to be the case, a vast proportion of C.G. Jung's work had yet to be published or even studied. I uncovered the identity and biography of Frank Miller, the subject of *Transformations and Symbols of the Libido*. My research continued with a study of *Memories, Dreams, Reflections*. I found the original manuscripts, editorial correspondences, and Jung's interviews with Aniela Jaffé, which formed the basis of the text. I established that, far from being an autobiography, the work was a biography, that on reading the first manuscripts, Jung had strongly objected to his misportrayal, and that his attempts to correct this were cut short by his death. I demonstrated that the Freudocentric legend of the origins of Jung's work – the view that the most important figure for Jung in the genesis of his work was Freud – had been critically fostered by the editing of this work. I published essays that demonstrated that this Freudocentric legend had led to the complete mislocation of Jung's work in intellectual history.

From 1993 until 2011, my work took place at the Wellcome Institute for the History of Medicine, which became the Wellcome Trust Centre for the History of Medicine, and formed an ideal context for it.

1994: In the course of editing Jung's 1932 seminar on "The Psychology of Kundalini Yoga", I started archival research in Switzerland. I discovered that Jung's manuscripts at the ETH had only just been catalogued in 1993, and they included more than 100 unpublished items, together with drafts and variants of published works that had not been studied, and thousands of unpublished correspondences. I commenced a collaboration with the Jung estate regarding bringing these works to publication.

1996: I discovered hitherto unknown transcriptions of *The Red Book* and commenced discussing its potential publication with the Jung estate the following year. On the basis of my presentations, reports and proposal, it was released for publication under my editorship in 2000.

1998: *Cult Fictions: Jung and the Founding of Analytical Psychology* utilised previously unknown archival materials to correct recent mystifications of the

DOI: 10.4324/9781003148982-10

founding of analytical psychology, in particular that it was in fact a religious cult. This work was the first micro-institutional study of Jung's emerging network during World War I, setting out the relations and tensions between Jung, his followers and his colleagues and the manner in which they began to establish the profession of analytical psychology and, in so doing, attempted to reform society.

2003: *Jung and the Making of Modern Psychology: The Dream of Science* set the genesis of Jung's work within a new account of the formation of the development of modern psychology and psychotherapy. This book reconstructed the emergence of Jung's work – extensively drawing for the first time upon a comprehensive study of his Nachlass – through the intersection of debates within fields such as philosophy, sociology, biology and anthropology, together with the new psychology, and reconstructed the reception of Jung's work in the human sciences together with its impact on the social and intellectual history of the twentieth century. I co-founded the Philemon Foundation, of which I am the general editor, with the aim of raising funds to enable Jung's unpublished works to be edited for publication. Unlike the *Collected Works*, these have been appearing in scholarly editions with contextual historical introductions and full apparatuses.

2005: *Jung stripped Bare, by his Biographers, Even.* This studied the biographical projects in Jung's lifetime, which culminated in *Memories, Dreams, Reflections*, together with the popular biographies that have appeared since his death. Through critically confronting the shortcomings of these biographies in the form of interpretive fallacies and factual errors, it presented an extended discussion of the relation between history, biography and fiction.

2006: I was appointed the Philemon Reader in Jung History at the Wellcome Trust Centre for the History of Medicine at UCL and became a professor in 2009. The Philemon chair lasted until 2017. Within this context, I have been supervising students working on dissertations on Jung history.

2009: *The Red Book: Liber Novus.* The introduction and apparatus situated this central book within Jung's biography, cultural and intellectual context and the evolution of his later work and indicated how the historiography of Jung studies should now be divided into "before" and "after" the publication of *Liber Novus*. I became acting director of the Wellcome Trust Centre for the History of Medicine at UCL.

2011: *Jung: A Biography in Books.* This book presented Jung's intellectual biography, tracing his pivotal encounters with books, and showed how, through his engagement with them, he formed a new conception of human nature. Commencing with his study of the classics of Western literature, this book demonstrated how he tried to transform the understanding of mythology and religion through psychology. It studied how the literary sources Jung drew upon informed his fantasies in *Liber Novus* and how, in reflecting upon them, he distilled ideas that led to a new psychology, through which he sought to illumine the history of human thought. A study of his alchemical notebooks showed how he came to understand the symbolic meaning of alchemy as self-development and how he sought to establish a cross-cultural psychology of higher development in collaboration with leading scholars of religion and mythology, which would revivify religious traditions and overcome the split in modern times between science and religion. In 2011, I established the UCL Centre for the History of the Psychological Disciplines, which later merged with the UCL Centre for Philosophy, Justice and Health to become the UCL Health Humanities Centre.

2013: *Lament of the Dead: Psychology After Jung's Red Book*. This sequence of dialogues with the late James Hillman reflected on the significance of *Liber Novus* for psychology. I moved to the School of European Languages, Culture and History (German). From 2015, I have been Vice Dean (International) of the Arts and Humanities Faculty.

2018: My students, in collaboration with students at the University of Strasbourg, established *Phânes: Journal for Jung History*, a multilingual, online open access journal.

2020: *Jung's The Black Books 1913–1932: Notebooks of Transformation*. The introduction and apparatus chart his attempt to resolve the twentieth-century crisis of meaning in his own person, and distil from this a means in psychotherapy that would enable others to do likewise. They show how *The Black Books* and *Liber Novus* together form the esoteric core of analytical psychology and enable its historical genesis to be studied; how the material up to 1916 illuminates the genesis of *Liber Novus*; how the material from 1916 charts his evolving understanding; how he sought to develop and embody the insights he had gained in his life, such as in the triangular relations with Emma Jung and Toni Wolff; and how his paintings from 1916 onwards should be understood in the context of the evolution of his personal cosmology.

From Neurosis to a New Cure of Souls

C.G. Jung's Remaking of the Psychotherapeutic Patient

Originally published in Davies, M.P. and S. Shamdasani, eds. *Medical Humanity and Inhumanity in the German-Speaking World*. London: UCL Press, 2020. Reprinted with permission.

In 1922, the ethnologist and linguist Jaime de Angulo issued a "challenge to all brother-neurotics—go, my brethren, go to the Mecca, I mean to Zürich, and drink from the fountain of life, all ye who are dead in your souls, go and seek new life."[1] It was, of course, to Jung that de Angulo was exhorting his "brother-neurotics" to go. By 1912, Jung's fame had spread, and an increasing number of neurotics wound their way to him. What de Angulo and his "brother-neurotics" were seeking in Jung's psychotherapy was no medical cure, but a way out of a widespread cultural and spiritual malaise.

Since its rise in the last quarter of the nineteenth century, in line with general medical practice, psychotherapy in its various forms had maintained a privative concept of health, that is, the absence of nervous and psychological disorders. This was linked with a negative notion of the aim of psychotherapy as being the removal of pathology and the restoration of normal living. While schools of psychotherapy had different conceptions of mental disorders, as well as of the means for their removal, this was generally one common denominator. From the time of the First World War onwards, Jung began to depart from this and to reformulate the practice of psychotherapy to have as its goal the higher spiritual development of the individual. This reformulation was to have far-reaching consequences for the subsequent development of psychotherapy, as well as for the plethora of humanistic, new age and alternative therapies that rose up. While claiming that his psychotherapy remained part of "medical psychology," this reformulation offered a new definition of the human, which many individuals adopted. Jung was not alone in proposing more melioristic possibilities for psychotherapy. From the 1930s onwards, a number of other figures in the field also did so. Significantly, these reformulations were coupled with competing conceptions of what it meant to be human. What follows, then, can be considered as a case study within a wider transformation of the field.[2]

This shift away from the then conventional medical view of the aims of psychotherapy opened the question of the relation of psychotherapy to religious practices. In 1904, the French psychologist Pierre Janet had made the observation that when patients found a friend or someone whom they could obey, their problems ceased. Priests had formerly fulfilled this function, and doctors could now do the same. Priests had done this in a haphazard manner and no longer had the authority that they once had. He noted that it was "a characteristic of our time that this work of moral direction has sometimes returned to the doctor, who is now often charged with this role of moral direction when the patient does not find enough support around him."[3] In 1912, Jung discussed the parallels between psychoanalysis and the practice of religious confession. He argued that the psychological value of religious confession lay in the fact that it enabled the sufferer to re-enter into the human community from isolation and to form a moral bond, which he identified with the psychoanalytic "transference." The moral value that the Catholic Church placed on confession was justified by the fact that "the greater part of humanity not only needs guidance, but wishes for nothing better than to be guided and held in tutelage."[4] Through confession, the priest stood in for the individual's parents and so helped them to free themselves from the family. For 1,500 years, this had functioned as an effective means of education. However, for contemporary, developed individuals, it had lost its educative value—"as soon as the Church proved incapable of maintaining her leadership in the intellectual sphere."[5] Modern individuals wanted understanding, without the sacrifice of the intellect. Their goal was to achieve moral autonomy and to be able to guide themselves. When faced with this demand, the doctor had to analyse the transference, which the priest did not have to do. Thus, in Jung's view, the decline of the confessional formed an essential context for the possibility of psychoanalysis, which presented itself as a modernised cure for souls.

If the doctor was now to take up the role increasingly being vacated by the priest, this reopened the question of the role of suggestion in psychotherapy. In the first decade of the twentieth century, a reaction set in against the use of suggestion and hypnosis in psychotherapy. "Catharsis," "interpretation," "persuasion" and "analysis" became the new buzzwords. Jacqueline Carroy has noted that, in the hypnosis literature, suggestion functioned as a heterodox, umbrella term which, as well as imperative suggestion, included paradoxical injunctions and interpretations.[6] In a similar manner, if one studies psychoanalytic and psychotherapeutic cases in the twentieth century, one finds that "interpretation" functioned in a similar catch-all manner. While the theoretical account of practices changed considerably, the same was not the case for the practices themselves, and under the rubric of interpretation in the psychoanalytic literature, it is not hard to find some of the best examples of authoritarian directives. Freud had claimed that the practice of psychoanalysis was free from suggestion. In 1913, Jung argued that this was simply an impossibility:

> It is unthinkable to critical understanding that suggestibility and suggestion can be avoided in the cathartic method. They are present everywhere . . . even with Dubois and the psychoanalysts, who all believe they are working purely rationally. *No technique and no self-effacement help here; the doctor works nolens volens, and perhaps most of all, through his personality, that means suggestively.*[7]

The therapist's conduct ineluctably became an exemplary paragon for the patient. Being impossible to escape, the only solution lay in attaining sufficient self-knowledge. Jung wrote, "I have had the opportunity of seeing many times that the analyst always gets just as far with his treatment as he has succeeded in his moral development."[8] The goal, however, lay not in directing the patient but in assisting the patient to attain self-governance and self-knowledge. We will shortly see how these issues played out in Jung's practice.

From 1913 onwards, Jung commenced in a process of self-experimentation that he termed his "confrontation with the unconscious" and his "confrontation with the soul." At the heart of this project was his attempt to get to know his own "myth" as a solution to the mythless predicament of secular modernity. This took the form of provoking an extended series of waking fantasies in himself. He elaborated, illustrated and commented on these fantasies in a work that he called *Liber Novus*, or *The Red Book*, which was at the centre of his later work.[9] This depicted the process through which he regained his soul and overcame the contemporary malaise of spiritual alienation, which was achieved through enabling the rebirth of a new image of God in his soul and developing a new world view in the form of a psychological and theological cosmology. *Liber Novus* presented the prototype of Jung's conception of the individuation process, which he held to be the universal form of individual psychological development.

However, there has been little study of what was taking place in Jung's practice during this critical period or how he attempted to develop a replicable form of psychotherapy from his own self-experimentation. In what follows, I intend to explore this through utilising unpublished letters and accounts of some of his patients. As Jung did not publish his case material or write about his practice other than in general terms, these documents allow us to fill this lacuna.

In retrospect, Jung stated that after his break with Freud, he found it necessary to develop a new attitude towards his patients:

> I decided for the present to wait presuppositionless for what they would tell by themselves. I also took account of what chance brought. It soon appeared that they spontaneously reported their dreams and phantasies and I only asked a few questions, 'What occurs to you in connection with that?' 'How do you understand that?' 'Where does that come from?' The interpretations rose by themselves from the answers and associations. I left all theoretical viewpoints by the side, and only helped the patients to understand the dream-images by themselves.[10]

This suggests that Jung's practice with his patients followed the same procedure with which he attempted to understand his own dreams and visions at this time: setting aside theoretical presuppositions to allow the images and figures to explain themselves. He maintained that it was for the sake of his patients that he undertook his self-exploration, as he thought that he could not expect them to do something that he did not dare to do himself. He made one other comment about his clinical work at this time:

> I have a medical diploma, I must help my patients, I have a wife and five children, I live at 228 Seestrasse in Küsnacht—these were actualities which made demands upon me. They proved to me day by day that I really existed. . . . So my family and my profession always remained a joyful reality and a guarantee that I was normal and really existed.[11]

Here, he states what his patients did for *him:* convince him of his normality. The general impression this gives is that his clinical practice was not seriously affected by the turmoil of his self-experimentation during this period.

In the autumn of 1911, the American psychoanalyst and neurologist James Jackson Putnam sent his cousin Fanny Bowditch Katz to be analysed by Jung. After the death of her father, Henry Bowditch, she had fallen into a prolonged depression. Katz wrote letters to Putnam detailing the development of the analysis, and Putnam replied back with advice. It is widespread today for therapists to be supervised, but it seems that Katz was one of the first supervised patients. Jung approved of this, and Katz would often read Jung her letters to Putnam for his approval. When Jung met Putnam, he discussed her situation with him. Katz's family seemed to be rather suspicious of Jung. On 10 December 1912, Putnam wrote to Katz: "I suppose it is not to be wondered that your nice aunt . . . should think Dr. Jung's ideas strange &

reprehensible. You know, I imagine, that even the majority of the doctors are very much down on the whole business."[12] At the same time, Putnam relayed advice to Jung via Katz: "Tell Dr. Jung you will get well & strong & he must find means to help you."[13] Putnam provided his own analysis of Jung to Katz:

> It is a fault in Dr. Jung [entre nous] that he is too self-assertive & I suspect that he is lacking in some needful kinds of imagination & that he is, indeed, a strong but vain person, who might & does do much good but might also tend to crush a patient. He is to be learned from but not followed too implicitly.[14]
>
> I suspect that Dr. Jung's very masterful ways may affect some of his patients more strongly than he realizes himself & you must not get dependent on him or hesitate to form critical judgements of him in your mind.[15]
>
> I cannot but suspect that you are suffering in part from the influence of Dr. Jung's personality & tendency to excessive too personal way of taking things. Perhaps I am wrong, but there will be no harm in realizing that he also is no God but a blind man trying to lead the blind, & that you are as much at liberty to criticize him as he is to criticize you.[16]

Putnam relayed Katz's account of her analysis with Jung to Ernest Jones, who was highly critical of Jung's procedures. As ever, indiscretion was the fundamental rule of psychoanalytic politics.[17]

Jung did not seem to be concerned with keeping strict confidentiality. At the Burgholzli hospital, it had been common procedure for psychiatrists to correspond with the families of patients. In the case of Katz, Jung continued in this vein, writing letters to Katz's mother reporting on her progress. In 1915, he informed her that her daughter needed to undergo a maturational process to reach the full independence necessary for health. He added that he could not describe this process to her, as it would require writing a large book.[18]

Jung was also not bound by the 50-minute hour. On one occasion, while he was on military service in 1915, he arranged to meet Katz to have a two-and-a-half-hour session at the train station.[19] James Kirsch, who had analysis with Jung at the end of the 1920s, recalled that some of his interviews with Jung took place walking in the hills around Küsnacht.[20] In the summer months, Jung would sometimes practice in his garden.

While he was analysing Katz, Jung sent her to be concurrently analysed by his assistant, Maria Moltzer.[21] At the beginning of 1913, Moltzer and Toni Wolff had been admitted as members of the Zürich Psychoanalytical Society as lay members.[22] When Moltzer started to practice, she was supervised by Jung. He described his supervision to the American psychiatrist Smith Ely Jeliffe:

> I trusted the cases entirely to her with the only condition, that in cases of difficulties she would consult me or send the patient to me in order to be controlled by myself. But this arrangement existed in the beginning only. Later on Miss M. worked quite independently and quite efficiently. Financially she is quite independent being paid directly by her patients. . . . I arranged weekly

meetings with my assistant, where everything was settled carefully and on an analytical basis.[23]

The practice of analysis in tandem subsequently became a standard feature of classical Jungian technique, it being held to be desirable for an individual to be analysed by a man and a woman.

Jung's self-exploration took the form of inducing and entering into waking fantasies, dialoguing with the characters that appeared, and drawing and painting the images that appeared.[24] He suggested these same practices to his patients. In 1916, he described his procedure in an unpublished paper, "The Transcendent Function."[25] This paper in effect charts how Jung was attempting to develop a generalisable psychotherapeutic method from his self-experimentation. He later termed this "active imagination." He noted that one commenced by concentrating on a particular mood and attempting to become as conscious as possible of all fantasies and associations which came up in connection with it. The aim was to allow fantasy free play, but without departing from the initial affect in a free associative process. This led to a concrete or symbolic expression of the mood, which had the result of bringing the affect nearer to consciousness, hence making it more understandable. The mere process of doing this could have a vitalising effect. Individuals could write, draw, paint or sculpt, depending on their propensities. Once these fantasies had been produced and embodied, two approaches were possible: creative formulation and understanding. Each needed the other, and both were necessary to produce the transcendent function, which arose out of the union of conscious and unconscious contents and resulted in a widening of consciousness.

In his practice at this time, Jung encouraged his patients to undertake similar forms of self-investigation. In her sessions with Katz, Moltzer talked openly about her own experiences and taught Katz about Jung's new conceptions. In one session, Katz noted in her diary that,

> In speaking of God, [Moltzer] spoke of Dr. Jung's conception of 'Abraxas' the Urlibido, which she also accepts; using the word Libido and Horme alike for the individual force. The Abraxas is the great cosmic force behind each God (the God embracing the devil is dualistic—Abraxas a monotheistic conception—the one power. Very difficult to understand and have remembered little.[26]

It is not surprising that Katz found this difficult to understand, for it appears that in this session Moltzer was giving her a digest of the first of Jung's *Septem Sermones ad Mortuos*. Like Jung, Moltzer had a book in which she wrote and painted. She called this her Bible and encouraged Katz to do the same. Katz noted in her diary, "Everyone must write his Bible and in working out mine I shall find my adaptation to R. [Rudolf Katz, her husband]."[27] Moltzer thought that it was only through art that one could constellate the unconscious.[28] Katz eventually returned to America, living to the age of 93. In 1956, she informed Jung that she owed her unusually good health and the originality of her silver jewellery to her years in Zürich.[29]

In 1912, Tina Keller was sent for analysis by her husband, Adolf Keller, one of the first pastors to become interested in psychoanalysis and a member of Jung's circle. Adolf Keller was the pastor of St Peter's Church in Zürich and had found psychoanalysis to be a valuable tool in pastoral counselling. In her childhood, Tina Keller had suffered from anxious fears, and these re-emerged in her marriage, despite it being a happy one. Adolf Keller asked Jung for advice, and he recommended analysis. Tina Keller began her analysis with Maria Moltzer. As a result of a dream, Moltzer sent her to Jung.[30] Keller recalled that Jung told her, "'you are very fortunate that you come to analysis after the Freudian ideas have been enlarged,' and I was quite sure that I would not have stayed in a Freudian analysis."[31] She described her situation in the following way:

> My husband's concern was that I should be freed from fear, but Dr. Jung knew he could not take my fears away. He said so to me and added that fear and anxiety were only symptoms, that I was in an 'individuation process' and the symptoms would only diminish as the individuation proceeded. . . . Dr. Jung challenged my faith and tried to expose my unconscious doubts. . . . He was sure that modern persons must come to a personal religious experience and such an experience can only come, when one has nothing to hold onto.[32]

From this it is clear that Jung conceived of the task of analysis as being more than just symptom removal: its aim was the higher development of the personality. For this to be possible, individuals needed direct religious experience. Nothing could be further from Freud's virulently atheistic attitude.

Jung not only encouraged his patients to talk spontaneously about their experiences but he spontaneously told them of his own. Patients appeared to have been quite aware of what Jung was undergoing. Keller recalled,

> At the time I was in analysis with Dr. Jung, he was still strongly under the impression of that period of irruption from the unconscious. . . . It was during the First World War and Dr. Jung would occasionally allude to his overwhelming experiences. Once he mentioned that they had caused his hair to begin to turn grey. . . . He often spoke of himself and his own experiences.[33]

Jung did not conceal the creative work of his ongoing self-experimentation from his patients:

> In those early days, when one arrived for the analytic hour, the so-called 'red book' often stood open on an easel. In it Dr. Jung had been painting or had just finished a picture. Sometimes he would show me what he had done and comment upon it. The careful and precise work he put into these pictures and into the illuminated text that accompanied them were a testimony to the importance of this undertaking. The master thus demonstrated to the student that psychic development is worth time and effort.[34]

On one such occasion, Jung showed her a painting in the *Red Book* and related it to his relations with his wife and Toni Wolff. Keller recalled,

> [Jung] said, 'see these three snakes that are intertwined. This is how we three struggle with this problem.' I can only say that it seemed to me very important that, even as a passing phenomenon, here three people were accepting a destiny which was not gone into just for their personal satisfaction.[35]

If the psychic process of the therapist affected the patient, Jung had no reluctance in openly sharing his. Keller noted,

> One felt accepted into the very special atmosphere of the discovery of the inner world and of its mystery. . . . Whenever Dr. Jung spoke of these experiences I could feel his emotion. Coming to analysis at that time one entered a very special atmosphere. One felt that Dr. Jung stood in awe before fragments that 'were coming to him,' and that he must try to understand, but that were quite beyond what the human brain can grasp. Everything was fluid, what he said was tentative, paradoxical and full of seeming contradictions.[36]

Jung developed a set of specific principles that he urged upon his patients. Keller noted,

> Dr. Jung insisted on preparation. We were taught to write out our dreams and association to each of its elements. . . . The most important technique I learned in the sessions with Dr. Jung was writing 'from the unconscious.' Early in my analysis Dr. Jung said, 'You must at once begin to prepare for the time you will no more be coming to me. Each time, as you are leaving, even as you are going downstairs, you have more questions. Write these down as if they were letters to me. You do not need to send these letters. When you ask a question, in the measure that you really want an answer, and you are not afraid of that answer, there is an answer deep inside you. Let it come up.' I tried and nothing came, and I told Dr. Jung. But he insisted. He even said, 'Surely you know how to pray!'[37]

The role of prayer as one of the sources for Jung's analytic technique has not been commented upon. It is important to realise that the psychology of prayer was an important subject in the psychology of religion and in psychical research. The new psychology of suggestion, autosuggestion and telepathy was invoked to explain prayer. Frederic Myers attempted to put forward a spiritual but non-theological definition of prayer or supplication, broadly defined as the appeal to the unseen. It was "an attempt to obtain benefits from unseen beings by an inward disposition of our own minds."[38] Judging by Keller's description of Jung's counsel, what seems to have been at issue here is a non-denominational form of prayer. The unconscious was the unseen, the higher power to which one appealed for instruction and healing.

Indications of Jung's interest in prayer may be found in his fantasies at the beginning of 1914. In a fantasy on 1 January 1914, Jung's 'I' found himself in a desert valley, where he met an anchorite called Ammonius.[39] The latter told him that he should not forget his morning prayer. Jung's 'I' realised that we had lost our prayers. In a fantasy of 14 January 1914, Jung's 'I' wanted to borrow a copy of *The Imitation of Christ,* with the "aim of prayer, or something similar," as there were moments when science left us sick.[40]

At the same time, Jung held back from advocating traditional prayer in sessions. One of his students, Kurt Binswanger, recalled, "[Alphonse] Maeder believed it to be good to pray with his patients during the (analytical) hour. And that was for Jung something he couldn't go on with."[41]

During the course of the analysis, Tina Keller felt love and hatred towards Jung:

> Dr. Jung never spoke of 'transference' but obliged me to face the fact that I was 'in love.' It would have been easier to use a technical term. Dr. Jung's theory was that I was 'in love' with some quality (or archetype) which he represented, and had touched in my psyche. If and in measure that I would be able to realize this quality or this unknown element in myself, then I would be free of him as a person.[42]

Not only did Jung dispense with technical language to describe his patient's relation to him, he appears to have done the same with respect to his relations to his patients and was quite open to speak of what he felt:

> He was convinced of the meaning of such a manifestation, and he said that what I brought was such an openness that he owed me some spiritual value that would fertilize my psyche and my 'individuation' would be a 'spiritual child.' This sounded good. He sincerely meant it, but it did not prove true.[43]

Here, Jung openly avows the active agency of the therapist in the therapeutic encounter, fertilising the patient's psyche and giving rise to the patient's individuation. After her analysis with Jung, Keller had analysis with Toni Wolff.

Far from being a solitary endeavour, Jung's confrontation with the unconscious was a collective endeavour, in which he took his patients along with him. Those around Jung formed an avant-garde group engaged in a social experiment that they hoped would transform their lives and the lives of those around them.[44] Keller noted,

> During the First World War, in the midst of the feeling of catastrophe, when cultural values were breaking down, when there was general consternation and disillusionment, a small group around Dr. Jung participated in his vision of an inner world unfolding. Many of us were later disappointed. The vision was too vast and leads into the future.[45]

Tina Keller subsequently became a psychotherapist. For decades, she was Jung's main representative in Geneva. She would turn to Jung for supervision. On one occasion, she discussed a borderline case she had taken on. Jung told her, "You have not the right to experiment in the same way as I have because I have now my name. If something happens to me, you see, it is different than if something happens to you."[46] Jung was quite aware of the experimental nature of his practice and of the protection accorded by his status and medical qualification. Another of Jung's patients during this period, Emil Medtner, claimed that were it not for Jung, he would have shared Friedrich Nietzsche's fate and "gone mad." Medtner likened analysis to what Goethe had once referred to as a "psychic cure in which insanity is let in to heal insanity."[47]

In 1913, Edith Rockefeller McCormick went to Zürich to have analysis with Jung, together with her husband. The McCormicks wrote letters home to Edith's father, John D. Rockefeller, apprising him of their progress and expressing their deep admiration for Jung. On 15 June 1915, Harold McCormick wrote,

> This is not a tabernacle of joy, but a shrine to which seekers only address themselves, and it was in this spirit that I have postponed again my sailing and Edith still finds herself held. With both of us, every day counts. This is not a place (the School of Zurich) which encourages remaining here beyond the right or normal time but the whole question is one of degree at best, for no one who is really interested in analytical psychology and finds it of help ever drops it, because if it is one thing,—it is to be lived, and the more one studies the more one is prepared to live on its basis. So one must strike out again in life else it (analytical psychology) defeats its own purpose. The fundamental idea of it is to teach one, one's self—and this is not always easy, and still more difficult, owing to conscious resistances, to follow one's path when it has been laid out by one's own self. But there is a natural tendency, which one must guard against, of preferring the ease of this life here to the hardships and difficulties of life and living in general, but neither Edith nor I have reached this point yet, and when it is reached I have no doubt it will be effectively met.[48]

This letter conveys that, for the McCormicks, as for many others during this period, Jung's analysis was becoming not only a form of therapy but also the basis for a new way of life grounded in psychology.

The first phase of Jung's self-experimentation had consisted in a "return" to himself, a reconnection with his soul. From Harold McCormick's letters, it appears that he was successful in aiding some of his patients to do likewise. On 1 September 1915, Harold McCormick wrote the following to John D. Rockefeller:

> We are doing our best and are deeply appreciating the opportunity of the work under the beautiful inspiration and guidance—only as to showing us ourselves and enabling us to better know ourselves—of Dr. Jung. It seems a trite thing to say, but I do most sincerely say that I am surprised how little

I have known myself heretofore or how little I have cared for the society & acquaintance and intimacy of myself. I am told there is a wealth of opportunity in this direction, without in any way meaning self-adulation.[49]

Their son, Fowler McCormick, also had analysis with Jung in the winter of 1916–1917. He recalled that, in many of the sessions he had, "Jung would occupy himself by carving in wood while we talked."[50]

We have seen that Jung recommended that his patients write letters to him without sending them. I have come across others who did just this.[51] The following is from such a letter by Cary de Angulo, which gives further indication of Jung's handling of the rapport. Cary de Angulo (née Fink) was of the first generation of women to take a medical degree in the United States, although she never practiced. After the collapse of her marriage to the brilliant linguist and ethnologist Jaime de Angulo, she went to Zürich to work with Jung in 1921. In 1923, she described their therapeutic relationship in the following way:

> The essential fact is that wandering about the universe completely detached, I have met you and entered into an indissoluble union with you. It took place automatically without any willing or not willing on my part just on account of your being what you are. To this 'you' I can write because this 'you' gives me a place in your life—a unique place of great intimacy and yet extreme aloofness. That is the way I define a symbolical relationship. I am at one and the same time inside your being and forever and completely separated from you. . . . Every hour I spend with you has holiness in it for me, not because I am worshipping you, but because I am reaching toward certain values which you express more patently than anyone else.[52]

Cary de Angulo was more receptive than Tina Keller to what Jung was proposing, and she sensitively describes the sincerity of the endeavour and the manner in which the aim was for her to recover her sense of religious values, rather than to worship Jung. Appreciating her intelligence and judgement, Jung turned to her for advice concerning the *Red Book*. She noted,

> You had the night before had a dream in which I appeared in a disguise and was to do work on the *Red Book* and you had been thinking about it all that day and during Dr. Wharton's hour preceding mine especially (pleasant for her I must say). . . . As you had said you had made up your mind to turn over to me all of your unconscious material represented by the *Red Book* etc. to see what I as a stranger and impartial observer would say about it. You thought I had a good critique and an impartial one. . . . For yourself, you said you had always known what to do with your ideas, but here you were baffled. When you approached them you became enmeshed as it were and could no longer be sure of anything. You were certain some of them had great importance, but you could not find the appropriate form—as they were now you said they might come out of a mad-house.[53]

Jung asked her to transcribe the *Red Book*. He saw this task as also having peda-gogical value. She noted that he said he "would explain things to me as I went along. . . . In this way we could come to discuss many things which never came up in my analysis and I could understand your ideas from the foundation."[54]

Jung also conducted analyses by correspondence. Jaime de Angulo sent his ex-wife his dreams. She discussed these in her sessions with Jung, and sent Jung's interpretations back to Jaime. In a session on 14 February 1924, she presented Jung with notes which Jaime de Angulo had written about himself and some dreams that he had sent. On the following day, she wrote to him Jung's general comments:

> He said that he would indeed want to 'moderate' you were you with him, and that the way he would do it would be to see that you understood thoroughly the concepts before you rushed ahead into the processes. . . . In as much as he is not in a position to put the brakes on you personally, he suggested that you read the 'Psychology of the Unconscious' again very carefully, and also the 'Types' making notes and discussions on the parts you do not understand, and sending these notes to me for criticism.[55]

She continued to give Jung's interpretations of four of his dreams. While Jung directed Jaime de Angulo to closely study his writings, this was not a general procedure. In the same letter, she conveyed Jung's advice concerning a case which Jaime de Angulo had taken on:

> [H]e said you should not by any means have tried to explain any theory to him, but if you were going to handle him as a case, the transference should have been made to do the ploughing of the ground, and the theory only administered with great caution and attention to his capacity to take it in.[56]

Patients in analysis with Jung quite naturally wrote to their friends about their experiences in Zürich. In the mid-1920s, the American theatre set designer Rob-ert Edmond Jones came to Jung for analysis. He wrote about his experiences to Mabel Dodge:

> I have been working with this man for two weeks and I have already begun to move in a world of the most ancient and magical visions of soul-states and the beginnings of Time. This is no psychoanalysis or any of those things. This man is a wise man possessed of the secrets. . . . This work is not merely curative. It is serene and austere and disciplinary. There is a good deal of Gurdjieff in it. I wish I could describe this experience to you but it is of no use. It is really more esoteric than anything else, an initiation into manhood. There is no trace of medicine or (therapeutics)? in it. A subtle deep terrible mystical journey, torments, vigils, illuminations. I think we have a very good

working combination. I got in right at the start by not hanging back the way lots of patients do; and it was such a blessed relief to me to find that I wasn't a homosexual and didn't have to be one of those. Jung says that I have the most remarkable gift for animating other people that he has ever seen. His nickname for me is Burster of Shells because I have yanked about half a dozen of his patients right out of their [shells] and made them admit. And he sometimes called me a Giver of Life.[57]

Dodge also received accounts from Mary Foote of her analysis with Jung. Drawn into the magic circle, she sent Foote her own dreams to take to be analysed by Jung.[58] These correspondence networks played a critical role in the dissemination of analysis and shaped the expectations of prospective patients. As Foote informed Dodge, "Jung doesn't remove your complexes & he thinks all progress comes from conflict so I suppose one will go on conflicting for the rest of one's life."[59] "Letters home" from Zürich did much to promote analysis in America and England and helped it to gain social acceptance. Through such trade routes, developments in the German-speaking world spread throughout the English-speaking world.

Jung's instructions to his patients on how to conduct active imagination were quite specific. To explain it, he would recount his own experiences. In 1926, Christiana Morgan came to Jung for analysis. She had been drawn to Jung's ideas upon reading *Psychological Types* and turned to Jung for assistance with her problems with relationships and her depressions. In a session in 1926, Christiana Morgan noted Jung's advice to her about how to produce visions:

> Well, you see these are too vague for me to be able to say much about them. They are only the beginning. You only use the retina of the eye at first in order to objectify. Then instead of keeping on trying to force the image out you just want to look in. Now when you see these images you want to hold them and see where they take you—how they change. And you want to try to get into the picture yourself—to become one of the actors. When I first began to do this I saw landscapes. Then I learned how to put myself into the landscape, and the figures would talk to me and I would answer them.[60]

Jung described his own experiments in detail to his patients and instructed them to follow suit. His role was one of supervising them in experimenting with their own stream of images. Morgan noted Jung saying,

> Now I feel as though I ought to say something to you about these phantasies. . . . The phantasies now seem to be rather thin and full of repetitions of the same motives. There isn't enough fire and heat in them. They ought to be more burning. . . . You must be in them more, that is you must be your own conscious critical self in them—imposing your own judgements and criticisms.[61]

Jung went so far as to suggest that his patients prepare their own *Red Books*. Morgan noted him saying,

> I should advise you to put it all down as beautifully as you can—in some beautifully bound book. It will seem as if you were making the visions banal—but then you need to do that—then you are freed from the power of them. If you do that with these eyes for instance they will cease to draw you. You should never try to make the visions come again. Think of it in your imagination and try to paint it. Then when these things are in some precious book you can go to the book & turn over the pages & for you it will be your church—your cathedral—the silent places of your spirit where you will find renewal. If anyone tells you that it is morbid or neurotic and you listen to them—then you will lose your soul—for in that book is your soul.[62]

With Morgan's permission, Jung used her material in an extended seminar, which ran from 1930 to 1934.[63] Morgan found Jung's treatment of her material inspiring:

> The seminar notes have arrived for which I thank you. I have read them—and I closed the book with a prayer—(a hymn) of gratefulness to you for not having detracted from—indeed for having enhanced—the august quality of those visions. I wish it were possible to convey how completely such an experience can change a life—how in fact, it works in actuality. How the meaning of life is the necessity to embody forth those very visions (or perhaps one should say to act under their sign)./I particularly liked all that you said about the animal face. I lost connection with it this winter.[64]

While patients such as these responded wholeheartedly to Jung's suggestions, others were more critical. In 1919, the English psychologist William McDougall went to have analysis with Jung. During the course of the analysis, McDougall, Jung and his assistant Peter Baynes went sailing together and had dinner together. Amy Allenby, a student of Jung's, later recalled,

> Baynes and Jung noticed that McDougall was firmly entrenched behind his persona, and that one could never get to the real person underneath. So Jung suggested that they should invite McDougall to an evening by the lake and ply him with wine until he would get a little drunk; they did, and it happened.[65]

By contemporary standards of psychotherapy, such practices would be seen as unprofessional "boundary breaking." Such a judgement is anachronistic. Jung never held such a conception of boundaries. In his view, there was no strict division between analysis and life. Analysis was conceived as leading to the psychological reformulation of society through fostering new attitudes and values in the individual. Foremost among these was freedom from hypocrisy, coupled with openness and honesty in personal relations.

McDougall was not convinced by his analysis. Shortly after, he wrote the following in one of his books:

> I have put myself into the hands of Doctor Jung and asked him to explore the depths of my mind, my 'collective unconscious'. . . . And the result is—I 'evermore came out by that same door wherein I went'. . . . I seem to find in myself traces or indications of Doctor Jung's 'archetypes', but faint and doubtful traces. Perhaps it is that I am too mongrel-bred to have clear-cut archetypes; perhaps my 'collective unconscious'—if I have one—is mixed and confused and blurred.[66]

In 1926, he published *An Outline of Abnormal Psychology*.[67] In his chapter on Jung's theories, he reproduced some of his dreams, Jung's analysis of them, and his own interpretations. Intrigued by this account, Smith Ely Jeliffe asked Jung for more information concerning his treatment of McDougall. Jung replied,

> I don't know whether I am bound to medical discretion in McDougall's case, as he designates himself as a hopelessly normal personality. I probably had no right to consider his case as one that would fall under the concept of medical discretion. There isn't much to be indiscreet about anyway. It was really as he states it: a very few dreams taken to Dr. Jung in order to have an argument about it, and withholding if possible all reactions which could be disagreeable. It was, as you suspect, a very modest number of conversations and anything else but a submission to the actual procedure of analysis of which, I'm afraid, Prof. McDougall has not the faintest idea. I like however his experiments with rats and wouldn't argue that point with him, but people who are absolutely innocent of psychology, I find, are usually profoundly convinced of their psychological competence.[68]

Jung's insistence that his patients prepare themselves for analysis also took the form of requiring patients to undergo analysis with one of his followers prior to seeing him and also of being tutored in analytical psychology. In the 1920s, Jung turned to Cary de Angulo to tutor some of his patients. On one occasion, he asked her to take on one of his patients, Dr Bond, for tutoring during his absence. As she was an "introvert of the nth degree," she needed much general preparatory knowledge.[69]

In addition to tutoring, preparation took the form of prior analyses with one of Jung's pupils. To the American writer Leonard Bacon, he wrote that patients had to first begin their analysis with one of his pupils so as to get a "decent preparation" before seeing him.[70]

The significance of preparation was that it enabled Jung to concentrate on fostering the higher development or individuation of his patients. From the 1920s, individuals did not come to Jung not knowing what to expect: they were selected and primed. The social role of the analytic patient—in this context, of a patient of Jung—had to be created. If they had extensive personal problems to sort out, Jung would generally leave this to his assistants. This indicates that what ensued was the result of quite unusual procedures. Of his practice, Jung noted that he had very few new cases and that most of them had had prior experience of psychotherapy. In 1954, he wrote that, just as with surgery, there was minor and major psychotherapy and that his concern was with the latter: "It is a question of a minority of patients with certain spiritual demands, and only these patients undergo a development which presents the doctor with problems of the nature described here."[71]

In his subsequent published writings, Jung insisted that his patients' individuation was not a product of suggestion but a natural spontaneous process, which was simply quickened by the analysis. Some saw it otherwise. Tina Keller recalled,

> I believe it was a kind of contagion because of the dynamic process that Dr. Jung was still involved in, and that those close to him were identifying with. This poses the question, whether a pioneer in an 'exceptional' state can safely work as a therapist? Or is there perhaps a special quality in such a man, so stimulating to the privileged persons, that the advantages outweigh the dangers?[72]

In her analysis with Jung, she, and others around her, was drawn into the process that Jung himself was undergoing. His experiment with himself was at the same time an experiment on them. In 1929, Jung explicitly described his aim as being one of bringing about "a psychic state in which my patient begins to experiment with his own being."[73] Their interactions with him played a critical role in establishing analytical psychology as a social movement. Through this, the results of Jung's self-experimentation began to have a transformative effect on an ever-growing number of people, as they took on his conceptions and let him change their lives. The willingness of a number of individuals to accept the invitation to experiment with their lives in such a manner and embrace his new conceptions convinced Jung that the latter were not merely idiosyncratic but replicable and had general significance.

The consequence of this expansion of the remit of psychotherapy beyond the cure of pathology was that what was formerly a "medical method of treatment" had become a "method of self-education," no longer bound to the consulting room.[74] This brought it into proximity with Eastern esoteric traditions, on the one hand, and European spiritual practices on the other. Consequently, Jung spent much time from the 1930s onwards engaged in the comparative study of these practices.[75] He maintained that his fantasies, and those of his patients, stemmed from mythopoetic imagination, which was missing from the present rational age. A reconnection with this could form the basis for cultural renewal. The task of moderns was one of establishing a dialogue with the contents of the collective unconscious and integrating them into consciousness. This was to play an important part in the popular "mythic revival." He held that cultural renewal could only come about through self-regeneration of the individual, in other words, through the individuation process. What he was proposing was a new "image of man." As he saw it, the task with which his patients were confronted was one of recovering a sense of meaning in their lives, made more pressing with the secularisation and rationalisation of contemporary culture. Consequently, he held that individuals who managed to recover a sense of meaning in their lives were healing not only themselves but also the culture. Thus, the aim of the therapeutic cure was not to help the patient adapt to existing social norms but to foster a process of self-realisation that would ultimately contribute to reshaping society. The psychotherapeutic patient had become the doctor of society.

Notes

1 Jaime de Angulo to Chauncey Goodrich, 28 August 1922, Goodrich papers, Bancroft Library, University of California at San Francisco.
2 On this wider context, see Shamdasani, "Psychotherapy in Society."
3 Janet, *Les obsessions et la psychasthénie, I,* 727.
4 Jung, *An Attempt at an Account of Psychoanalytic Theory, CW* 4, §433.
5 Ibid., §434.
6 Carroy, *Hypnose, Suggestion Etpsychologie,* 179–200.
7 Jung, "Timely Psychotherapeutic Questions," *CW* 4, §584 (emphasis in original). On Jung's use and understanding of hypnosis and suggestion, see Shamdasani, "The Magical Method That Works in the Dark."
8 Jung, Ibid., §587.
9 Jung, *The Red Book.*
10 Jaffé and Jung, *Memories, Dreams, Reflections,* 194.
11 Ibid., 214.
12 Putnam to Bowditch Katz, 10 December 1912, Katz papers, Countway Library of Medicine.
13 Putnam to Bowditch Katz, 12 December 1912.
14 Putnam to Bowditch Katz, 7 January 1912.
15 Putnam to Bowditch Katz, 10 December 1912.
16 Putnam to Bowditch Katz, 10 December 1913.
17 Putnam cited a reply from Jones in an undated letter to Bowditch Katz.
18 Jung to Mrs Katz, 27 February 1912.
19 Jung to Bowditch Katz, 11 January 1915.
20 James Kirsch, interview with Gene Nameche, 1968, Jung Biographical Archive, Countway Library of Medicine.
21 On Bowditch Katz's analyses, see also Taylor, "C.G. Jung and the Boston Psychopathologists 1902–1912." On Bowditch Katz, Moltzer and Jung, see Shamdasani, *Cult Fictions.*
22 30 January 1913, "Protokolle des Psychoanalytischen Vereins, " archives of the Psychological Club, Zürich.
23 Jung to Jelliffe, July 1915, in Burnham and McGuire, *Jelliffe,* 198.
24 On the evolution of the techniques of Jung's self-experimentation, see Shamdasani, "Jung's Practice of the Image."
25 Jung, "The Transcendent Function," *CW* 8, §§170–171.
26 Bowditch Katz, entry for August 1917, Diary, Katz papers.
27 17 August 1917, Diary.
28 7 May 1917, Diary.
29 Fanny Bowditch Katz to Jung, 17 January 1956, Jung archive, Swiss Federal Institute of Technology, Zürich, Switzerland.
30 Swan, *The Memoir of Tina Keller-Jenny,* 17.
31 Ibid., 19.

32 Keller, "C.G. Jung," 5.
33 Keller, "Recollections of My Encounter with Dr. Jung," A2.
34 Swan, *The Memoir of Tina Keller-Jenny*, 21.
35 Tina Keller interview with Gene Nameche, 1969, R.D. Laing papers, University of Glasgow, Scotland, 27.
36 Keller, "Recollections of My Encounter with Dr. Jung," B12, A2.
37 Swan, *The Memoir of Tina Keller-Jenny*, 23.
38 Myers, *Human Personality and its Survival after Bodily Death*, Vol. 2, 310.
39 Jung, *The Red Book*, 269.
40 Ibid., 292.
41 Kurt Binswanger, interview with Gene Nameche, Jung Biographical Archive, Countway Library of Medicine, 14.
42 Keller, "Recollections of My Encounter with Dr. Jung," B19.
43 Ibid., B19.
44 For a study of another important case at this time, see De Moura, "Learning from the Patient."
45 Keller, "Recollections of My Encounter with Dr. Jung," A5.
46 Tina Keller interview with Gene Nameche, 18.
47 Cited in Ljunggren, *The Russian Mephisto*, 91.
48 Harold McCormick to John D. Rockefeller, 15 June 1915, Rockefeller Archive Centre, Terrytown, NY.
49 Harold McCormick to John D. Rockefeller, 1 September 1915, Rockefeller Archive Centre.
50 Fowler McCormick interview with Gene Nameche, Jung Biographical Archive, Countway Library of Medicine, 8.
51 One example being Rivkah Scharf (I thank Nomi Kluger Nash for enabling access to her papers).
52 Cary Baynes (née de Angulo), 14 January 1923, letter drafts, Baynes papers, Contemporary Medical Archives, Wellcome Library, London.
53 26 January 1924, letter drafts.
54 Ibid.
55 Cary de Angulo to Jaime de Angulo, 15 February 1924, Cary Baynes papers.
56 Cary de Angulo to Jaime de Angulo, 15 February 1924.
57 Robert Edmond Jones to Mabel Dodge, 1926, Dodge papers, Beinecke library, Yale University.
58 Mary Foote to Mabel Dodge, November 1925, Dodge papers. On Mary Foote, see Trousdell, "The Lives of Mary Foote."
59 Mary Foote to Mabel Dodge, 1929.
60 Christiana Morgan, 8 July 1926, analysis notebooks, Countway Library of Medicine.
61 Analysis notebooks, 12 October 1926.
62 Analysis notebooks, 12 July 1926.
63 Jung, *Visions*.
64 Morgan to Jung, 31 June 1931, Jung Archive, Swiss Federal Institute of Technology, Zürich, Switzerland.
65 Amy Allenby, interview with Gene Nameche, Jung Biographical Archive, Countway Library of Medicine, 3.
66 McDougall, *National Welfare and National Decay*, 134.
67 McDougall, *An Outline of Abnormal Psychology*, 181–205.
68 Jung to Jeliffe, 7 June 1932, in Burnham and McGuire, *Jeliffe*, 326.
69 Jung to Cary de Angulo, 17 August 1925, Baynes papers.
70 Jung to Leonard Bacon, 26 July 1926, Bacon papers, Beinecke Library, Yale University.
71 Jung, *Mysterium Coniunctionis*, *CW* 14, §514.
72 Keller, "Recollections of My Encounter with Dr. Jung," B17–18.

73 Jung, "The Aims of Psychotherapy," *CW* 16, §99.
74 Jung, "The Problems of Modern Psychotherapy," *CW* 16, §174.
75 For the former, see Jung, *The Psychology of Kundalini Yoga.*

Bibliography

Burnham, John C. and William McGuire, eds. *Jelliffe: American Psychoanalyst and Physician; and His Correspondence with Sigmund Freud and C.G. Jung.* Chicago: University of Chicago Press, 1983.

Carroy, Jacqueline. *Hypnose, suggestion et psychologie: [invention de sujets.* Paris: Presses Universitaires de France, 1991.

De Moura, Vicente. 'Learning from the Patient: The East, Synchronicity and Transference in the History of an Unknown Case of C.G. Jung', *Journal of Analytical Psychology* 59, no. 3 (2014): 391–409.

Jaffé, Aniela and C.G. Jung. *Memories, Dreams, Reflections,* translated by Richard Winston and Clara Winston. London: Fontana, 1990.

Janet, Pierre. *Les obsessions et la psychasthénie, I.* Paris: Alcan, 1903.

Jung, C.G. *The Psychology of Kundalini Yoga: Notes of the Seminar Given in 1932,* edited by Sonu Shamdasani. Princeton: Princeton University Press, 1996.

Jung, C.G. *Visions: Notes of the Seminar Given in 1930–1934,* edited by Claire Douglas. Princeton: Princeton University Press, 1997.

Jung, C.G. *The Red Book. Liber Novus,* edited by Sonu Shamdasani; translated by Mark Kyburz, John Peck and Sonu Shamdasani. New York: W.W. Norton, 2009.

Keller, Tina. 'C.G. Jung: Some Memories and Reflections', *Inward Light* 35 (1972): 1–18.

Ljunggren, Magnus. *The Russian Mephisto: A Study of the Life and Work of Emilii Medtner.* Stockholm: Almqvist and Wiksell International, 1994.

McDougall, William. *National Welfare and National Decay.* London: Methuen, 1921.

McDougall, William. *An Outline of Abnormal Psychology.* London: Methuen, 1926.

Myers, Frederic W.H. *Human Personality and Its Survival of Bodily Death.* London: Longmans, 1903.

Shamdasani, Sonu. *Cult Fictions: C.G. Jung and the Founding of Analytical Psychology.* London: Routledge, 1998.

Shamdasani, Sonu. 'The Magical Method That Works in the Dark', *Journal of Jungian Theory and Practice* 3 (2001): 5–17.

Shamdasani, Sonu. 'Jung's Practice of the Image', *Journal of Sandplay Therapy* 24, no. 1 (2015): 7–21.

Shamdasani, Sonu. 'Psychotherapy in Society: Historical Reflections'. In *Exploring Transcultural Histories of Psychotherapy*, edited by Sonu Shamdasani and Del Loewenthal, 8–23. London: Routledge, 2020.

Swan, Wendy K., ed. *The Memoir of Tina Keller-Jenny: A Lifelong Confrontation with the Psychology of C.G. Jung.* New Orleans: Spring Journal Books, 2011.

Taylor, Eugene. 'C.G. Jung and the Boston Psychopathologists 1902–1912'. In *Carl Jung and Soul Psychology,* edited by E. Mark Stern, 131–144. New York: Haworth Press, 1986.

Trousdell, Richard. 'The Lives of Mary Foote: Painter and Jungian', *Journal of Analytical Psychology* 61, no. 5 (2016): 588–606.

Chapter 10

Heyong Shen

I am Heyong Shen; I grew up in Heze in Shandong province, China, close to the hometown of Confucius and near the holy Tai mountain and the 72 springs of Jinan.

I became full professor of psychology in 1996 and became a Jungian analyst (IAAP) and sandplay therapist (ISST) in 2003. Now I am the president of the China Society for Analytical Psychology and the China Society for Sandplay Therapy.

Supported by IAAP and ISST, I have organized eight international Conferences for Analytical Psychology and Chinese Culture every two or three years since 1998. The theme of the eighth conference was "Enlightenment and Individuation: East and West" (2018).

I was a speaker at the Eranos East and West Roundtable Conferences (1997, 2007, 2019); all three speeches related to the theme psychology of the heart.

Psychology of the heart is based on Chinese culture and integrated with Jungian analysis. As C.G. Jung said in *The Red Book*: "There is a knowledge of the heart that gives deeper insight." "But how can I attain the knowledge of the heart?" Jung continued: "You can attain this knowledge only by living your life to the full."

I wrote some articles focused on the significance of psychology of the heart in the 1980s, published the book *Psychology of the Heart* in 2001, and used them as the basis for the Fay Lecture in 2018: "Psychology of the Heart, and the Heart of Jungian Analysis."

I very much appreciate Dr. Joe Henderson, Mario Jacoby, Thomas Kirsch, Murray Stein, John Beebe, and David Rosen, as well as Chinese philosophers Liu Dajun, Wu Yi, Yan Zexian, Chen Bing, and Hu Fuchen, who gave me great support for the psychology of the heart.

I am the chief editor of the Chinese translation of the *Collected Works* of C.G. Jung. Our team has translated over 100 books of Jung and Jungian psychology into Chinese in the last 20 years.

My graduate study was on Buddhism and psychoanalysis in 1984. The research of my Ph.D. dissertation was on psychological field theory (Kurt Lewin) and Gestalt psychology. I have published many papers and books on these topics.

I was Fulbright scholar in residence (1996–1997) for the research and teaching of Chinese psychology at UNO/UCLA (USA) and visiting scholar for the research of group dynamics at Southern Illinois University (1993–1994). I trained Jungian

DOI: 10.4324/9781003148982-11

analysis at the Zürich C.G. Jung Institute, Kusnacht, and at the San Francisco C.G. Jung Institute (1997–2002).

My recent publications include the following: "C.G. Jung and Chinese Culture" (2018), "Psychology of the Heart" (Fey Lecture, 2020), "Why Is the Red Book Red?" (in Murray Stein and Thomas Arzt, eds. *Jung's Red Book for our Time: Searching for Soul under Postmodern Conditions*. Asheville, NC: Chiron Publications, 2017), "The image and the meaning of the Chinese character for 'enlightenment'" (*Journal of Analytical Psychology*, 2019), "Representations and symbols of Kuafu's myth in Analytical Psychology and Chinese culture: History vs. contemporary, consciousness vs. unconscious, collective vs. individual" (*Culture & Psychology*, 2019), "Images of Chinese Sandplay: The Garden of the Heart & Soul" (in Dyane N. Sherwood, ed. *Into the Heart of Sandplay*. Oberlin, OH: Analytical Psychology Press, 2018), "Mythodrama, the Meaning of Myth, Archetype and Healing in Chinese Context" (*The Japanese Journal of Play Therapy, 2017*), "The Missing Women of China" (in Carta, S., ed. *The Analyst in Polis*. Volume II, 2017), "Behind the Mask of China: The Continuing Trauma of the Cultural Revolution" (in Carta, S., ed. *The Analyst In Polis*. Volume I, 2017), "The Dao of Anima Mundi: I Ching and Jungian Analysis, the Way and the Meaning" (Einsiedeln, Switzerland: Daimon Publishers, 2017), "Garden of the Heart and Soul, Working with Orphans in China – Symbolic and Clinical Reflections" (in Carta, S., ed. *The Analyst in Polis*. Volume III, 2020).

Over the last 10 years, I gave several plenary speeches for IAAP and ISST conferences, was a speaker for Eranos East and West Round Table Conferences, Fay Lecture, and Vatican Forum, and gave lectures at Roma University, Italy, Bar-Ilan University, Israel, Zürich University, Switzerland, University of Washington, Seattle, WA, University of Tehran, Iran, and Kyoto University, Japan.

I am the founding president of the Oriental Academy for Psychology of the Heart and have set up three institutes for analytical psychology and Chinese culture in three universities (South China Normal University, Fudan University, and the City University of Macao). Over 1,000 graduate students have completed research focused on Jungian analysis and depth psychology for their master's degrees and Ph.Ds.

Our team set up the "Garden of the Heart & Soul" cherish program of psychological support for orphans in 2007. Our volunteers went to Wenchuan in 2008 and to Yushu in 2010 for earthquake relief. To date we have built 86 workstations all over the mainland of China specifically for the psychological needs of orphans.

When Covid-19 broke out in Wuhan, China, at the beginning of 2020, we set up "Garden of the Heart & Soul 2020 online" on 26 January 2020 to provide psychological services for the public; over 10,000 people visited the website in the first few months.

The "Garden of the Heart & Soul" is our practice of Jungian analysis and the psychology of the heart. As Jung expressed, one can attain the knowledge of the heart only by living one's life to the full. The heart is essential for life, so the psychology of the heart keeps one giving, relating and living. Heart and soul are the basis for personal, interpersonal and spiritual life, as well as for individuation and transformation.

The Dao of Anima Mundi

I Ching and Jungian Analysis, the Way and the Meaning

Originally published in *Anima Mundi in Transition: Cultural, Clinical & Professional Challenges*, edited by Emilija Kiehl and Margaret Klenck. Einsiedeln, Switzerland: Daimon Verlag, 2017. Reprinted with permission.

Certain Chinese philosophical ideas inform this chapter. I am going to discuss the ancient, ineffable notion of "Dao" as an archetype, with emphasis on the goal of embracing "the heart of Dao", together with the meaning pointed to by Confucius in introducing the term "zhong" ("equilibrium") as the psychological path to the state of harmony implied by the word Dao. I will also mention "shi" ("timing", which in a parallel way spans both the Greek notion of Kairos and the Jungian notion of synchronicity) and will link zhong to shi to discuss "shi-zhong" [an "equilibrium with time" achieved through a heartfelt influence often best achieved through wu wei (acting without acting)] as we often must as analysts. I need such ideas to speak in a Chinese way to the theme of this chapter, which has been stated in Jungian Latin: "The Dao of Anima Mundi."

The Mysterious Heart of Dao, the Subtle Words With Great Meaning

Let us start with the Dao (or Tao). This is not only the Great Watercourse Way of Taoism. It is also the goal of the rational Confucian path of "faithfulness and forbearance" (which never forgets that we all have the "same heart") and the intuitive genius of the Buddhist focus on the "middle way (madhyamā-pratipad)" and of Buddhism's profound respect for "suchness (tathātā)." Even more, Dao is the reality whose manifold meanings are contained within and conveyed by *I Ching* to the psyches of those who consult this wise Chinese oracle. The image of Dao in a Chinese bronze inscription is shown in Figure 10.1.

Figure 10.1 San family plate, late Zhou Dynasty.

For me, however, *I Ching* itself, the book that, thanks to Jung, sits on so many people's bookshelves, is the embodiment of Dao. Jung was sure that Confucius himself had written in the *I Ching – Xi Ci* ("The Great Commentary"): "*I Ching* is made on the principles of heaven and earth, therefore it contains all the rules and ways from heaven to earth . . . to have the knowledge of all, and serve the world with Dao" (Huisheng, 2008, pp. 372–373).

Jung thus did not overstate when he observed, "In Chinese philosophy one of the oldest and most central ideas is that of Tao, which the Jesuits translated as 'God'." But this is only correct for the Western way of thinking. Other translations of Tao (or Dao), such as "providence" and the like, are merely makeshift. Richard Wilhelm brilliantly interprets Tao as "meaning." "The concept of Tao pervades the whole philosophical thought of China" (C.G. Jung, *CW* 8, para. 917).

Jung points out that "Lao Tzu described 'Dao' as such in the famous *Tao Te Ching*":

> There is something formless yet complete
> That existed before heaven and earth.
> How still! How empty!
> Dependent on nothing, unchanging,
> All pervading, unfailing.
> One may think of it as the mother of all things under heaven.
> I do not know its name, but I call it "Meaning" (Dao).
> If I had to give it a name, I should call it "The Great" [Ch. XXV]
> (C.G. Jung, *CW* 8, para. 918)

The word "name" as used here in Wilhelm's rendering of the Chinese text is often formed by two characters, only one of which really means "name" in the secular Western sense of "signifier." The other character means the more ambiguous term "word", as it used in the last sentence by Lao Tzu quoted here. For example, Lao Tzu, whose common name is "Er" ("ear"), has the styled word "Dan" ("big ears"). Similarly, the styled word "Dao" is the beautifully symbolic "meaning", which includes the idea of finding the mean, but its common name, "Da" ("great"), points to its value and why we should want to revere it. The basis of this evaluation is unpacked more fully if we look closer at the word Da.

The Chinese character Da (great), from its image on the Oracle Bone Inscriptions in which it was first found, is the image of a man—a person standing tall and stretching out, thus called "Da-Ren" (great man).

The image of Da (great) in Chinese looks simple, but it conveys the symbolic meaning of transforming and attaining what is beyond man. And in such an image, just as Lao Tzu said, "[t]he great square shows no corner" and "the great imagery has no form" (Huisheng, 1999, pp. 84–85). From great and (moving or transforming) "nothingness" (such as "wu wei"/no action, and "wu wo"/"no self"/Anatta), we reach the transcendent function and transformation.

Figure 10.2 The image of "great" Da

In *I Ching,* we can read another meaning in the word great: the great man (Da-Ren), an idea which both Richard Wilhelm and C.G. Jung appreciate very much.

> A great man is he whose virtues are in accord with heaven and earth, whose brightness is in accord to the sun and the moon, whose order matches the four seasons, and who listens to the spirits for the fortune and misfortune.
>
> (Huisheng, 2008, pp. 14–15. *Tao Te Ching*, Chapter 25)

I must say, I have always viewed this passage from the *I Ching* as Chinese philosophy's description of the individuation process.

But there is as much differentiation of this idea in the rest of Chinese philosophy as we find within our own psychology in the works of von Franz, Neumann or Edinger. For instance, the aforementioned quote from Lao Tzu by Jung is in the first half of *Tao Te Ching*'s Chapter 25. The second half goes thus:

> Great (Da) is also called Shi (i.e. constantly on the move). Shi is also called Yuan (i.e. far-reaching), and Yuan is also called Fan (i.e. returning to the very beginning). Therefore, the Dao (the Meaning and the Way) is great, the Heaven is great, the Earth is great, the Man is also great. In the universe there are four greats, and the Man is one of the four. The Man copies the Earth as example, the Earth copies the Heaven as example, the Heaven copies the Dao as example, and the Dao just copies the Great Nature.
>
> (Huisheng, 1999, pp. 50–51. *Tao Te Ching*. Chapter 25)

If I were to try to put this in the language of analytical psychology, then I would say, Dao is great because, like the self, it is a container of everything. Indeed, a Chinese proverb says, "The capacity of containing makes greatness." But of course Lao Tzu has added the thought that only through greatness may things transform. This has profound implications for our understanding of individuation, including the individuation that sometimes will not happen because the patient cannot embrace his or her capacity to take their place among the greats in life.

When I see texts related to Dao, *I Ching* and Jung's interpretation of them, I recall the theme of this Conference, "Anima Mundi in transition: Cultural, Clinical and

Professional Challenges." It is these very challenges that require us to be great men and women to serve those forces in the universe that are driving anima mundi's transition into Tao, if only we will allow them to speak to us. We ourselves came to Kyoto, Japan, in a similar way that Obama recently went to Hiroshima: to strive to foster the relationship between the East, the West and Nature. We do this too when we explore together the clinical and professional challenges of our field in today's rapidly changing and increasingly dangerous world.

I use "Dao Xin Wei Wei" ("the mysterious heart of Dao") in Chinese to express my understanding of "the world soul"—anima mundi, really the "soul of the universe"—and I mention both the soul's mystery and its reach to get to the heart of this Conference.

Dao Xin Wei Wei (the mysterious heart of Dao) comes from a "16-character scripture" recorded in *Shang Shu* (one of the five classic books of ancient Chinese literature). The full text is as follows:

> The heart of man is perilous,
> the heart of Dao is mysterious;
> be refined and be focused,
> and to hold the honest Mean.
>
> (Wang Shixun and Wang Cuiye, 2012, p 361)

It is said that this scripture has been passed on from the ancient Emperors Yao (about 2350 BC), Shun and Yu generation after generation.[1]

The mysterious heart of Dao may also be known as "the obscure and vague way" or "the formless and soundless great path." This is exactly the connotation of Dao used by Jung—its wonderful evocation of the not knowing, which is known so well by analysts in their way of helping patients to gain insight into the collective unconscious and, thus, into their place within the archetypal image of anima mundi in its present moment of transition.

Within this quatrain of four lines, each composed of four characters, which begins with "The heart of man is perilous", we are given a 16-character scripture that expresses the fundamental idea of "holding the two extremes while employing the middle course or unity", which is the method of clinical practice utilized by C.G. Jung that may be referred to as the "transcendent function" but is really an invitation to "active imagination"—a journey that is, in Dao, to realize the self that has always, mysteriously, been there.

In Jung's opinion, the archetypal image of Dao contains the integration of the conscious and unconscious, the wholeness of yin and yang. Jung says,

> Out of this union emerge new situations and new conscious attitudes. I have therefore called the union of opposites the "transcendent function." This rounding out of the personality into a whole may well be the goal of any psychotherapy that claims to be more than a mere cure of symptoms.
>
> (C.G. Jung, *CW* 9i, para. 524).

The Metaphor of He Tu, the Image of *I Ching*

In his 1935 Tavistock Lectures, Jung stated (on ancient Chinese philosophy),

> The ideal condition is named Tao, and it consists of the complete harmony between heaven and earth. Figure 13 represents the symbol for Tao. The condition of Tao is the beginning of the world where nothing has yet begun—and it is also the condition to be achieved by the attitude of superior wisdom. The idea of the union of the two opposite principles, of male and female, is an archetypal image.
>
> (C.G. Jung, *CW* 18, para. 262)

The Chinese Tai Chi diagram referenced here and used by Jung is shown in Figure 10.3.

As stated in *I Ching – Xi Ci*, "equal parts of Yin and Yang is called Dao" (Huisheng, 2008, pp. 376–377). So, too, in Chuang Tzu's comments on *I Ching*: "*I Ching* is about the way of Yin and Yang" (Wang Rongpei, 1999, pp. 584–585).

Jung met Richard Wilhelm at the opening ceremony of Count Keyserling's School of Wisdom in Darmstadt, Germany. This was in November 1920. The two men must have "clicked", because Jung then invited Wilhelm to give a seminar on *I Ching* at the Psychology Club in Zürich in December 1921.[2] Jung had already grasped that Richard Wilhelm's great contribution was bringing the meaning of *I Ching* and, through it, passing on the flame of Chinese culture (the living germ of the Chinese spirit) to the West.

Jung is quite clear about this: in explaining the "blocking of libido" in *Symbols of Transformation* (1912), Jung writes, "The ancient Chinese philosophy of the *I Ching* devised some brilliant images for this state of affairs" (C.G. Jung, *CW* 5, para. 250). Also, in Part VI "The Battle for Deliverance From the Mother" of Volume 2

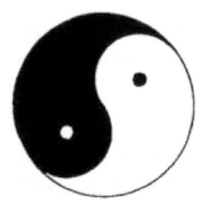

Figure 10.3 Chinese Tai Chi diagram used by Jung.

of *Symbols of Transformation*, Jung used the legend of the dragon-headed horse, He Tu (river map), and *I Ching* to analyze the symbol of the horse. He describes it thus: "The *I Ching* is supposed to have been brought to China by a horse that had the magic signs/the 'river map' on his coat" (C.G. Jung, *CW* 5, para. 423).

"He Tu" (river map) and "Luo Shu" (Luo script) are the origins and the first images of *I Ching*. Legend has it that in the ancient days during Fuxi's time, a dragon-headed horse emerged from the Yellow River near Luoyang with He Tu, and a turtle spirit emerged from the Luo Shui River with Luo Shu on its back. Fuxi then evolved Bagua (the Eight Trigrams) and the rules of Wu Xing (the Five Elements) from them, thus originating *I Ching*.

In the classic scriptures from the pre-Qin period,[3] there are many records of He Tu and Luo Shu. As written in *I Ching – Xi Ci*: "Map from the River, Script from Luo Shui, the saints follow them." China's He Tu and Luo Shu are shown in Figure 10.4.

However, He Tu and Luo Shu are not just legends: their ancient history and actual existence have been repeatedly confirmed by modern archaeological discoveries. In 1987, a jade turtle with a carved jade piece was unearthed at the Ling-jia-tan site at Hanshan, Anhui Province; it has been dated back to the Neolithic Period 5,000 years ago. The jade piece was carved with primordial Bagua charts and placed in between the ventral and dorsal sides of the jade turtle, as if re-enacting the legend of He Tu and Luo Shu being carried by spirits (see Figure 10.5).

In 1930, Jung gave a more detailed analysis of the He Tu images and *I Ching* in a seminar about mandala:

> The "River Map" is one of the legendary foundations of the I Ching, which in its present form derives partly from the twelfth century B.C. According to

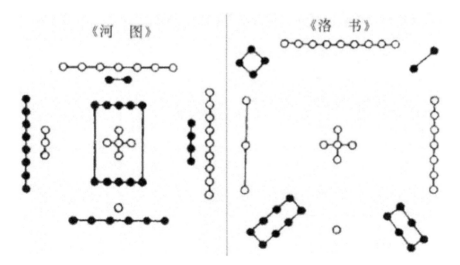

《河　图》　　　　《洛　书》

Figure 10.4 China's He Tu and Luo Shu.

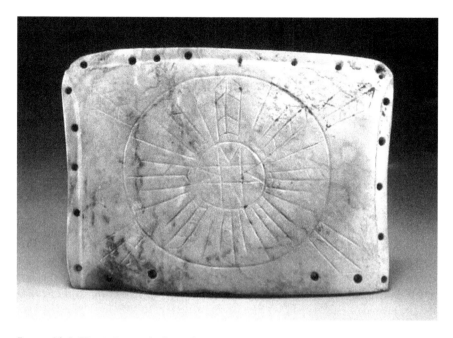

Figure 10.5 The jade turtle from Ling-jia-tan.

the legend, a dragon dredged the magical signs of the "River Map" from a river. On it the sages discovered the drawing, and in the drawing the laws of the world-order. This drawing, in accordance with its extreme age, shows the knotted cords that signify numbers. These numbers have the usual primitive character of qualities, chiefly masculine and feminine. All uneven numbers are masculine, even numbers feminine.

(C.G. Jung, *CW* 9i, para. 642)

The He Tu that Jung used in his book is shown in Figure 10.6.

About He Tu, Jung commented as follows, using the Qian hexagram:

Qian in the middle is the heaven, which then originates the four virtues, such as the movement of heaven is full of power. So now we have:

Qian: self-generated creative energy
Heng: all-pervading power
Yuan: generative power
Li: beneficent power
Zhen: unchangeable, determinative power

(C.G. Jung, *CW* 9i, para. 640)

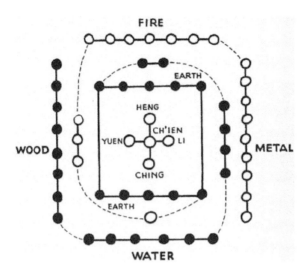

Figure 10.6 The He Tu used by Jung in "Concerning Mandala Symbolism."

He Tu is presented in the form of an image which holds logic and is formed by numbers. Image, logic and number are crucial to *I Ching*. But of equal importance is the "Chi" in *I Ching* described by Jung, although the English expression he used was "power" or "energy." He Tu tells us that numbers are based on Chi. Chi channels Dao and touches the heart of Dao. Here is the connection to the mysterious heart of Dao and to anima mundi. He Tu and Luo Shu are both primal archetypal images and the inspirations contained therein. Ancient minds and their archetypal images are held in He Tu's and Luo Shu's circles and dots and the links in between (Figure 10.7).

As shown in Figure 10.7, in the middle of He Tu are the numbers 5 and 10; each group of numbers on the four sides subtracts to 5, and the middle numbers also give 5 and 15. The middle of Luo Shu is also 5, and the horizontal, vertical and diagonal sums are all 15. Thus, in the archetypal images of He Tu and Luo Shu, "wu" (5) is the center. The oracle bone inscription for the Chinese character 5 (wu) is shown in Figure 10.8.

The image in Figure 10.8 conveys the symbolic meaning of "crossing noon", and the "knotted point" indicates the core and the middle number. Not only does it contain all of both yin and yang, but it is also the foundation of the Five Elements (Wu Xing); its logic holds the wonders of the numbers of heaven and earth. It is also the embodiment of the equilibrium (zhong) within "to hold the honest Mean", the utmost Dao.

Therefore, the wu (5) or center of He Tu is also referred to as "where the heart of Dao is", representing "the heart of heaven and earth." In the Chinese context, the

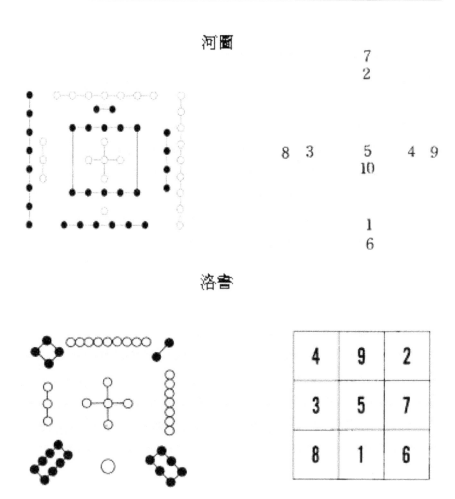

河圖

7
2

8　3　　5　　4　9
10

1
6

洛書

Figure 10.7 He Tu's and Luo Shu's circles and dots and the links in between.

Figure 10.8 The Fuxi Primordial Hexagrams of *I Ching* and the King Wen Manifested Hexagrams

heart of heaven and earth is the heart of the universe; for example, Lu Jiuyuan (1139–1193, idealist neo-Confucian philosopher) once said "my heart is the universe."

I see the wu (5) in the middle of He Tu as part of wu ("I" or "self") in Chinese. wu (I/self) may be taken as self, as Jung once quoted Chuang-tzu's "I (wu) lost myself" (or I lost my ego) in the *Secret of the Golden Flower*. When the ego of consciousness surrenders, the self from the heart begins to emerge; so when wu (I/self) meets the heart, the "enlightenment"[4] comes. As a result, we have the "psychology of the heart", based on Chinese culture combined with analytical psychology.

Hence, from wu (5) to wu (I/self), and from wu (I/self) to wu (enlightenment);[5] only by the heart can we receive the meaning of the images. The mysterious heart of Dao shall bring us the heart of the universe (anima mundi). In "Psychology and Alchemy", Jung wrote, "The idea of the *anima mundi* coincides with that of the collective unconscious whose centre is the self" (C.G. Jung, *CW* 12, para. 265).

On the basis of the archetypal images of He Tu and Luo Shu, Chinese sages inferred the Fuxi primordial hexagrams of *I Ching* and the King Wen manifested hexagrams. The mystery of these diagrams and the structure and pattern within *I Ching* are all from the archetypal images of He Tu and Luo Shu—from them, we have equilibrium (zhong) and to hold the equilibrium and the movements of the heart of the universe and the Chi it contains, as well as time and equilibrium with time.

We can read on the back cover of the English translation of *I Ching*: "The I Ching, or Book of Changes, represents one of the first efforts of the human mind to place itself in the universe." "Its central themes, set forth in imagery of singular force and originality, is the continuous change and transformation underlying all existence" (Wilhelm, 1950).

For Chinese philosophers, especially Taoists, these archetypal images contain the "returning to one's true nature" and the "unity of heaven and man" that they pursue, and they hold the way, the method and meaning of returning from "acquired" to "innate."

In *Memories, Dreams, Reflections*, Jung writes,

> This raised the question of the unity which must compensate this diversity, and it led me directly to the Chinese concept of Tao. . . . It was only after I had reached the central point in my thinking and in my researches, namely, the concept of the self, that I once more found my way back to the world.
>
> (C.G. Jung, 1965, p. 208)

Shi-Zhong and Gan-Ying, Equilibrium With Time and Synchronicity

What *I Ching* brings to Jung, or what Jung brings to *I Ching*, has another crucial meaning relevant to this equilibrium and to hold the equilibrium, which is time—the synchronicity developed by Jung.

For Jung, synchronicity is at once the embodiment of the way, and the meaning of *I Ching* is as a guide to knowing how to proceed to walk on this way. As

Jung said, "The method [of *I Ching*], like all divinatory or intuitive techniques, is based on an acausal or synchronistic connective principle" (C.G. Jung, *CW* 8, para. 866). He further explains:

> I first used this term in my memorial address for Richard Wilhelm (delivered May 10, 1930, in Munich). The address later appeared as an appendix to *The Secret of the Golden Flower*, where I said: "The science of the *I Ching* is not based on the causality principle, but on a principle (hitherto unnamed because not met with among us) which I have tentatively called the synchronistic principle".
>
> (C.G. Jung, *CW* 15, para. 81)

When Jung expressed his understanding of synchronicity and explained its meaning, he not only quoted *I Ching* but also used the Chinese "Dao", citing Chapters 25, 24, 11, 14, 21, 37, 73, etc. from *Tao Te Ching* in sequence. For example, Jung said:

> "Nothing" is evidently " 'meaning" or "purpose", and it is only called Nothing because it does not appear in the world of the senses, but is only its organizer. Lao-tzu says:
> "Because the eye gazes but can catch no glimpse of it,
> It is called elusive.
> Because the ear listens but cannot hear it,
> It is called the rarefied.
> Because the hand feels for it but cannot find it. It is called the infinitesimal.
> These are called the shapeless shapes,
> Forms without form, Vague semblances".
>
> (C.G. Jung, *CW* 8, para. 920)

Thus, the heart of Dao is mysterious. The way and the meaning of the Dao are not for the eye and ear, but for the heart.

Jung stated that "the development of Chinese philosophy produced from the significance of the magical the 'concept' of Tao, of meaningful coincidence, but no causality based science" (C.G. Jung, *CW* 8, para. 941).

After quoting Lao Tzu's *Tao Te Ching* in an explanation of synchronicity, Jung refers to Chuang Tzu:

> Chuang-tzu (a contemporary of Plato's) says of the psychological premises on which Tao is based: "The state in which ego and non-ego are no longer opposed is called the pivot of Tao." If you have insight, says Chuang-tzu, "you use your inner eye, your inner ear, to pierce to the heart of things, and have no need of intellectual knowledge." This is obviously an allusion to the absolute knowledge of the unconscious, and to the presence in the microcosm of macrocosmic events.
>
> (C.G. Jung, *CW* 8, para. 923)

"The fasting of the heart" by Chuang Tzu has a resonance for me that the words of Mountain Lake about "thinking with one's heart" might have had for Jung[6]; these were the keywords that inspired me and planted the seed in a dream I had back in 1993, which later grew to become the "psychology of the heart." The dream came to me after I spent several months of self-analysis in the forest of Southern Illinois in the United States. In the dream, I pulled off my head, put it on the table, looked at the head and thought as a dialogue between the head and the heart emerged. What Chuang Tzu called the fasting of the heart" echoes in Jung's writing on synchronicity: "the intellect should not seek to lead a separate existence, thus the soul (the Heart) can become empty and absorb the whole world. It is Tao that fills this emptiness" (C.G. Jung, *CW* 8, para. 923). What Jung describes here is exactly the meaning of the fasting of the heart" (Chuang Tzu, Chapter 4: Ways of the Human World).

On Dr. Henderson's desk, there was a card. There were two Chinese characters on the card: "timing" and "chance." All around these two characters was handwriting in fine print; these were notes of understandings and insights on timing by Dr. Henderson.

I asked him where he learned of *I Ching*. Dr. Henderson said that he learned about it from Jung. He was inspired by Jung and went on to study *I Ching*. I then asked Dr. Henderson what the meaning of *I Ching* was to him. He answered that, for him, the most important meaning of *I Ching* was timing: to investigate it in depth and in the moment, to follow the flow and gain equilibrium with time. That is very true. The three basic meanings of *I Ching*—what is changing, what is unchanging, and what is simple—are all related to time. Only with the right timing can we attain equilibrium, be simple in the face of change and therefore be able to feel securely held in what cannot change, the self.

The Dao in *I Ching* is profound. To sum it up, we may call it equilibrium with time. For many traditional Chinese philosophers, this is the core spirit of *I Ching*. All of the hexagrams are reflections of time, and all of the 384 Yao lines are how things change in accord with time. What equilibrium with time reflects is changing with time to follow Dao. In this way, we accept time, of which so many of us are usually terrified.

In recent years, I have been drawing upon a notion of heartfelt gratitude as a key to my increasing acceptance of time. I have been using "Gan" ("heartfelt influence") and "Gan-Ying" ("heartfelt influence" and "responding from the heart") to understand and interpret "synchronicity" as the images and meaning expressed by the Xian hexagram (31, The Influence) and the Zhongfu hexagram (61, The Inner Truth). Just as the I Ching says, "Yi, no thinking, no action, heartfelt influence that connects the world. If not for Yi being the greatest spirit in the world, it cannot be so" (Huisheng, 2008, pp. 392–393).

To Jung, *I Ching* is a book that has its own life. Perhaps this life of Yi can also allow us to feel the aliveness of anima mundi in the face of its transitions.

The Soul Flower, Images of *I Ching* and Meaning

One thing of particular importance is that Jung has integrated *I Ching* into the expression and practice of analytical psychology—we see it in his clinical cases, his active imagination and the process of individuation.

In "A study in the Process of Individuation", Jung began with a quote from Chapter 21 of *Tao Te Ching*:

> Tao's working of things is vague and obscure.
>   Obscure! Oh vague!
>   In it are images.
>   Vague! Oh obscure!
>   In it are things.
>   Profound! Oh dark indeed!
>   In it is seed.
>   Its seed is very truth.
>   In it is trustworthiness.
>   From the earliest Beginning until today
>   Its name is not lacking
>   By which to fathom the Beginning of all things.
>   How do I know it is the Beginning of all things?
>   Through *it!*

(C.G. Jung, CW 9i, para. 525)

However, there is one more sentence of eight characters (in Chinese) before Jung's quote in this chapter: "The form of the grandest virtue follows only Dao" (Kong De Zhi Rong, Wei Dao Shi Cong) (Huisheng, 1999, pp. 42–43).

If we look at this from the perspective of analytical psychology, and according to the images of the eight Chinese characters, then "the form of the grandest virtue follows only Dao" may be explained as such: the grandest virtue is a great container, the capacity of containing makes greatness, only through greatness may things be contained, and only from Dao, the way and the meaning will individuation be reached. Thus, this Chapter 21 of *Tao Te Ching* and its description of "Dao"—the things, the seed, the truth and the trustworthiness—is it not an inspiration to feel and to reflect on anima mundi?

Jung provided 24 paintings by his patient Miss X in "A Study in the Process of Individuation." The "soul flower" first appeared in the ninth painting (Figure 10.9). On this Jung wrote, "In Picture 9 we see for the first time the blue 'soul-flower,' on a red background, also described as such by Miss X" (C.G. Jung, *CW* 9i, para. 596).

For me, as I came to face this soul flower many times while working on this chapter, I seemed to see—or feel—the "Magnolia" from Jung's Liverpool dream in 1927 and the *Secret of the Golden Flower* by Jung and Wilhelm (1928). So this soul flower is like the "suchness" (Jung would have said "just-so-ness") of the Flower Garland World (the Jewel Net of Indras of the Huayen World), which displays the equilibrium with time we are urged toward by the *I Ching*. Surely this image is also a vivid manifestation of the mysterious heart of Dao, one that allows us to feel its extraordinarily open connection to anima mundi.

We can see how Jung expressed his feeling for the living reality imaged in this painting within the unusual passion he summoned to describe the person who had created this image in "A Study in the Process of Individuation": "Her heart overflowing with loving kindness . . . with compassion . . . with joyfulness . . . with equanimity" (C.G. Jung, *CW* 9i, para. 596). Jung added, lest we mistake his patient's arrival at the core of her introverted feeling as merely the achievement of a sentimental view of life, that,

> The underlying thought is clear: no white without black, and no holiness without the devil. Opposites are brothers, and the Oriental [person] seeks to liberate himself from them by his nirdvandva ("free from the two") and his neti neti ("not this, not that"), or else he puts up with them in some mysterious fashion, as in Taoism.
>
> (C.G. Jung, *CW* 9i, para. 597)

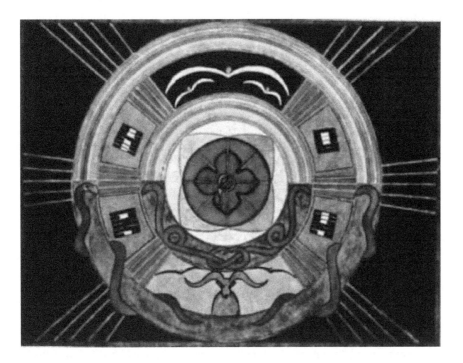

Figure 10.9 Soul flower

In this painting, Miss X, though not herself an Oriental person, used four hexagrams from *I Ching* around the soul flower: upper left, Yu (enthusiasm, hexagram 16, thunder earth providing for); upper right, Sun (decrease, hexagram 41, mountain swamp diminishing); lower right, Sheng (pushing upward, hexagram 46, earth wind ascending); lower left, Ding (cauldron, hexagram 50, fire wind holding). Jung described, "The connection with the East is deliberately stressed by the patient, through her painting into the mandala four hexagrams from the *I Ching*" (C.G. Jung, *CW* 9i, para. 597).

Jung interpreted and analyzed the hexagrams one by one in his "A Study in the Process of Individuation." The key in which, and the meaning contained in all of the hexagrams, is also the images and inspiration they draw from the old Chinese notions of equilibrium, timing and equilibrium with time that eventually entered philosophy in a more codified way with Confucius.

The essence of the thought embodied in the *I Ching* is such: To act in undue time is excessive, to act in due time is equilibrium. Decreases and increases depend on time, so too do providing for and ascending. Grand success holding in the cauldron will respond when gain equilibrium.

Jung wrote,

> The phases and aspects of my patient's inner process of development can therefore express themselves easily in the language of the *I Ching*, because it too is based on the psychology of the individuation process that forms one of the main interests of Taoism and of Zen Buddhism.
>
> (C.G. Jung, *CW* 9i, para. 602)

Jung discussed the case with the following analysis:

> Miss X's mandala, on the other hand, comprises and contains the opposites, as a result, we may suppose, of the support afforded by the Chinese doctrine of Yang and Yin, the two metaphysical principles whose co-operation makes the world go round. The hexagrams, with their firm (yang) and yielding (yin) lines, illustrate certain phases of this process. . . . Thus the Oriental truth insinuates itself and makes possible—at least by symbolic anticipation—a union of opposites within the irrational life process formulated by the *I Ching*.
>
> (C.G. Jung, *CW* 9i, para. 603)

As Jung was working on the foreword for the English-language version of Wilhelm's translation of the *I Ching*, which finally appeared in 1950, he decided to invite the *I Ching* to describe how it felt about being translated thus and drew the Ding hexagram (cauldron).

It was as though *I Ching*, already embodied in the image of Ding, decided to identify itself to Jung as a way of entering into a conversation with him. For Jung, on the other hand, to converse with *I Ching* was like linking himself up with "spiritual agencies" in a particularly lively active imagination. He saw *I Ching* as having its own life and respected it as he would a god. As many religions teach, when supplicants place god in their heart, god will respond to them. As Confucius said, "Make sacrifices to the dead as if they were present, make sacrifices to the spirits as if the spirits were present" (Yang Bojung and Arthur Waley, 1999, pp. 24–25). Or, as the inscription on the lintel of Jung's house stated: "Summoned and unsummoned, God will be present."

I call this Gan-Ying (heartfelt influence and responding from the heart) and see it as the first principle of psychology of the heart. And of course it is also the embodiment of the mysterious heart of Dao" and related to the faithfulness and forbearance by Confucius, to the with all of one's heart by Mencius, to emptying one's heart-mind by Lao Tzu, to the art of heart by Guan Zhong, to the fasting of heart by Chuang Tzu, to the heart tradition of Zen Buddhism and to Huineng's nature of self.

The Mysterious Heart of Dao, Heartfelt Influence and Response

The archetypal images of *I Ching*, such as the hexagrams Xian (influence) and Ding (cauldron), are also closely related to the development of analytical psychology in China. We used the hexagram Xian (31, influence) for the First International Conference of Analytical Psychology and Chinese Culture in 1998. The archetypal image of Xian became the theme and initiation. Just as the Tuan commentary of Xian says,

> *Xian* means *gan* (heartfelt influence, stimulate), heaven and earth stimulate each other, and all things take shape and come into being. The holy man stimulates the hearts of men, and the world attains peace and rest. If we contemplate the out-going stimulating influences, we can know the nature of heaven and earth and all beings.
>
> (Wilhelm, 1950, p. 541)

In 2006, after the Third International Conference of Analytical Psychology and Chinese Culture, we (along with Murray Stein, John Beebe, Joe Cambray, Linda Carter and others) visited Wilhelm's former residence. We also visited Quindao, the homeland of Lao Nai Xuan, Wilhelm's teacher of *I Ching*. Under the t1,000-year-old elm tree in the Temple of Supreme Purity on Mount Lao, we divined an answer to the question, "What is the future of analytical psychology in China?" The response from *I Ching* was the hexagram Ding, the cauldron (50), with the third line changing it into the hexagram Weiji, before completion (64). There was much to consider in that change, but I would like to focus here on what was unchanging in it. We start with a container that is itself in flow and undergoing vicissitudes.

In the image of the Ding hexagram is fire over wood; thus, the superior man consolidates his fate by making his position correct. The cauldron is standing, so it settles the heart and puts it at ease. The seed is refined to consolidate the fate. Chinese alchemy has long had the way of "Refinement of Essential Matter into Vital Breath."

Thus we were told, once again, as we incubated one part of the future of analytical psychology in Asia, that making one's position correct is the way to reach equilibrium with what we must work on at a particular time and that consolidating one's fate in the same process is the way to reach harmony. This means realizing that even when the state of equilibrium and harmony are truly understood, and in this way brought to conscious realization, only with time will they lead to any lasting equilibrium. In 2008, a powerful earthquake (8.0) hit the southwest of China, like "The Tong (copper) Mountain shaking at the West, and the Ling (spiritual) bell resonating at East."[7] Members of our Chinese Federation of Analytical Psychology went to the earthquake zone and set up the Garden of the Heart & Soul for psychological relief. Now, we have 76 workstations with thousands of volunteers in the orphanages of China.

In 2013, the Sixth International Conference of Analytical Psychology and Chinese Culture was held in Qingdao with the theme: "Wilhelm and *I Ching*, Jung and *Red Book*." Murray Stein and the *Red Book* drama group came and performed their enactment of Jung's confrontation with the unconscious as recorded in *Liber Novus*. Again, we visited Wilhelm's former residence and Lao Nai Xuan's homeland at Mount Lao. Again, under that same 1,000-year-old elm tree, when Paul Brutsche spoke, it was as though he spoke with the voice of Jung, as though he felt that this second home of Richard Wilhelm had an atmosphere of "another Bollingen." At that moment, the elm tree responded; the sound of the falling leaves was like music from nature and heaven.

That moment brought what we feel about *I Ching*'s equilibrium with time; from this, we seemed to have had the experience of the mysterious heart of Dao.

I am not superstitious, but I knew in the presence of Murray Stein, Paul Brutsche, John Hill, Dariane Pictet and others that the moment we shared, the experience of being so near to the actual standpoint of Richard Wilhelm, and the feeling of being together in the same spirit with the same heart is what Jung really means by "synchronicity", which for me is Gan-Ying (heartfelt influence and responding from the heart) literally entering the mysterious heart of Dao.

Now, in closing, I think it is good to see Jung's words:

> Anyone who, like myself, has had the rare good fortune to experience in association with Wilhelm the divinatory power of the *I Ching* cannot remain ignorant of the fact that we have here an Archimedean point from which our Western attitude of mind could be lifted off its foundations.
>
> (C.G. Jung, *CW* 15, para. 78)

He continues,

> What is even more important is that he has inoculated us with the living germ of the Chinese spirit, capable of working a fundamental change in our view of the world. We are no longer reduced to being admiring or critical observers, but find ourselves partaking of the spirit of the East to the extent that we succeed in experiencing the living power of the *I Ching*.
>
> (C.G. Jung, *CW* 15, para. 78)

And then Jung says,

> We must continue Wilhelm's work of translation in a wider sense if we wish to show ourselves worthy pupils of the master. The central concept of Chinese philosophy is *tao*, which Wilhelm translated as "meaning." Just as Wilhelm gave the spiritual treasure of the East a European meaning, so we should translate this meaning into life. To do this—that is, to realize *tao*—would be the true task of the pupil.
>
> (C.G. Jung, CW 15, para. 89)

And now my own words: "The Dao of Anima Mundi: *I Ching* and Jungian Analysis, the Way and the Meaning." I can only hope that we, here at this conference, can find it in us to feel "The Dao of Anima Mundi"—if so, then *I Ching* and Jungian analysis will have come together, in a Chinese way, to understand how at this time of transition we can still find the way and the meaning that put us in harmony with time.

Acknowledgments

This chapter is based on a research project supported by the Chinese National Social Science Foundation (16ASH009). My thanks to John Beebe, who edited the paper with his profound understanding of Chinese philosophy and *I Ching*.

Notes

1 Although there have been doubts regarding when was Shang Shu written, the ancient texts recently presented in the bamboo manuscript at Tsinghua University give sufficient support to the 16-character scripture I quoted.
2 In *Memories, Dreams, Reflections*, we read that Jung first invited Richard Wilhelm to the Psychology Club in Zürich in 1923. Thanks to Tom Kirsch, Ulrich Hoerni and Thomas Fisher, we know that the exact date was 15 December 1921. "This is confirmed by the existing lists of talks held at the Club since its beginning" (letter from Thomas Fisher to Heyong Shen).
3 The pre-Qin period usually means the history before 221 BC in China, particularly the Spring–Autumn and the Warring States periods (770–221 BC).
4 The image of the Chinese character for enlightenment is the image of the heart and the image of wu (I/self) together.
5 In Chinese, the characters for I or self and enlightenment are based on the number 5 (wu) and have similar pronunciations.
6 See Jung's conversation with the Native American elder, Mountain Lake, in 1924, recorded in Jung (1989). *Memories, Dreams, Reflections*. New York: Vintage Books, p. 247.
7 From "A New Account of Talks of the World." Joseph Needham quoted the story in his *Science and Civilization in China*. Mr. Yin from Chinchow, who is reported to have asked a monk (Hui Yuan), "What is really the fundamental idea of the I Ching?" To which the monk is said to have replied: "The fundamental idea of the I Ching can be expressed in one single word, Gan, Heartfelt Influence", just like "The Tong (copper) Mountain shaking at the West, and the Ling (spiritual) bell resonating at East."

References

Confucius. (1992). *The Confucian Analects* (James Legge, Trans.). Changsha: Hunan Publication.

Huisheng, F. (Trans.). (1999). *Laozi (Tao Te Ching)*. Changsha: Hunan People's Publishing House.

Huisheng, F. (Trans.). (2008). *I Ching, the Chou Book of Changes*. Changsha: Hunan People's Publishing House.

Jung, C.G. *CW* 5.

Jung, C.G. *CW* 8.

Jung, C.G. *CW* 9i.

Jung, C.G. *CW* 12.

Jung, C.G. *CW* 15.

Jung, C.G. *CW* 18.

Jung, C.G. (1965). *Memories, Dreams, Reflections*. New York: Vintage Books.

Lao Zi. (1994) *Tao Te Ching* (Arthur Waley, Trans.). Changsha: Hunan Publication.

Luo Zhiye (Trans.). (1997). *Shan Shu, the Book of History*. Changsha: Hunan Publication.

Wang Rongpei (Trans.). (1999). *Zhuangzi*. Changsha: Hunan People's Publishing House.

Wang Shixun, and Wang Cuiye (Trans.). (2012). *Shang Shu/the Book of History*. Beijing. Zhonghua Book Company.

Wilhelm, R. (1950). *I Ching or Book of Changes* (Cary F. Baynes, Trans.). New York: Princeton University Press.

Yang Bojung and Arthur Waley. (1999). *The Analects*. Changsha: Hunan People's Publishing House.

Zhuang Zi. (1997). *Chuang Tzu* (Wang Yongpei, Trans.). Changsha: Hunan Publication.

Chapter 11

Thomas Singer

I am a psychiatrist and Jungian psychoanalyst who was born in St. Louis, Missouri, where my family settled as part of the German-Jewish immigration to America in response to the political and economic upheaval in Germany in the 1840s. In fact, ancestors on both my mother's and father's sides of the family were German-Jewish immigrants, with my mother's family settling in Louisville, Kentucky, and my father's family settling in St. Louis, Missouri. They were part of a German-Jewish mercantile tribe that, over the generations, fared well in America and achieved economic and social success that most likely exceeded their initial expectations. In a way, they lived and contributed to the "American dream." Their business interests were wed to philanthropic activities as well, and members on both sides of my family participated in the founding of Jewish hospitals in St. Louis and Louisville. My great-grandfather on my mother's side founded a distillery in Louisville, and their Barkhouse Brothers' Gold Dust Kentucky Bourbon became the most popular whiskey sold west of the Mississippi beginning in the 1870s. My grandfather on my father's side started selling shoes around the age of 13 before the turn of the twentieth century, and he loved to tell the story of how he went to his boss and asked if he could sell the damaged shoes remaindered in a warehouse. He traveled throughout southern Illinois and emptied the two floors of shoes.

It was typical for members of this German-Jewish tribe to place the highest value on education, business, and philanthropy. They embraced the liberal causes of their eras. Both my mother and father shared in this tradition, although like many of their peers they had moved away from a Jewish identification religiously, but not culturally. My father was a businessman and a leader in the St. Louis community as president of St. Louis Children's Hospital and served on other boards. He was very active in the Jewish movement to help European Jews find safety in the 1930s and 1940s. He was not a Zionist, as he, along with many of his well-educated Jewish peers, favored advancing Jewry worldwide rather than creating what they thought was a separatist Zionist state. This was not atypical for that time. Both my father and my mother did not like the idea of Jews keeping themselves separate from the rest of the community, although often such separatism was the only way to survive virulent anti-Semitism. My mother was very active in the arts and ran a gallery specializing in contemporary prints from the late

DOI: 10.4324/9781003148982-12

1960s for close to 40 years. She was a creative force in promoting the visual arts in the community and curated sculpture shows at St. Louis institutions such as the world-famous Shaw's Botanical Garden. This background emphasizing culture, education, service, and a world view enhanced by extensive travels was my inheritance. And it all seemed very natural to me.

In spite of this description of success and well-being that was also part of the post–World War II 1950s in which I was a young boy, there was a sense of unease beneath the surface. Both of my parents underwent Freudian psychoanalysis for very real underlying distress, even though psychoanalysis was also de rigueur for their group. My mother lost twins to serious ulcerative colitis, from which she almost died when I was eight—which was just about the time I announced I wanted to be a doctor. And my father, a very learned, introverted man was an only child, whose older brother died in his second year. He suffered from what then was called obsessive compulsive neurosis. In my senior year of high school, at a fine, old private boys' day school in St. Louis that both my father and older brother had attended, I ended up writing a senior thesis on Camus' *The Stranger*, *The Plague*, and *The Fall*. I was already feeling the sense that something wasn't quite right in myself and in our American culture, despite the sense of outward success and well-being. I graduated from St. Louis Country Day School in 1960 and attended Princeton University, where I majored in religion and European literature. I was surely searching for something that was missing in my home and my culture with regard to spirit. A summer "grand tour" with friends between my junior and senior years ending in Greece changed my life. I climbed Mt. Lykabettos in the heart of Athens on my first day in Greece and devoured Kazantzakis' *Zorba the Greek* at the top. My life was never the same afterwards. I ended up taking a "year off" and teaching English in Athens before going to medical school at Yale. If Greece introduced me to Zoe, Yale introduced me to Thanatos. A big dream from that time seemed to give a vision of my past and future life.

> I am a German sailor on a World War II destroyer. I work in the boiler room. A torpedo hits and destroys the ship. I am blown out of a huge hole in the front of the ship and die. But then I am reborn and proceed to live two lives, that of an experimental jet pilot and that of a farmer.

Sometimes I think that the dream predicted the course of my life. The experimental jet pilot can be seen as the intuitive flights of a Jungian analyst that have been the source of creative energy for much of my adult professional life. And the life of the farmer perhaps refers to my grounding marriage to my wife Jane, who is a horticulturist and garden designer. Our marriage of intuition and sensation has been fruitful in so many ways, not the least of which is that she grounds my intuitive flights with practical, earthly realities and does not indulge my mother complex seeking adoration and praise. Jane has very little interest in my Jungian pursuits, and that is probably the best for both of us. We have four grown children, all of whom live close by and who have turned out to be thoughtful and loving people.

In my training at the C.G. Jung Institute in San Francisco, I was able to know some great analysts/people, including Joe Henderson, John Perry, Joe Wheelwright, Thomas Kirsch, Kay Bradway, Jane Wheelwright, John Beebe, Jean Kirsch, Iden Goodman, and others. They were all extraordinary individuals, but I ended up feeling that there was not much for me to create because they had already discovered everything there was to know that was important. It wasn't until my 60s that I began to find my own creative voice as a writer, and I have been extraordinarily lucky over the past 20 years to have remained relatively healthy and have been able to explore my own ideas and visions in articles and books, which have been an enormous source of energy and curiosity for me. Working with Sam Kimbles to develop the concept of the "cultural complex" opened up a door of research and world travels in my mind and psyche that has resulted in books that I have edited on Australia, Latin America, Europe, the United States, and Far East Asian countries. This work has been perfectly suited to what most interests me. Equally exciting has been developing a series of conferences and books on ancient Greece and the modern psyche, which is the direct result of my having been reborn in Greece as a young man. Also sharing the heart of these professional and personal interests has been my work with the Archive for Research in Archetypal Symbolism (ARAS), which places the symbolic image at the center of the creative imagination. I feel enormously grateful to have been able to live a full and creative family and professional life.

A Personal Meditation on Politics and the American Soul

This chapter was originally published in 2007 by Spring Journal Inc., in *Spring, A Journal of Archetype and Culture*, Volume 78: A Personal Meditation on Politics & the American Soul.

Introduction

An invitation to write about politics and the American soul should cause anyone with common sense to turn and run in the opposite direction, in the same way that seeing an advertisement for the "soul of a BMW" or hearing Cadillac's newly trademarked slogan—"Life. Liberty. And The Pursuit"™—induces nausea. The language of soul and politics has been so co-opted by a vast public relations machine, which instantaneously turns everything, including soul, into a marketable commodity, that there are probably only a handful of us foolish enough to tackle the subject.

The purpose of this chapter is to be more impressionistic and evocative than precisely descriptive of the relationship between the American soul and politics—partly because it is so hard to give specific definitions to such essentially indefinable realities. It may be helpful to think of soul as having both a function and a content. As a function and not a specific content, we experience soul as emotional, embodied, psychic movement.

Soul, as a function of psychic movement, can legitimately attach itself to various contents—landscape, people, events, eras, values. One can think of our individual and collective souls as being that psychic function that creates and contains the playing fields for the endless encounters between instinct and spirit. And because of the elusive nature of soul as a function or a content and the essential unknowability of whether there is even such a thing as a collective soul, our topic begs to find a hook in a specific time and place.

Such a hook presented itself to me in 2004 when I was asked to moderate a conference on the theme of "The Soul of America" at the San Francisco Jung Institute. The topic was as overwhelming to me then as it is now. At the time, a deep divide in the American political psyche took on a simplistic but potent symbolic form in the image of the red and blue states. It was natural for the conference's topic of "The Soul of America" to veer toward a discussion of "the political fight for the soul of America."

As a Northern Californian for the past 35 years, with deep roots in both the Midwest and East coast, I chafe at the one-sidedness of most characterizations of members of one political, religious, ethnic, racial, or regional group by another. Living in a liberal region with progressive politics, I did not want to get up and proclaim that the Democrats had an inside track on the "real" soul of America or that Bush was an "idiot." Both were too easy, because those were the opinions of almost everyone in the audience and, for that matter, of almost everyone I know. The fact is that no one group in America has an exclusive claim to either the "soul of America" or being "idiots," even though one side will usually claim soul for itself and idiocy for its rival. (In the political rhetoric of the last few decades, the right has been most effective at staking out "the soul of America" for itself and far less stupid than most on the left have claimed.)

It is very easy to project soul into politics and politics into soul. Indeed, I believe it is the first task of an inquiry such as this to try to differentiate soul from politics. This differentiation begins with the acknowledgment that soul and politics get mixed up with each other all the time in the collective psyche and in the intermingling of myth, politics, and psyche in our cultural unconscious.[1] With the goal of differentiation in mind, the first part of this chapter will address the topic of "The Soul of America," and the second part will address "Politics and The Soul of America."

PART ONE: WHAT IS THE SOUL OF AMERICA?

And if the soul
is to know itself
it must look into a soul:
the stranger and enemy, we've seen him in the mirror.[2]

I start with these lines from George Seferis's poem "Argonauts" because I believe that each of us discovers different bits and pieces of "the soul of America" as the personal journeys of our individual lives interface with the unfolding story of our nation's soul journey. When we inquire about the soul of America, I think we need to keep in mind that we are talking about a living interface between the experience of our individual souls and that of the national soul. And if looking into the depths of our personal souls often reveals mysteries, ambiguities, and contradictions, how much more complex is it to reflect on the nature of our American soul? We should begin this inquiry with the recognition that we discover the soul of America only as we discover the story of our own souls. If the Hindus speak of *Atman* and *Brahman*, perhaps we should think about an intermediary zone and speak of the individual soul and the group soul.

Let me give you a brief example that illustrates the importance of this semipermeable membrane or interface between personal soul and collective soul. John Perry, a well-known Jungian analyst of an earlier generation, once told me the story of his meeting, as a young man, with Jung in 1936. On one of his journeys to America, Jung had visited the house of John Perry's father in Providence, RI. Perry's father served there as a Bishop in the Episcopal Church. Conversation with Jung at the Perry house touched on the Native American Indian's role in the story of America and the need for modern man to connect with the "archaic man" inside. Jung expressed his opinion that to connect with the soul of America one needed to connect with the American Indian. That night, a young John Perry dreamed that he was standing by the fireplace in the living room with his hand on the mantelpiece. A bare-chested American Indian appeared in the fireplace and threw a tomahawk directly at him. In a startled response, Perry managed to catch the tomahawk in his hands.[3] One way to think about this dream is to say that the soul of John Perry was introduced to the soul of America in his meeting with a Native American.

Not all of us have such extraordinary meetings between our individual soul and the soul of our country, but each of us is certainly startled when some aspect of America's soul appears to us in our own psychic house. In this context of the encounter of personal soul with national soul, I want to relate a story of my own unexpected personal soul meeting with a part of our nation's soul.

In July 2004, just a few months prior to the national elections later that fall, I traveled with my family from San Francisco to Alton, IL. This journey helped give me an inkling of how to speak about what the phrase "soul of America" evokes in me without falling into the easy trap, at a time of presidential elections, of identifying soul with one political group or another. It is no accident that my own musings about "the American soul" began with a personal, physical journey halfway across the country, since so much of what we think of as "the soul of America" is embedded in journey—whether it be from a foreign land to America, from East to West to open the continent, or from West to East in search of our roots. The "journey" is at the heart of the "soul of America," and my journey to the Midwest in July 2004 was no exception.

Alton sits on the bluffs of the Mississippi River, just below where the Mississippi and Missouri Rivers come together (see Figure 11.1). It is a proud old river town that celebrates its history of having been a safe haven for abolitionists in the pre–Civil War era, as well as having been the site of the famous Lincoln-Douglas debates. I had traveled to Alton with my wife and children in order to bring home the ashes of my mother-in-law, Agnes, who had died in the San Francisco Bay Area

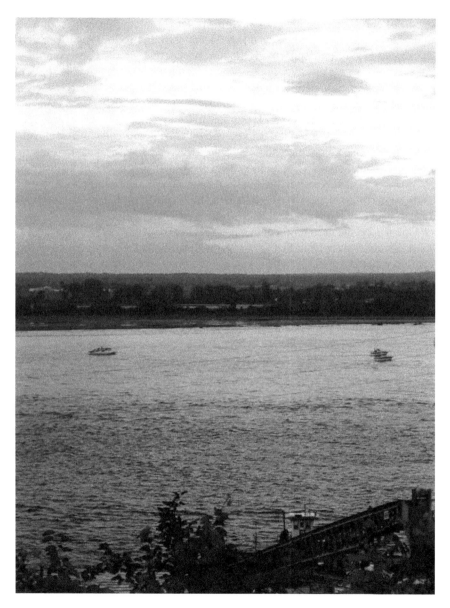

Figure 11.1 A view of Alton, IL, across the Mississippi.

earlier in the spring. Alton was the resting place of Agnes's ancestors, her child-hood home, and the home where she had raised her own family. Such homecomings remind us that the soul connects the material and the spiritual realms just as the Mississippi River connects north and south, east and west in the heart of the country.

If you grow up in the Midwest, as I did, the Mississippi River reflects the soul of the country. The river's journey is the soul's journey, as Huck Finn and Tom Sawyer taught us in our youth. The grandeur of the river and the fertile valleys surrounding it make it a real, a symbolic, and a spiritual heartland all at the same time—a flowing source of vast generosity and security. It is not an exaggeration to compare the coming together of the Missouri and Mississippi with the confluence of other great rivers of the world, such as the Tigris and Euphrates. Proud civiliza-tions flourish in the fertile valleys and lowlands at the confluence of great rivers, and we were returning Agnes to the generous source of her origins, where her personal soul might join the American soul in its return to the origin of all souls.

On July 3, 2004, having carried Agnes's ashes halfway across the country to her homeland beside the river, we traveled to the Alton Cemetery for a memorial service to honor this profoundly kind and decent woman. Agnes was widely known as "Saint Agnes" because she was like the river—vast in her giving and compas-sion, both to her family and friends in her personal life and to her patients in her professional life as a nurse. From the photo I took that day in the sublime cemetery (Figure 11.2), you can see why I began to get fleeting recollections and intimations of Walt Whitman's *Leaves of Grass* as we placed Agnes's ashes in the grave next to her husband's. The cemetery's green canopy of trees and carpet of grass were both a soothing balm and a clear call to my soul, which felt deeply linked to the soul of my mother-in-law and, as Walt Whitman put it, the souls of "black folks . . . White, Kanuck, Tuckhoe, Congressman." I felt my soul resonating with the soul of the river and the soul of the town and the soul of my mother-in-law, all participating in the uniquely Midwestern incarnation of the American soul. Here is how Whitman wrote about leaves of grass, the death of old and young alike, and the meeting of individual soul and the American soul in his long poem "Song of Myself:"

1
I celebrate myself, and sing myself,
And what I assume you shall assume,
For every atom belonging to me as good belongs to you.
I loafe and invite my soul,
I lean and loafe at my ease observing a spear of summer grass.
My tongue, every atom of my blood, form'd from this soil, this air,
Born here of parents born here from parents the same, and their parents the
    same,

. . .
31
I believe a leaf of grass is no less than the journey-work of the stars.[4]

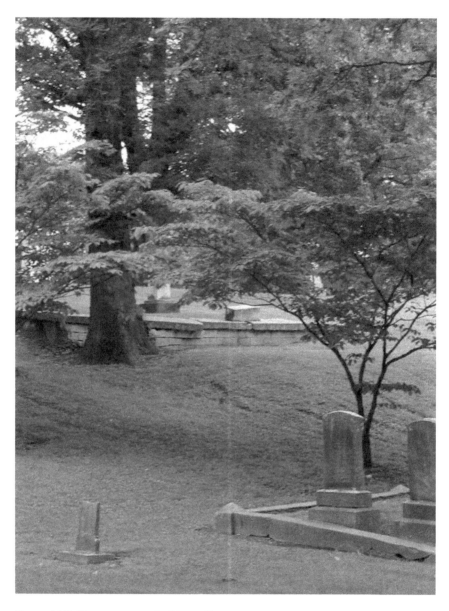

Figure 11.2 The cemetery in Alton, IL.

In Section 21 of "Song of Myself," Whitman proclaims himself the bard of the American soul when he writes, "I am the poet of the Body and I am the poet of the Soul."[5] He is writing of the body and the soul of America, which he likens to a blade of grass whose very existence mirrors the "journey-work of the stars" in its immortality. At Agnes's service, "a blade of grass" allowed me to participate for a moment in the immortality of her soul and the American soul.

On July 4, the day following Agnes's memorial service, my family went down to the Mississippi River to join in the holiday's festivities. We were at peace with ourselves and open to participating in the celebration of our nation's birth in the knowledge that we had truly accomplished the purpose of our ritual journey home. If you have not celebrated the Fourth of July by the banks of the Mississippi, I urge you to do so before you become a leaf of grass. Quite unexpectedly, I discovered there another forgotten part of Whitman's "Song of Myself" whispering to my soul as I wandered among the day's celebrants—adults guzzling beer and listening to rock and roll music as the children danced and played and jumped up and down by the river's edge.

32
I think I could turn and live with animals, they are so placid and self-contain'd,
I stand and look at them long and long.
They do not sweat and whine about their condition,
They do not lie awake in the dark and weep for their sins,
They do not make me sick discussing their duty to God,
Not one is dissatisfied, not one is demented with the mania of owning things,
Not one kneels to another, nor to his kind that lived thousands of years ago,
Not one is respectable or unhappy over the whole earth.
. . .
52
The spotted hawk swoops by and accuses me, he complains of my gab and my
    loitering.
I too am not a bit tamed, I too am untranslatable,
I sound my barbaric yawp over the roofs of the world.[6]
I too am not a bit tamed, I too am untranslatable,
I sound my barbaric yawp over the roofs of the world.

What is a "barbaric yawp?" Why did the quintessential poet of the American soul, Walt Whitman, link the "barbaric yawp" to the American soul? There are two parts to Whitman's phrase, a phrase that now brings up some 110,000 "hits" on a Google Internet search. "Barbaric" means "without civilizing influences, uncivilized, primitive," and a "yawp" is a "loud, harsh cry." Neither "barbaric" nor "yawp" suggests a civilized approach to things. Taken together, they signify a primitive enthusiasm in the form of a nonverbal cry from the essential nature of a living being. In Whitman's imagination, the essence of the American soul is neither civilized nor verbal. The "barbaric yawp" is the fierce "voice" of a soul that is essentially unrestrained and exulting in its self-expression.

George W. Bush's Texas swagger and his inarticulate utterances are heard by many in America as some sort of cry from our country's "body and soul." One has to accept the fact that he and those who follow him are as much a part of the American soul and its "barbaric yawp" as our more progressive sensibilities. My linking of George W. Bush to the "barbaric yawp" is intended to be both ironic and absolutely serious simultaneously. Who are we to know what or who contains the "barbaric yawp?" Who has a legitimate claim on the American soul? Again, what is the American soul?

Steven Herrmann, a Jungian with a deep scholarly interest in Whitman, wrote to me:

> Whitman's "yawp" is a *conscious* cry from the Soul of America to make the barbarian in American political democracy conscious! The "barbaric yawp" is Whitman's call from the depths of the American Soul to awaken the possibility of hope in a brighter future for American democracy.

Hermann went on to write:

> The aim of Whitman's "barbaric yawp" was to sound a new heroic message of "Happiness," Hope, and "Nativity" over the roofs of the world, to sound a primal cry which must remain essentially "unsaid" because it rests at the core of the American soul and cannot be found in "any dictionary, utterance, symbol" [*Leaves,* Section # 50]. The "barbaric yawp" is a metaphorical utterance for something "untranslatable," a primal cry from the depths of the American Soul for the emergence of man as a spiritual human being in whom the aims of liberty and equality have been fully realized and in whom the opposites of love and violence, friendship and war, have been unified at a higher political field of order than anything we have formerly seen in America. His "yawp" is an affect state, a spiritual cry of "Joy" and "Happiness" prior to the emergence of language.[7]

As Hermann notes, Whitman's image of man's emergence as a spiritual being

> refers to a person that can realize his earthly existence within the context of his total life pattern, including his depths of erotic passion. Whitman's barbarian is both a spiritual and a sexual being. He is not split inside, but whole and conscious of his full instinctive nature and lives it out according to the preference of his Soul.

In contemporary America, Whitman's "barbaric yawp" is as inclusive of the violence found in the television show *The Sopranos* as it is of the unitary vision of Martin Luther King's "I Have a Dream." This suggests expanding our national imagination to embrace the American soul's "barbaric yawp" as both vulgar and compassionate at the same time. It was the genius of Whitman to see in "the barbaric yawp" of the American soul the capacity for an interconnected transcendent unity.

This section on the soul of America would not be complete without mentioning one final example of how glimpses of the American soul come through individual encounters that open up a window or interface between the individual soul and the

larger, collective soul of the group. As she was gestating a novel on slavery, freedom, and the black experience, Toni Morrison tells us in her Preface to *Beloved,*
she met her main character in the following way:

> I sat on the porch, rocking in a swing, looking at giant stones piled up to take
> the river's occasional fist. Above the stones is a path through the lawn, but
> interrupted by an ironwood gazebo situated under a cluster of trees and in
> deep shade.
>
>   She walked out of the water, climbed the rocks, and leaned against the
> gazebo. Nice hat.
>
>   So she [Beloved] was there from the beginning, and except for me, eve-
> rybody (the characters) knew it—a sentence that later became "The women
> in the house knew it." The figure most central to the story would have to be
> her, the murdered, not the murderer, the one who lost everything and had no
> say in any of it.[8]

Like Perry's American Indian with the tomahawk, this is a soul figure that appears
out of nowhere, or as Jungians might say "out of the unconscious"—personal,
cultural, and collective. She emerges out of the water and presents herself to Toni
Morrison, who is trying to figure out how to create a novel based on the true story
of "Margaret Garner, a young mother who, having escaped slavery, was arrested
for killing one of her children (and trying to kill the others) rather than let them be
returned to the owner's plantation."[9]

The soul figure with the "nice hat" who greets Toni Morrison becomes the
central character in her novel, *Beloved.* Beloved is the soul of a murdered inno-
cent, which becomes a conduit for the voices of all of the other black people who
perished in slavery and its aftermath. These collective voices are as deep a part of
the American soul as John Perry's American Indian or Walt Whitman's barbaric
yawp. Here is how another character from the novel, Stamp Paid, understands the
collective "roaring" soul sound that surrounds the house where Beloved has taken
up residence with her mother:

> [H]e believed the undecipherable language clamoring around the house was
> the mumbling of the black and angry dead. Very few had died in bed, like
> Baby Suggs, and none that he knew of, including Baby, had lived a liva-
> ble life. Even the educated colored: the long-school people, the doctors, the
> teachers, the paper-writers and businessmen had a hard row to hoe. In addi-
> tion to having to use their heads to get ahead, they had the weight of the whole
> race sitting there. You needed two heads for that. Whitepeople believed that
> whatever the manners, under every dark skin was a jungle. Swift unnaviga-
> ble waters, swinging screaming baboons, sleeping snakes, red gums ready
> for their sweet white blood. In a way, he thought, they were right. The more
> coloredpeople spent their strength trying to convince them how gentle they
> were, how clever and loving, how human, the more they used themselves up

to persuade whites of something Negroes believed could not be questioned, the deeper and more tangled the jungle grew inside.

But it wasn't the jungle blacks brought with them to this place from the other (livable) place. It was the jungle whitefolks planted in them. And it grew. It spread. In, through and after life, it spread, until it invaded the whites who had made it. Touched them every one. Changed and altered them. Made them bloody, silly, worse than even they wanted to be, so scared were they of the jungle they had made. The screaming baboon lived under their own white skin; the red gums were their own.

Meantime, the secret spread of this new kind of whitefolks' jungle was hidden, silent, except once in a while when you could hear its mumbling in places like 124.[10]

The "undecipherable language" that Morrison describes in her novel is as much a voice of the American soul as Whitman's primal barbaric yawp. It is filled with the "roaring" sound of the "black and angry dead" and the "mumbling" sound of the white race's collective projection onto blacks, which is portrayed as the "whitefolks' jungle" of "swift unnavigable waters, swinging screaming baboons, sleeping snakes, red gums ready for their sweet white blood." Beloved becomes the spokesperson for a part of our American soul that is as much with us today as when Margaret Garner murdered her baby girl rather than return her to slavery.

Like any other soul, the American soul seeks incarnation in a specific place, specific time, specific event, and even a specific person or groups of people. This specificity of incarnation loves location and the right person(s) at the right moment. This very specificity means that many places and times in American history can claim some piece of the American soul as their own. At the same time, the American soul should not be thought of as bound to any particular person or group, any special place on the continent, or any unique time in our nation's history. As a whole, the American soul is much broader than its particularity and specificity, reaching as far back as the American Indians' migration across the Bering Strait and as far forward as one can imagine hearing Whitman's barbaric yawp.

PART TWO: HOW DOES THE AMERICAN SOUL EXPRESS ITSELF IN POLITICS?

> We all have complexes; it is a highly banal and uninteresting fact. . . . It is only interesting to know what people do with their complexes; that is the practical question which matters.[11]

In the second section of this chapter, I want to add "politics" to the already fermenting "soul-of-America" brew that I have been stirring. The first ingredient for the political part of this American soul concoction that comes to mind is a strangely beautiful book by Doris Lessing, *Briefing for a Descent into Hell*.[12] The central part of the novel takes its lead from the Platonic myth that this world is only a veiled shadow of the world of ideal forms. Indeed, the main character, Charles Watkins, leads us on a science-fiction journey of his inner world, in which he discovers that each individual soul is briefed before its descent to earth and its human incarnation through birth on earth. Earth itself is described as a "poisonous hell" for which the soul needs to be prepared. This is the "briefing" of the soul, just as birth as a human is the "descent."

For many Jungians, the inner world is primary and participation in the politics of the earthly realm is in fact a "poisonous hell." Some prefer to avoid politics altogether in favor of other, "deeper" soul work. We all know something about the soul's disillusionment when it participates in the everyday politics of institutional life—be it in the Jungian community or national presidential elections. In my own personal experience, I came away from intense engagement in Senator Bill Bradley's 2000 campaign for the Democratic Party's nomination for president feeling burned by the "poisonous hell" of earthly politics. Out of that experience (which I am sure is matched by many similar experiences among this book's readers in the political arena), I would like to share some reflections on how I am currently thinking about the relationship between politics and the American soul.

First, I do not think that the soul of America is to be located in identification with one party or the other. Neither party possesses the soul of America. Presumably, the soul of a right-wing fundamentalist is as engaged with the journey of the American soul as the soul of a progressive liberal. Nor do I think the soul of America is located in one specific issue or another, whether it be abortion, immigration, discrimination based on race or other differences, gay marriage, the environment, the war in Iraq, or a host of other compelling issues.

Usually, a discussion of politics focuses on the rough and tumble of political struggle, 95% of which is about how to gain and exercise power. But I am going to turn the traditional discussion of politics as it relates to power a bit upside down in this meditation and focus not on Machiavelli but on some basic, recurring collective psychological themes and tensions that have coursed through our political history. These recurring themes embody deep-seated conflicts in our nation's psyche, in which neither side of the ambivalences and tensions has an exclusive claim on meaning or correctness. Both sides have a legitimate claim to soul.

The psychological form in which these recurring conflicts take shape over generations is what I have been exploring in the concept of "cultural complexes."[13] Each culture has its own version of how to work out basic human tensions and conflicts. The uniqueness of a culture's way of experiencing these basic human problems becomes embodied in its cultural complexes, which then play themselves out in political life. Sunnis or Shi'ites do not have the same way of dealing with their problems as Midwesterners or Southerners.

In speaking about individual complexes as revealed by the Word Association Test, Jung wrote, "Our destinies are as a rule the outcome of our psychological tendencies."[14] Another way of saying this is that our personal complexes are the hand that Fate has dealt us. How we play the hand that Fate has dealt us, or what we do with our personal complexes, determines who we become as individuals. Jung put it rather bluntly: "We all have complexes; it is a highly banal and uninteresting fact. . . . It is only interesting to know what people do with their complexes; that is the practical question which matters."[15] I believe that the same is true of our cultural complexes. What we do with our cultural complexes determines not only who we become as a people but the destiny of the American soul. A good deal of our working out (or not working out) of our cultural complexes occurs in the political arena.

Cultural complexes, underpinned by archetypal patterns, form the core of those highly charged struggles that have defined who we are as an American people throughout our national history. Such cultural complexes accrue a memory of their own, a point of view of their own, and a tendency to collect new experiences in contemporary life that validate their unchanging points of view. Cultural complexes also tend to fire off autonomously and with deep emotion when an event triggers them. We know that a cultural complex may well be on the scene when there is a highly aroused emotional reaction to current events. Emotional reactivity of the collective psyche is the calling card of a cultural complex.

For instance, our more than 300-year conflict around race, as mirrored in the clamoring voices of *Beloved* in the first section of this chapter, is an example of an entrenched cultural complex that is always ready to detonate in the psyches of whites and blacks.

My thesis, then, is that the American soul is embedded in our various cultural complexes. Furthermore, our cultural complexes are what give political life its dynamism and its content. Both the energy and the issues of political debate spring from the autonomous, highly charged emotional material of our core cultural complexes. Political life is the natural social arena in which cultural complexes play themselves out. We forge the American soul in our struggle with our cultural complexes. In the political arena, cultural complexes seem mostly to generate heat, division, and hatred; they are inflammatory and polarizing; they usually end in a stalemate without any resolution, only to recur in the next election or the next generation; sometimes they are ignored or kept unconscious for decades; occasionally they can be worked out slowly in engagement, compromise, reconciliation, and healing after generations of recurring battle. In short, they behave like complexes.

We might now reframe the question about the relationship of politics to the American soul as follows: "What are we doing with our cultural complexes in political life?" Or perhaps the question may be better phrased, "What are our cultural complexes doing with us in our political life?" In order to explore those questions, we need to ask, "What are our primary cultural complexes?" As a way of answering these questions, I would like to offer a list of themes or "relationships" around which cultural complexes have formed in the American psyche over the course of our nation's history.

As I briefly consider each of these relationships, I will refer to "soul-making" and whether it appears to be happening around specific cultural complexes. I imagine soul-making as potentially occurring when there is a legitimate claim for something of deepest human value on both sides of a conflict that has come alive in the collective psyche and has been engaged in the political arena. I hope that the reader will keep in mind that the seven American cultural complexes that I outline here interweave with one another in a tangled skein and are by no means as clear or as simple as I sketch them.

Our Relationship to Money, Commerce, and Consumer Goods

Core Attitude of Cultural Complex

One of the highest values in American society has been the accumulation of personal wealth and material goods, often at the expense of or in disregard for the common good. This complex emphasizes individual achievement in the material world. On the positive side of this complex is the promised opportunity for every person to maximize his or her material well-being. The negative side of this cultural complex emphasizes our collective and individual right to eat the world, own the world, amass personal wealth, and continuously increase the gross national product. In the name of participating in the American Dream, consumerism has become almost synonymous with the highest good.[16]

Specific Current Political Issue: Campaign Finance Reform

In an attempt to curb the equation of material wealth with the common good, recent attempts have been made to introduce campaign finance reform as a way of equalizing the role of money in a democratic society. These attempts have been "dead on arrival" and have been undermined by both parties. On this issue, there is no soul-making occurring in either major political party. There is little meaningful engagement in the political arena with the overemphasis on money and consumerism in our civic life or in our political life. We are soul-dead with regard to active, conscious engagement of this cultural complex. Our collective psyche is consumed by its consumerism. (Al-Qaeda was very conscious of this when it attacked the World Trade Center.)

Our Relationship to the Natural Environment

Core Attitude of Cultural Complex

Historically, we have been a country of vast and seemingly unlimited natural resources. This has fostered a cultural complex based on the belief that this blessing entitles us to everything we want and that we own everything in the natural world. A growing number of people have come to understand that stewardship is the responsibility that goes along with the privilege of vast but dwindling natural resources.

Specific Current Political Issues

There are a host of ongoing political debates related to the environment that suggest soul-making is going on with regard to this cultural complex. These include policy conflicts about global warming, clean air and water, the limitation of natural resources, and the desire to use those limited resources wisely.

Our Relationship to the Human Community, Including Family Life, Social Life, and the Life Cycle From Conception to Death

Core Attitude of Cultural Complex

This country was built on a belief in the inalienable rights and freedoms of the individual as much as it was on utopian communalism. A core American cultural complex spins out of the unending dynamic tension between the myth of the self-sufficient individual in opposition to the welfare of the community as a whole and the reality of the community's responsibility to the individual. The good of the whole and all of its members is endlessly challenged by the rights of the individual.

Specific Current Political Issues

This cultural complex is ubiquitous in our political debates and makes itself known in all sorts of issues that range from the right to bear arms and taxation to national health-care policy and how to fund pensions and Social Security. Again, national soul-making appears to be going on in the engagement of this cultural complex. The debate over the rights and responsibilities of the individual in relation to the needs of the collective and its responsibilities to all of its members engages citizens across the political spectrum.

Our Relationship to the Spiritual Realm

Core Attitude of Cultural Complex

Our Puritan heritage launched our country both in dissent and in a tradition of strict belief in moralistic behavior. The belief that America has a special relationship to God fuels our sense of national entitlement, which is matched only by our strong tradition of religious dissent, which drives our national skepticism about privileged authority, divine or otherwise. Out of these twin foundational attitudes grew our tradition of the separation of church and state. Inclusive pluralism and dogmatic fundamentalism are the vying poles of a uniquely American cultural complex that is the psychological inheritance of our religious traditions. As in many other countries, the archetypal split between good and evil in our collective psyche projects itself onto many political issues, from the clash over abortion to the debate about the war in Iraq.

Specific Current Political Issue: Abortion

Perhaps about as much soul-making has been going on around this issue as around any in recent political history. Although the issue has generated murderous heat, it has also raised fundamental questions about the nature of soul and life, which, to my mind, are part of any healthy debate in society. The clash of religious fundamentalism with the rights of a woman to make choices about her own body in a society that values the separation of church and state cuts across so many of our cultural complexes that I think it forces everyone to sort out what he or she believes on an incredibly difficult series of issues. That is soul-making. It has turned many things upside down in our society. For instance, conservatives most often align themselves with the rights of the self-sufficient individual and progressives tend to side with the needs of all in the community. But on the issue of abortion, progressives uphold the right to individual choice, while conservatives argue for a community value that applies to all.

Our Relationship to Race, Ethnicity, and Gender— All of the "Others"

Core Attitude of Cultural Complex

There have been two distinct poles in the American cultural complex with regard to race, ethnicity, and gender. As much as in any other country in the world, inclusiveness in terms of race, ethnicity, and gender has been part of our national character and its proud "melting-pot" history. But ever since the nation's inception, the radioactive background behind the apparent embrace of diversity has been the premise that white, Anglo-Saxon, heterosexual men were destined to dominate the nation.

Specific Current Political Issues: Same-Sex Marriage and Immigration

The powerful unconscious hold of the cultural complex of discrimination on the basis of sex, race, ethnicity, and age has been challenged on multiple levels simultaneously in the past several decades. Indeed, the assault on the established complex has been so thorough that the new cultural complex replacing it—"political correctness"—has itself become the dominant persona of the collective, behind which lurks the shadow of stereotyping on the basis of differences. In a sense, white male dominance and the embracing of diversity can be thought of as two sides of the same coin of this cultural complex. But, most importantly for our discussion, soul-making in the collective psyche is occurring at unprecedented speed with regard to the active engagement of this complex in such potent current political issues as same-sex marriage and immigration, and in the fact that, for the first time in American history, a black man, a woman, and a Mormon are running simultaneously for the presidential nomination.

Our Relationship to Speed, Height, Youth, Progress, and Celebrity

Core Attitude of Cultural Complex

As the "new land," America has always been identified with what is new—a new land with new people and new ideas, faster, higher, younger, ever progressing, ever renewing itself. The wedding of celebrity, charisma, and ingenuity are forever the hope of the American Dream and American politics. The new land gave substance to the belief in our nation's unique destiny, poignantly portrayed in John Gast's *American Progress* from 1872 (Figure 11.3). This wonderful illustration shows an archetypal anima figure who serves as a symbolic image of the American soul's identification with "Progress." "She"—the American soul as Progress—floats at the core of a national cultural complex of entitlement, exceptionalism, and the American Dream.

Specific Current Political Issue: Stem Cell Research

This political debate has tremendous potential for soul-making in the collective psyche because it pits what is "God-given" against what is "new." Surely, there is soul on both sides of the debate. Our addiction to creating something newer, quicker, easier, and better is a source of American ingenuity and prosperity. It endlessly challenges what has existed for a long time, if not forever. For many, what has existed forever is good enough, and for some it is even God's will.

Our Relationship to the World Beyond Our Borders

Core Attitude of Cultural Complex

The theme of the freedom of the individual vs. the individual's responsibility to the whole is writ large in the cultural complex of our relationship to the broader world beyond American borders. In this case, our nation arrogates for itself, as a nation, the same rights as the individual, whose freedom it sees as paramount. As an "individual" nation, we place our economic and security interests, for the most part, above our responsibility to the global community as a whole. The tension between the freedom of the individual and the individual's responsibility to the whole in this complex joins forces with another cultural complex—our sense of entitlement, which comes from our view of ourselves as exceptional and therefore as knowing what is best for the world. These two cultural complexes are acted out in peculiar ways—we wage war in other parts of the world in the name of individual freedoms just as easily as we retreat from broader engagement in the world in the name of individualistic isolationism, which renounces responsibility to the broader whole.

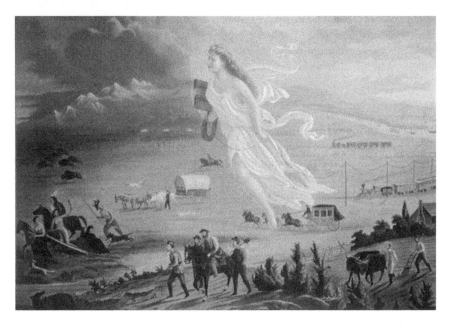

Figure 11.3 John Gast's *American Progress* (1872). In John Gast's *American Progress*, a diaphanously and scantily clad woman, representing America, floats westward through the air with the "Star of Empire" on her forehead. She has left the cities of the East behind and the wide Mississippi, and still her course is westward. In her right hand, she carries a schoolbook, a testimonial to the National Enlightenment, while in her left she trails the slender wires of the telegraph, which will bind the nation together. Fleeing her approach are Indians, buffalo, wild horses, bears, and other game, all of which disappear into the storm and waves of the Pacific Coast. They flee the wondrous vision—the star "is too much for them."

Source: Adapted from a contemporary description of Gast's painting, written by George Crofutt, who distributed his engraving of it widely. http://www.csubak.edu/~gsantos/ img0061.html.

Specific Current Political Issues

The American-led war in Iraq is a horrific contemporary example of how a cultural complex (or more than one cultural complex) can seize the collective psyche and come alive in politics. Part of the motivation for waging this war grew out of a deep-seated American belief that affirms the unique destiny of our people as guardians of democratic principles and therefore as exceptional, blessed by God with endless opportunity, and perhaps even eternal youth and immortality as a nation. The conduct of the Iraq War has revealed the flaws in a cultural complex that puts the nation's rugged individualism ahead of a sense of responsibility to and participation in the global community. The experiences of the wars in Vietnam and now Iraq have begun the slow process of challenging these core beliefs that sit at the heart of those fundamental American cultural complexes in which our fierce individualism joins forces with our sense of entitlement and exceptionalism. As the deflation of bankrupt policies settles into the collective psyche, one hopes that this terrible misadventure has had its soul-making impact on the body politic.

Conclusion

In each of the broad areas that I have characterized as cultural complexes, a set of specific issues takes center stage at any given time in the political life of our country. In the great crucible of politics, where our core cultural complexes enter the political life of the nation, the American soul is forged and crucified—made, remade, unmade, made again—over and over. These autonomous psychological clusters of memory, affect, and repetitive historical behavior seize our collective psyche in an endless round of racial strife, economic striving, gender warfare, and unending worship of technology, progress, speed, height, information, youth, innocence, moral simplicity, heroic achievement, and insatiable consumerism, all of which have addicted the entire nation—Democrats, Republicans, independents, and the uncommitted alike. It is the "barbaric yawp" of the American soul embodied in political life.

Signs of soul life can clearly be detected in the growing conflict around our relationship to the natural environment. Such signs can also be detected in the intensifying struggles and rapidly changing collective attitudes toward race, gender, and sexual identity. In these particular cultural complexes, the American soul seems to be transforming itself through highly engaged political activity. On the other hand, our country is so addicted to money, to speed, to youth, to consumerism, and to progress that our collective soul seems lost or invisible in our possession by these complexes. Our national politics with regard to these possessions seems hopelessly unengaged and unconscious. Lively debate on the current political issues generated by these underlying cultural complexes that course through our history like an underground river is essential to the continuing growth of our collective psyche and our individual souls as well.

The politics of the day that challenge our more entrenched cultural complexes are met with the same kind of fierce resistance from groups that an analyst encounters when asking a patient to take on or confront a personal complex—or that the ego faces when it encounters the unconscious resistance of an entrenched complex, which it does its best to keep from being known or made conscious. Frankly, I was surprised, in taking this most approximate inventory of our cultural complexes, that I reached the conclusion that soul-making activity is taking place in so many areas of our political life. At the outset of writing this chapter, I would have said that there was little happening in our political life that suggested soul. Of course, many readers may disagree with my conclusions.

Many in our country would prefer that the sound of our national soul be less of a yawp and closer to the "om" of Hinduism. "Om" evokes compassion, peace, reverence, and unity. To make a bad pun, om is a far cry from Whitman's primal barbaric yawp. But the reality is that the sound of the American soul is more messy than om, and when the barbaric yawp sounds its discordant note in politics, it is rarely unifying or resonant of deep compassion. Rather, at its best, it vibrates with dynamism, energy, and the promise of renewal. Perhaps we should be most afraid of the time in our country when the mix of politics and soul has left us so deadened by disillusionment and distrust that we are unable even to hear the barbaric yawp.

Notes

1 Thomas Singer, ed., *The Vision Thing: Myth, Politics and Psyche in the World* (London and New York: Routledge, 2000).
2 George Seferis, "Argonauts," in *Collected Poems: 1924–1955,* trans., ed., and intro by Edmund Keeley and Philip Sherrard (Princeton, NJ: Princeton University Press, 1967), p. 9.
3 Personal communication from John Perry.
4 Walt Whitman, "Song of Myself," in *Walt Whitman: The Complete Poems* (London: Penguin Books, 2004), pp. 63, 68–69, 93.
5 Ibid., p. 83.
6 Ibid., pp. 94, 124, emphasis added.
7 Personal communication from Steven Herrmann.
8 Toni Morrison, *Beloved* (New York: Vintage Books, 1987), p. xviii.
9 Ibid., p. xvii.
10 Ibid., p. 234.
11 C. G. Jung, *Analytical Psychology: Its Theory and Practice,* The Tavistock Lectures, Lecture 3 (New York: Vintage Books, 1968), p. 94.
12 Doris Lessing, *Briefing for a Descent into Hell* (London: Vintage Books, 1981).
13 See Thomas Singer, "The Cultural Complex and Archetypal Defenses of the Collective Spirit: Baby Zeus, Elian Gonzales, Constantine's Sword, and Other Holy Wars," *The San Francisco Library Journal* 20, no. 4 (2002): 4–28; Thomas Singer, "Cultural Complexes and Archetypal Defenses of the Group Spirit," in *Terror, Violence and the Impulse to Destroy,* ed. John Beebe (Zürich: Daimon Verlag, 2003), pp. 191–209; and Thomas Singer and Samuel L. Kimbles, eds., *The Cultural Complex: Contemporary Jungian Perspectives on Psyche and Society* (London and New York: Brunner-Routledge, 2004).
14 C. G. Jung, "Freud and Psychoanalysis," *The Collected Works of C. G. Jung,* Vol. 4., trans. R. F. C. Hull (Princeton, NJ: Princeton University Press, 1961), para. 309.
15 C. G. Jung, *Analytical Psychology: Its Theory and Practice,* The Tavistock Lectures, Lecture 3 (New York: Pantheon Books, 1968), p. 94.
16 Jack Beatty, *Age of Betrayal: The Triumph of Money in America, 1865–1900* (New York: Alfred Knopf, 2007).

Selected Bibliography

Beatty, Jack. *Age of Betrayal: The Triumph of Money in America, 1865–1900.* New York: Alfred Knopf, 2007.
Gellert, M. *The Fate of America: An Inquiry into National Character.* Washington, DC: Brassey's Inc., 2001.
Henderson, J. "The Archetype of Culture." In *The Archetype.* Proceedings of the 2nd International Congress for Analytical Psychology. Ed. Adolf Guggenbuhl-Craig. Basel and New York: S. Karger, 1962/1964.

Henderson, J. "The Cultural Unconscious." In *Shadow and Self: Selected Papers in Analytical Psychology*. Wilmette, IL: Chiron Publications, 1990, pp. 103–113.

Herrmann, Steven. "The Cultural Complex in Walt Whitman." *The San Francisco Jung Institute Library Journal* 23, no. 4 (2004): 34–62.

Herrmann, Steven. "Walt Whitman and the Homoerotic Imagination." *The Jung Journal Culture and Psyche* 1, no. 2 (2007): 16–47.

Jung, C. G. *Freud and Psychoanalysis*. Princeton, NJ: Princeton University Press, 1961.

Jung, C. G. *Analytical Psychology: Its Theory and Practice*. The Tavistock Lectures. New York: Pantheon Books, 1968.

Kalsched, D. *The Inner World of Trauma: Archetypal Defenses of the Personal Spirit*. London and New York: Routledge, 1996.

Kimbles, Samuel L. "The Cultural Complex and the Myth of Invisibility." In *The Vision Thing*. Ed. Thomas Singer. London: Routledge, 2000, pp. 157–169.

Lessing, Doris. *Briefing for a Descent into Hell*. London: Vintage Books, 1981.

Morrison, Toni. *Beloved*. New York: Vintage Books, 1987.

Packer, George. *The Assassins' Gate: America in Iraq*. New York: Farrar, Strauss and Giroux, 2005.

Perry, J. "Emotions and Object Relations." *The Journal of Analytical Psychology* 15, no. 1 (1970): 1–12.

Samuels, Andrew. *The Political Psyche*. London and New York: Routledge, 1993.

Seferis, George. *Collected Poems: 1924–1955*. Trans., ed., and intro. Edmund Keeley and Philip Sherrard. Princeton, NJ: Princeton University Press, 1967.

Singer, Thomas, ed. *The Vision Thing: Myth, Politics and Psyche in the World*. London and New York: Routledge, 2000.

Singer, Thomas. "The Cultural Complex and Archetypal Defenses of the Collective Spirit: Baby Zeus, Elian Gonzales, Constantine's Sword, and Other Holy Wars." *The San Francisco Library Journal* 20, no. 4 (2002): 4–28.

Singer, Thomas. "Cultural Complexes and Archetypal Defenses of the Group Spirit." In *Terror, Violence and the Impulse to Destroy*. Ed. John Beebe. Zürich: Daimon Verlag, 2003, pp. 191–209.

Singer, Thomas and Samuel L. Kimbles, eds. *The Cultural Complex: Contemporary Jungian Perspectives on Psyche and Society*. London and New York: Brunner-Routledge, 2004.

Chapter 12

Murray Stein

As I get older – I am now in the middle of my eighth decade – and look back to evaluate the motivations, passions, and activities that have driven and sustained me consistently through my life, I ask, "Are they the same today as they were before?"

I realize that one of my greatest pleasures has been the joy of learning, and this remains as compelling and sustaining as ever. I have also realized in retrospect that my teachers in high school, at universities, and at the Jung Institute in Zürich have been marvelous guides into the life of the mind. Reading and learning have given me great pleasure and joy in the past, as they still do in the present.

What about aesthetics? I wouldn't say that I absolutely live for beauty in the way an aesthete like Oscar Wilde did, but it is important to me nevertheless, even if at a more moderate level. I don't think I would want to live in an ugly world. I am not a true stoic, although it is in my blood from my mother's side of the family, who were German Baptist pioneers in the wilderness of nineteenth-century Saskatchewan, Canada. I look for beauty and find it in many places: in nature, in the beautiful city of Zürich at certain times of day in the calendar year (especially the fall and winter), in music and art, in cinema, in noble animals. I am fascinated with the human face, and when a smile opens a somber face wide and makes the eyes sparkle, I feel joy in my whole being

Nowadays the prospect of becoming "enlightened" attracts my attention and interest more than it did in the past. Can one justifiably anticipate growing in wisdom with age? I don't think it is automatic or a given of human nature, because many people have died in advanced age without the grace of discernible enlightenment. This development seems to depend on cultivating mindfulness and imagination in a specific way. I follow the instructions for active imagination as I've learned about them in Jung's writings and studied how this process develops in *The Red Book*. And dreams, my own and those of others who share theirs with me, often bring me to a flash of enlightenment. They suggest enlightenment, if in a realm beyond ego consciousness.

I must also mention the importance of "service" in my life. This is an abiding motivation that keeps me going, even when the waves are high and the troughs between them are deep. From my father and mother I inherited an indefatigable

DOI: 10.4324/9781003148982-13

sense of service. My father was a pastor, and the last words I heard him speak as he lay dying and some fellow pastors were visiting him in hospital were "I would still like to be of service!" He said this with tears in his eyes. I have had the same sense of willing obligation to serve a community, and in my case it has been the community of Jungians worldwide.

A most important item, which is the foundation of a satisfying life for me, is relationships – family, wife, children, friends, colleagues, students, analysands, and neighbors. If any one of these is disturbed, especially the close ones, I quickly lose a zest for life. My emotional stability depends absolutely on close and harmonious relationships. On this everything else depends.

I have used the phrase *amor fati* over the years to express a particular feeling I often have about my life. With all its twists and turns, beginnings and endings, openings and closings of doors and windows of opportunity, my life has shown a distinct pattern of meaningful coincidences. I call this grace. For instance, my interest in Jungian psychology began by chance in a conversation at a garden party on a Sunday afternoon in 1968. After that, I became fascinated by Jung's mind and attitude toward life. A year after my first chance encounter with Jung's writings, I found myself enrolled in the training program at the Jung Institute in Zürich to become a Jungian analyst. In retrospect, I would say that most, if not all, of the most important decisions in my life have had the element of synchronicity at their center.

Age intensifies one's focus on the center and brings the essential matters and values more clearly to the fore. It is a return to the self. For me, these later years have been a time of gathering in and subjecting the contents accumulated previously from so many sources to a process of distillation. One hopes a *grand cru* will come of it.

Murray Stein, Ph.D. Goldiwil, Switzerland 2020

On Jung's View of the Self—An Investigation

Originally published in (2008) *Journal of Analytical Psychology* 53, 3, 305–327. Reprinted with permission.

Jung's Self-Concept—Scale and Perspective

One does become weary dealing the question of whether the term "self" should be capitalized. I have struggled with this for years and gone back and forth. My fond hope is that, in this investigation, I will be able to conclude once and for all: there is one self only, not two. And let us not capitalize it, lest we confuse the self with Divinity. I have to add at the outset that I think "self" is an excellent term for what it is meant to denote, a real stroke of genius on Jung's part. Why? Because it is at once personal and impersonal, individual and universal. This is important because to tilt too far one way or the other would destroy its ability to capture the full scope of the meaning and psychological value it has when it retains this paradoxical unity.

Let me begin by observing that it is generally recognized by anyone even a little familiar with Jung's writings that he drew a critically important distinction between the meaning of the terms ego and self. On this point, the author was clear and consistent throughout. The distinction is a matter of scale and perspective. As a term, self refers to a psychic domain that encompasses all aspects of the ego complex and the surrounding penumbra of actual and potential consciousness, and it surpasses this nexus of psychic material in several respects: its range and scope of reference is greater in extension, in that it subsumes all conscious and unconscious levels and aspects of the psyche under its aegis. Its texture is there-fore also more complex, because it embraces all of the polarities and tensions within the psyche as a whole, not only those within consciousness and the ego complex, and its center of gravity transcends the conscious-unconscious divide. The self is responsible for the unity of the psyche as a whole, whereas the ego complex provides some measure of unity only for consciousness. The relation of these terms—ego and self—is that of a part to the whole. The ego is a part of the self, so one should be careful not to think of them as two separate and distinct psychic territories. When I say "I", it is the self speaking, but not the whole self, just the part I am speaking for at the moment. That would be the ego.

For the adult personality, the ego is defined as the center of consciousness and, therefore, also as the subject within the self-conscious person, while the self is defined as a virtual center and also (paradoxically) as the circumference of the whole psyche, conscious and unconscious, and the source of its full potential and state of unity. The self accounts for the unity of the personality before the ego is formed, as well as for its unity as a whole after ego formation and development have taken place.

With the notion of self, moreover, Jung was reaching intuitively and theoreti-cally for a psychological dimension that far exceeds the limits of individuals' usual *conscious* self-awareness, identity, sense of self, and experience of psychic reality. It is this notion in particular that constitutes the essential link between analytical psychology and explicitly religious forms of spirituality because it stretches to infinity. The "self" term takes our thinking beyond an everyday secular range of self-knowledge—be it ever so psychoanalytically well informed about complexes, instincts, archetypal images, phantasies, alpha function and beta particles, etc.—toward the unknown within, toward the mystery of existence, toward a personal relation to and possible inclusion in the infinite, and toward the *numinosum*. All of this comes under the heading of the self in analytical psychology. Within the ego complex we are focused, defined, and somewhat cognizant of our thoughts, feel-ings, and the grounds for our emotional conditions; we claim an identity more or less unified and singular, a sense of self that is bounded and unique. As the self, on the contrary, we are utterly indeterminate, infinitely potential, never fully realized, and linked to (even fused with) the Divine. The self links the ego complex to ultimate wholeness. It encompasses all of the psyche's inherent inner oppositions and obscurities, the shadows, and the numerous contradictions and riddles with which one has to live with respect to subtle and ever shifting foci of ego identity and identification. The self arches high up, rising above the abysses that cut through the personality, linking and containing the persona and the shadow (good and bad), the gendered ego complex and the anima-animus (masculine and feminine), and conscious and unconscious. Self is what we are above, beneath, and beyond all identities, identifications, and partial personalities—personal, cultural, historical, engendered, and moral. It is what we are when all that we know or suspect that we are is added together, *plus* what we are when all of that is stripped away— a surplus of psyche. We can extinguish the ego, but it is doubtful that we can kill the self. It is especially this *extra* that we want to investigate when we direct our attention to the self. And this is the task I have set for myself in this chapter.

An Ontological Grounding for the Self

Jung's *Mysterium Coniunctionis* is a late literary and theoretical meditation on the self. In it, albeit in obscure and indirect terms, he summarizes his reflections on the self as psychic totality and provides hints that would indicate a much larger than individual and personal, indeed an ontological and even metaphysical, grounding for the self. As the title indicates, the work is concerned especially with the self's polarities, as well as with the prospect for overcoming the psyche's chief divide, that between the conscious and the unconscious. At the outset, Jung boldly announces the *Gegensatzstruktur der Psyche* ("the polaristic structure of the psyche") as a given (Jung 1955/56, p. 15). (I will let Jung speak in his native German occasionally because the translation of some of these passages is a problem, and inevitably, as in all translations, there are some misleading errors.) The opus of alchemy was to unite the opposites, Jung declares, and this too is the goal of analysis. From here on, however, his way forward is anything but direct.

Mysterium is, like the psyche itself, replete with ambiguities, and for the translator it is a full-blown nightmare. My text for this chapter happens to be one of the thorny passages, in which Jung states a connection between the self and Divinity. It is one of many passages in Jung's works that link the human and the Divine; it is a particularly telling one, and one that happened to produce a mistranslation.

In the chapter titled "Luna," where Jung explores the symbolism of the moon with particular reference to the larger symbolism of the feminine in alchemy, there is a subsection called "The Dog." The image of the dog brings up for Jung the paradoxical definition of the self as something at once noble and base, as though one could think of it as the greatest treasure and a curse at the same time. In the original German, Jung writes, "*Der Hundesohn des KALID ist der hochgepriesene 'Sohn der Philosophen,' und damit wird die Ambiguität dieser Gestalt hervorgehoben: sie ist hellstes Licht und tiefste Nacht zugleich, also eine vollkommene coincidentia oppositorum, als welche die Göttlichkeit das Selbst ausdrückt*" (Jung 1955/56, para. 171).

Hull translates this as follows: "Kalid's 'son of the dog' is the same as the much extolled 'son of the philosophers.' The ambiguity of this figure is thus stressed: it is at once bright as day and dark as night, a perfect *coincidentia oppositorum* expressing the divine nature of the self" (para. 176 in the English version). "Son of the philosophers" is for Jung, as we know, an alchemical term that represents the self. Because "son of the philosophers" is designated by Kalid as "son of a dog," its ambiguity is evident. For the Arab author Kalid, "son of a dog" would be a curse; on the other hand, "son of the philosophers" is a most high and noble designation. Hence Jung's comment: it is the brightest light and the deepest night at the same time, a perfect "coincidence of opposites." The tension could not be greater within something at once so fine and so despicable, and yet at the same time this image depicts exactly what Jung is writing about in this book: the self as a union of opposites.

Then comes this treacherous German phrase: "*als welche die Göttlichkeit das Selbst ausdrückt.*" Hull translates this as "expressing the divine nature of the self." This is a misleading translation. More accurately, it would read, "as the Divinity expresses the self" or "as the self expresses the Divinity," but definitely NOT "expressing the divine nature of the self." Literally, *ausdrückt* means "expresses" (*aus* = ex; *drückt* = presses; my image for this is a hen laying an egg, "pressing it out"). It does not indicate identity of the two terms. The relation between them is not identity but a type of "expression" of one the other. I suspect Jung would have it both ways: the self expresses the Divinity AND the Divinity expresses the self. The relation is indicated in the term "expresses." It is a close relationship but not an identity.

As Jung announced at the beginning of *Mysterium*, the psyche is structured as a polarity, and now he adds that this structure is in some sense related to the Godhead. The structure of self-division into conscious and unconscious components, for instance, and into ego and shadow, noble and base, and high and low, is not only human but also Divine. The one reflects, or expresses, the other. The self is an expression of something beyond itself (*die Göttlichkeit*), but it is not identical with it or necessarily of the same substance. This will be important for any discussion of the self as a psychological and human factor, for if the self is seen as divine, the psychological self becomes critically removed from historical processes in the individual, a floating specter within the messiness of finite lived life.

It is no doubt significant that Jung uses the term *die Göttlichkeit* here rather than the simpler *Gott* (God). The term *die Göttlichkeit*[1] does not translate easily into English. It is a noun made from an adjective: *göttlich* = divine-like, like a deity, made of divine substance, or having the quality of divinity. *Die Göttlichkeit* does not refer to a specific god or goddess. As a noun, the attribute is made into a substance, as when we make the move in English from high to Highness, as in "Her Highness." A quality is turned into a substance, a being with a specific quality. *Göttlichkeit* is the quality that all of the specific gods and goddesses hold in common, something in which they all participate. *Göttlichkeit* is the quality that makes them divine and distinguishes them from non-divine beings.

Jung is not *equating* self with Divinity in this passage, nor is he saying that the self is divine; instead, he is bringing the terms into relation with one another. The idea is that *die Göttlichkeit* mirrors the self in the common pattern of *coincidentia oppositorum*. This is a non- or post-traditional restatement of the familiar biblical idea that humankind is created in the image of God (Genesis 1:27—"So God created man in his own image, in the image of God he created him; male and female he created them"). Jung clearly states a strong and intimate relation between the self and *die Göttlichkeit* (both as defined by the phrase, *coincidentia oppositorum*), but they are not identical. Jung is not reducing one to the other, of which he has been often accused by theologians and psychoanalysts.

Psychology or Theology?

Nevertheless, quite a few questions call for attention as one reflects on this passage. Is Jung subtly subsuming psychology under theology and setting up a kind of theologically based psychology with the Imago Dei doctrine as its centerpiece? Clearly, he is not borrowing the standard Christian version of the God image in this reference to *die Göttlichkeit*. For classical Christian theology, God is pure light and goodness, and in Him there is no darkness or shadow at all. This was the very doctrine to which Jung objected so frequently in his writings on Christianity, furiously disputing the *privatio boni* doctrine of evil[2] and critiquing the Christ image as one-sided because it splits off and leaves out the darkness of the shadow as represented in Satan. Jung argued that the Christian doctrine of God chooses to privilege one side of *die Göttlichkeit*, the light aspect, and to repress the other features. Jung's image of Divinity as "the brightest light and the deepest night at the same time, a perfect *coincidentia oppositorum*" is much closer as a figure to Abraxas, the deity he referenced in *Septem Sermones ad Mortuos* in 1916: "Abraxas begetteth truth and lying, good and evil, light and darkness, in the same word and in the same act" (Jung 1963, pp. 383–384). The Divinity that Jung finds in the form of *coincidentia oppositorum* is inclusive of the opposites good and evil, light and dark.

Given Jung's many references to Kant, it would be safer to assume that, for him, psychology supersedes theology and can therefore inform theology about the nature of ultimate reality, i.e., Divinity. It can, for example, guide theology away from one-sidedly privileging the light over the dark, which has been endemic to the three great monotheistic traditions. It is precisely this pull toward the tilting of God images in the direction of perfection, which reflects lopsided social and cultural biases as well, that has rendered these traditions passé and outmoded in the modern world.

It is also certainly not the case, however, that Jung was espousing a purely humanistic critique of religious faith and belief. In a vituperative exchange with the Jewish philosopher and theologian Martin Buber, who had accused him of being one of the chief figures responsible for the decline of religious faith in modernity, Jung explains his position on the relation of psychology to the articles of religious belief:

The fact is that the ego is confronted with psychic powers which from ancient times have borne sacred names, and because of these they have always been identified with metaphysical beings. Analysis of the unconscious has long since demonstrated the existence of the powers in the form of archetypal images which, be it noted, *are not identical with the corresponding intellectual concepts*. One can, of course, believe that the concepts of the conscious mind are, through the inspiration of the Holy Ghost, direct and correct representations of their metaphysical referent. But this conviction is possible only for one who already possesses the gift of faith. Unfortunately I cannot boast of this possession. . . . What I have described is a psychic factor only, but one which exerts a considerable influence on the conscious mind. Thanks to its autonomy, it forms the counterposition to the subjective ego because it is a piece of the *objective psyche*. It can therefore be designated as a "Thou."

(Jung 1952b, para. 1505)

Further,

The so-called "forces of the unconscious" are not intellectual concepts that can be arbitrarily manipulated, but dangerous antagonists which can, among other things, work frightful devastation in the economy of the personality. They are everything one could wish for or fear in a psychic "Thou."

(Ibid., para. 1504)

Here Jung is, of course, picking up on Buber's use of the term "Thou" to describe a certain type of relationship with a living other. Too often, to call these factors "merely psychic" reduces them to names and concepts and misses their living power and forcefulness, which Jung wants to emphasize.

The Self as Imago Dei

If *die Göttlichkeit* is only a reference to an extra-egoic *psychological* force—a living and dynamic factor, as Jung stresses in the preceding quotes—and indeed exclusively and without remainder refers to the most elemental and all-encompassing force that humans are capable of experiencing, imagining, conceiving, and projecting, i.e., the ultimate God image, this would reduce, that is, confine, it to the *psychological*, the archetype of the self. And the self *is* in Jung's view exactly such an ultimate central archetype of order and, clearly, in his view a *coincidentia oppositorum*. The monotheistic God image—provided it is not rendered insufficient and one-sided by idealizing defenses or is not simply the one God image that manages to gain priority and pre-eminence from among a plethora of them—is precisely such an inclusive figure and, therefore, an image of the self archetype. The gods and goddesses of polytheism, on the other hand, are lesser or subsidiary psychic forces, which in the end are united in and governed by the ultimate archetype of unity, the self. They represent the anima-animus level of the psyche, while the God image of the monotheisms represents the self, the ultimate psychic ground from which the lesser figures spring and by which they are united and controlled.

However, the term self is also meant to transcend the monotheistic God image, which *inevitably* tends toward one-sidedness and partiality. Jung says that he chose the term self

> in accordance with Eastern philosophy, which for centuries has occupied itself with the problems that arise when even the gods cease to incarnate. The philosophy of the Upanishads corresponds to a psychology that long ago recognized the relativity of the gods. This is not to be confused with a stupid error like atheism.[3]

Here the archetype of the self would be seen as the psychic agency responsible for any and every type of unifying image, theory, plan, or fantasy. In other words, it is the bottom line of any type of emergent orderedness.

This line of thought, however, would seem to contradict the view that Jung appears to express in *Mysterium*, namely, that the self is an expression of *die Göttlichkeit*, provided we take this translation option. If the self is an Imago Dei, the Dei of which it is an image must be greater, a deeper mystery, a more encompassing reality than it by itself encompasses. If some kind of congruence exists between the structure of the self and the dei of which it is an imago, and both can be said to be a coincidence of opposites, a composite of the brightest light and densest darkness, then they reflect one another. As such, one can read traits of the one off of the other. Because humans can know only what lies within the capacity of the psyche (this is Jung's basic epistemological position) and cannot step out of the psyche to know things as they are in themselves and in absolute, ontological truth-metaphysical terms, when we imagine the final and ultimate reality (*die Göttlichkeit*) and place this figure into the abysmal unknown and unknowable beyond, what we find is what we also recognize the self to be: a *coincidentia oppositorum*. Jung's is different from the traditional doctrinal argument in that it works both ways. It moves from the idea of the Imago Dei implanted in the human psyche to a vision of the originating Creator and then forward from the Creator to statements about the self. In his famous *Answer to Job*, Jung asserts that the Deity gains consciousness of Itself by gazing into its human mirror image. There is a two-way passage of information.

What is being advocated is a remarkably un-Protestant-like state of continuity and mirroring between the supernatural Divinity and the human self. For Protestant theology, God is radically other than human. Jung would say that the standard Protestant estimate of the human is limited to ego consciousness and that he is moving vastly beyond this in his explorations of the infinite unconscious. Jung is proposing a kind of depth psychology in which the master feature of the human psyche, the archetype of the self, can be located and taken up as "Divinity within." On the one hand, the self is grounded in *die Göttlichkeit*; on the other hand, *die Göttlichkeit* is grounded in the human psyche as the self archetype. The mystery of *die Göttlichkeit* as *unerforschliche Wesen* ("unfathomable being") is retained because the human mind cannot be certain that all is revealed in the psyche or that consciousness can ever apprehend the whole of reality, psychic or otherwise.

I cite another instance of the Imago Dei idea in Jung's writing. In one passage in the fierce exchange of 1952 with Martin Buber, who had characterized Jung as a modern Gnostic and in fact named him as a secret devotee of Abraxas, a God image that, as we have seen, fits the pattern of *coincidentia oppositorum* accurately, Jung replied with tongue in cheek:

> Here, just for once, and as an exception, I shall indulge in transcendental speculation and even in "poetry": God has indeed made an inconceivably sublime and mysteriously contradictory image of himself, without the help of man, and implanted it in man's unconscious as an archetype, an ἀρχέτυπον φως, archetypal light: not in order that theologians of all times and places should be at one another's throats, but in order that the unpresumptuous man might glimpse an image, in the stillness of his soul, that is akin to him and is wrought of his own psychic substance. This image contains everything he will ever imagine concerning his gods or concerning the ground of his psyche.
>
> (Jung 1952b, para. 1508)

The idea here is identical to that expressed in *Mysterium*, written at about the same time, in the phrase: "*als welche die Göttlichkeit das Selbst ausdrückt.*" In both instances, *die Göttlichkeit* (or "God," as he says to Buber) plants the Imago Dei (as ἀρχέτυπον φως or archetypal light in the reply to Buber) within the human psyche. Expressed in the psyche as an archetype, the self is the source and the point of origin of all humanly elaborated mythologies and theologies, even if it is not necessarily a complete or accurate description of "the unfathomable Being" itself. The self, as the fundamental psychic ground of all human images and ideas of deity, is itself grounded in Divinity. As Jung says, this is "poetry," but this poetry speaks a deep truth about Jung's vision.

The relation between psychology and religion was also the basic theme under discussion in Jung's correspondence with the English Roman Catholic theologian Victor White. In one letter, Jung, responding to an article White had published on Gnosticism, tells White that he had asked himself:

> *Have I faith or a faith or not?* I have always been unable to produce faith and I have tried so hard, that I finally did not know any more, what faith is or means. . . . The equivalent of faith with me is what I would call *Respect*. I have respect of the Christian Truth. Thus it seems to come down to an involuntary assumption in me, that there is something to the dogmatic truth, something *indefinable* to begin with. Yet I feel respect for it, although I don't really understand it. But I can say, my lifework is essentially an attempt to understand what others apparently can believe. . . . My respect is—mind you—involuntary; it is a "datum" of irrational nature. This is the nearest I can get to what appears to me as faith."
>
> (Lammers and Cunningham 2007, p. 119)

This project of seeking to understand what others can believe, which Jung claims here as his "lifework," is a driving force behind his various explorations of the self.

The Self, the Body, the "World"

If the self is conceived as an Imago Dei in the form of a *coincidentia oppositorum*, as Jung says in *Mysterium*, what about its relation to the body and the natural world? Is the self a cutoff, purely spiritual entity housed within an alien material form as the ancient Gnostics held, or is it much more intimately embedded in, and conditioned by, the social and cultural world and in fact fully at home in the human body? The view of the self as Imago Dei could pose a problem if the psyche is seen as somehow essentially unattached and transcendent to concrete life in the flesh.

Jung advanced a possible answer to this question in a late theoretical paper, "On the Nature of the Psyche":

> Since psyche and matter are contained in one and the same world, and moreover are in continuous contact with one another and ultimately rest on irrepresentable, transcendental factors, it is not only possible but fairly probable, even, that psyche and matter are two different aspects of one and the same thing.
>
> (Jung 1946/1954, para. 418)

In this and other works of the same late period in his life, such as "Synchronicity: An Acausal Connecting Principle" (Jung 1952a), Jung was conceptualizing a model for a unified field theory of psyche-soma-world, an essential unity of mind and matter, in which the archetypal patterns that emerge in the psyche are samples of patterns found throughout nature. *Die Göttlichkeit* would therefore be seen as an immanent player in the world of material objects and processes and not be an arm's-length observer as traditional theology would have it. The self as Imago Dei, too, is both material and spiritual. Marialuisa Donati has expounded on this in her paper, "Beyond synchronicity: the worldview of Carl Gustav Jung and Wolfgang Pauli," which she concludes with the following statement:

> As a result of their discussion of synchronicity, Pauli and Jung's investigation crosses the limits of single sciences such as physics and psychology, in order to take its place within the wider realm of the philosophy of nature. . . . Jung and Pauli's discussions on synchronicity shed light on the special need for a philosophy of nature today, emerging from a theoretical revision of the relation between mind and matter.
>
> (Donati 2004, p. 728)

In this regard, Jung was not in agreement in the least with the ancient Gnostic analysis of the human soul's state of bitter alienation in a hostile material universe.

If there is no break between the psyche and the material world, a persistent danger lurks that the psyche will be reduced to matter as an epiphenomenon of brain chemistry. Is the self "expressed" by *die Göttlichkeit* or by the neurons of the brain? Could it be that the brain, consisting of 100 billion neurons working (still so mysteriously) in millions of organized networks, is being reflected in the self concept that Jung puts forward as the containing, organizing, centering foundation of the psyche? Or if not only the brain, then the whole neuroanatomy? Is the Imago Dei in fact an image of our neuroanatomy rather than an expression of Divinity? Or can it be both, because in Jung's late view spirit and matter are two sides of a single reality?

Should *die Göttlichkeit* be found out to be the neuronal basis of the mind and the Imago Dei its psychic image, even this reduction, as radical and still improbable as it seems, would leave open the question: Does an even more fundamental pattern-generating factor underlie this base of the psyche? Is there a spirit-matter patterning energy that is active beneath this basement in what has classically been referred to as the *unus mundus*? Jung clearly thought that his studies on synchronistic phenomena pointed in this direction. Perhaps the self as we know it in the psychological realm is, even if it rests and depends critically on a neuroanatomical base, still a more or less reliable mirror of a general pattern in reality as such, that is, in the Divinity. In Jung's writings we find the persistent intuition that a mysterious force is at work behind the scenes, putting its imprint on body and soul and creating the pattern of "*coincidentia oppositorum, als welche die Göttlichkeit das Selbst ausdrückt.*" Jung often speaks of the hidden hand that guides our destiny in the course of individuation.

To extend this line of thought, one can venture that the Divinity that expresses itself in the human psyche with a psychological self also leaves imprints in the material world generally—in all animals, plants, man-made objects, and the cosmos. The human self would be but one instance of the Imago Dei in all things. Joseph Cambray has taken up the discussion of emergence and complexity theory in the natural sciences and specifically of "complex adaptive systems" (CAS) to reflect on the constellation of archetypal patterns in the psyche (Cambray 2004) and further to note that such patterns may be of the scale-free network variety, thus finding homologous expression throughout the natural world. "Complex systems," he writes, speaking of the psyche as such a system,

> tend to exhibit "scale-free" features, showing similar patterns in a homologous series, or nested emergent phenomena. . . . The self-organization manifesting in CAS appears transcendent from what is known about the behavior of the individual agents (and transcendent from the perspective of consciousness if the system is biological, including human).
>
> (Cambray 2004, p. 231)

George Hogenson has similarly argued that symbol formation, of which the Imago Dei would be an example, can in contemporary scientific terms be best explained using "operative concepts. . . [like] dynamic self-organization, self-organizing criticality, fractals, and power laws" (Hogenson 2006, p. 156). These modern analytic tools would allow for a reasonable contemporary scientific account of "the interface of dream, symbol, and the material world that Jung intuited" (Ibid., 165). Referencing the research on dreaming by Harvard neuropsychologist Carl Anderson, Hogenson observes that

> what is important about the fractal nature of the REM sleep brain patterns is that they follow a power law distribution with precisely the same mathematical structure as "the flow of the Nile, light from quasars, ion channel currents, neuronal firing patterns, earthquake distribution, electrical current fluctuations in man-made devices, inter-car-intervals in expressway traffic, and in variations in sound intensity in all melodic music."
>
> (Ibid.)

All of this tends to confirm the notion that the Imago Dei in the human psyche, the self, rests for its constellation in a particular person upon transcendent self-organizing dynamics within the universe as such, which we could perhaps agree to call *die Göttlichkeit* if we mean by that the dynamic instigator and organizer. The human psyche thus stands in profound continuity with the world, as does the world with the psyche. This is what Jung intuited in his notion of psyche and matter being two sides of a single reality.

The Self Under Development

It might be wrongfully concluded that once the Imago Dei takes form in a human being and is constellated as a core self, it resembles a static construct embedded in this discrete particle of flesh, perhaps repeating the same old songs from birth to death, but changing fundamentally. On the other hand, developmental psychology has long held that the human psyche is not a static entity but undergoes gradual and rapid developmental shifts throughout an individual's entire lifetime. Stages of the development of the ego and self have been discovered and discussed by Freud, Jung, Fordham, Erikson, Piaget, Klein, Winnicott, and a host of other theoreticians. Fordham speaks of de-integration and re-integration processes in the self that account for the building up of ego consciousness, but do these bring about essential change or development in the self per se? Does the self change as a result of lifelong individuation? And if so, how does this affect its transcendent source, *die Göttlichkeit*? Is the transcendent somehow also brought into a developmental process as the Imago Dei emerges in an individual person's life?

To forestall the notion that we are dealing with static entities when speaking of ego and self, Jung describes, a few pages later in the same section of *Mysterium* "The Dog," two main steps, or phases, in the alchemical (i.e., the psychological) opus that lead to the full emergence of the alchemical *lapis* (i.e., the self), which is the goal of the process. Psychologically, this work requires overcoming the radical polarity in the psyche between conscious and unconscious, a polarity that is endemic to the human personality and comes about naturally in the course of earlier developments of ego consciousness. It amounts to a division within the self. Jung is speaking here of a further stage of individuation after the ego has been formed, persona identity has been achieved, and the consolidation of conscious personality and character structure has been put into place and lived. Using the imagery of alchemy, he writes,

> [There are] two main divisions of the work, the *opus ad album et ad rubeum*. The former is the *opus Lunai*, the latter the *opus Solis*. Psychologically they correspond to the constellation of unconscious contents in the first part of the analytical process and to the integration of these contents in actual life. . . . The psychological parallel is the transformation of both the unconscious and the conscious, a fact known to everyone who methodically "has it out" with his unconscious.
>
> (Jung 1955/1956, para. 181)

The first piece of the analytic work (the Lunar opus—whitening) is the exposure of unconscious contents, which is followed by the integration of these contents into conscious and practical living (the Solar opus—reddening). First, there is the discovery phase, bringing up contents of the unconscious into consciousness—Jung names hypochondriacal obsessions, phobias, and delusions, as well as dreams, phantasies, and creative forerunners. These must be "whitened," that is taken into the light of consciousness and accepted fully for what they are. Once these aspects of the self are made thoroughly conscious, the assimilation of them and their meaning into practical life can begin.

Together, these two phases of the work were seen to bring about the transformation not only of consciousness but also of the unconscious. In his seminal paper, "The Practical Use of Dream-Analysis," Jung speaks of "mutual penetration of conscious and unconscious, and not—as is commonly thought and practiced—a one-sided evaluation, interpretation, and deformation of unconscious contents by the conscious mind" (Jung 1934, para. 327). This mutual penetration changes both sides of the equation, conscious and unconscious. The point here is that the self as psychic totality is actually a work in process, not an inner object simply waiting to become raised up into visibility. Emergence of the self is a lifelong process continuing into old age, especially if the work of making it conscious is deliberately undertaken. The Imago Dei develops in the course of individuation.

Nevertheless, no matter how far the development toward consciousness may advance, a region of mystery remains. A few lines later in *Mysterium*, Jung writes, "the salvation (*salus*) is one, just as the thing (*res*) is one . . . it is the fact of the self, that indescribable wholeness of people that *cannot be made visible* but is indispensable as an intuitive concept" (Jung 1955/1956, para. 181, emphasis added). Jung designates the self here as "a fact" (*eine Tatsache*) that surpasses description. As a fact, it is indisputable and psychically real, and so one *can* speak of "an experience of the self" or "the self as experience." But, even as one recognizes and names the self as a "fact," it remains paradoxically out of reach as an intuitive concept (*intuitiver Begriff*). Intuitive concepts reach for the unknown and the ineffable, which in itself remains forever beyond the ego's grasp. The self is an aporia, an insoluble contradiction. This should serve to keep one clear of literalism and dogmatism.

Experiencing the Self

How, then, can we speak of experiencing the self, this Imago Dei, a transcendent psychological fact or concept, and of bringing it into view at least partially within our limited conscious horizons? What does it mean to *experience* the self? Can we observe the self from the vantage point of ego consciousness?

Jung himself seemed to regard religious experiences as equivalent to and synonymous with experiences of the self. In his view, an experience of the self is a religious experience and vice versa. An account of these as found in all of the cultures of the world would describe the self archetype from various cultural and traditional vantage points.

Rudolf Otto classically described this type of experience in his book *Das Heilige* (*The Idea of the Holy*—a preferable translation would be simply, *The Holy*). From that extremely influential work, which was explicitly about *religious* experience and which Otto claimed was a unique kind of experience—*sui generis*—Jung borrowed the terms *numinosum* and numinous to describe the experience of the archetypal images of the collective unconscious, most importantly including that of the self. Otto defined the numinous as a *mysterium tremendum*. Jung in turn regarded the numinous experience of the Holy as the religious expression of the psychological experience of the self because the self is so deeply related to *die Göttlichkeit*. It is the same experience with a different name. Religious persons beg to differ, understandably, and claim that their experiences point beyond the Imago Dei to the Dei itself, beyond the subjective to the objective. As a psychologist, Jung stopped short of ontological or metaphysical claims of this sort, but he could relate to them in his feelings as a human being and as the subject of similar experiences.

The religions of the world provide for their adherents a host of images, ideas, and names that may evoke the experience of the Holy in one or another mental or physical form. Each tradition shows a wide variety of religious experience. Religious icons, for example, are entrances to an experience of the numinous, as are prayer, meditation, ritual actions, and pilgrimages, and so, we must now add, are active imagination, intersubjective dialogue, and intimate psychophysical communion. All of these can lead to numinous experiences, to experiences of a *mysterium tremendum*, and to a sense of awe that one may justifiably name an experience of the self. I want to argue, however, that this is only one type of experience of the self.

There is another category of experience that we may name an experience of the self, and this has to do with energy flow and overcoming or transcending the barrier between conscious and unconscious aspects of the psyche. This type does not have much to do with religious awe and numinosity, although Otto does write about "The Element of 'Energy' or Urgency" in *Das Heilige*, but can be described instead as moments of abandon and psychic fullness, when physical and psychic energy flow freely and without obstruction into a channel formed by an impersonal "director," which is not the self-conscious, intentional, willful ego. Such moments are generally not without tightly prescribed form, although the form may be largely unconscious to the actor. Indeed, most frequently they are highly and formally structured and articulated with extraordinary finesse and refinement. A convincing religious ritual, for instance, is both indelibly scripted by tradition and learned by practice, but in the moment of performance it is filled with a flow of energy and spontaneous emotion that generates numinosity. So too with art. At St. Petersburg's Mariinsky Theater, the star ballerinas, who dance with and far beyond "technique," pouring their whole beings into well-practiced and deeply ingrained habitual forms, incarnate the self in their effortless-looking movements. Those who can deeply see this and take it in also experience the self in and through them. It is a complete psychic and physical involvement without inhibition or restraint, holding back nothing, the full all-out abandonment to an impersonal form and style, which makes it "of the self" and not "of the ego." Sometimes we talk, read, run, work, play, cook, and eat like this. Life in the self means overcoming the divide between conscious and unconscious, being both at once. In this we also participate in the fullness of *die Göttlichkeit* as immanent within the space and time limitations of our physical world. One can think of incarnation of the Divine in these grace-filled and full-bodied moments.

Like the more familiar numinous experiences described as religious, these are also experiences of the Imago Dei expressed by *die Göttlichkeit*, and they can take place in social settings or in solitude, when mental activity, feeling, and behavior become uninhibited and lead to unconsciously scripted unions and conjunctions—physical, psychological, and spiritual. One may come to these in "dialogues" that become "monologues with two voices" (duets); in reveries whether alone or with another; in solitary walks in nature or through urban landscapes when one's self-consciousness as a separate individual fades away and one becomes united with the surroundings; in athletic or artistic creation that "happens," beyond technique and conscious determination; and in dreams that are symbolic and numinous. Here the ego joins with the self and becomes one with the Imago Dei, approximating or perhaps even becoming fully fused with *die Göttlichkeit* behind it.

A third category of experiences of the self, in my opinion, consists of the conscious containment of opposites (for example, the sublime and the shabby—the perfection of the Mariinsky Theater and the trashy parking lot behind the St. Petersburg Hotel) in a single, undivided image. Jung draws on alchemy for this in the image of Kalid's "son of the dog," who is also the "son of the philosophers." For the individual, this has to do with the immensely difficult task of holding in conscious awareness a fuller and more objective perception of oneself than is normal, which integrates in a single sense of self, or self-image, the persona and the shadow (good and bad, light and dark, angel and animal), the gender-identified ego and the otherwise-gendered subpersonality within (a syzygy), and the superior with the inferior psychological functions and attitudes. This is heightened or expanded self-consciousness, as well as full self-acceptance. It denotes psychological maturity, which may ripen with age and result in psychic objectivity about oneself, others, and the world at large.

Conclusion

"Yesterday I had a marvelous dream," Jung writes to Fr. Victor White at the end of 1946 as he is recovering from a heart attack.

> One bluish diamondlike star high in heaven, reflected in a round, quiet pool—heaven above, heaven below. The imago Dei in the darkness of the Earth, this is myself. The dream meant a great consolation. I am no more a black and endless sea of misery and suffering but a certain amount thereof contained in a divine vessel.
>
> (Lammers and Cunningham 2007, p. 60)

It was from experiences such as this that Jung drew when he penned enigmatic phrases like the one in *Mysterium*, "*als welche die Göttlichkeit das Selbst ausdrückt.*" The Divinity, symbolized by a bluish star, is reflected in the endless sea of misery within the darkness of the experienced world, and here it expresses itself in a form, as Imago Dei, reflected within the psyche. This imago is the sacred vessel that contains all of our self-contradictions, polarized partial personalities, and confusing emotional states. It gives our specific individual life its impersonal divine form and meaning. To hold this vessel firmly in the mirror of consciousness must be counted as an experience of the self. This is what remains when all of the specific contents and personal structures of one's psychic identity are erased. It is the surplus factor, the soul itself.

Notes

1 I find 17 instances of the use of this and a related term (*das Göttliche*) in the *GW*, but this is the only place in which Jung uses it as an active noun, as the subject of an action. Otherwise it is used adjectively. There are, on the other hand, many dozens of instances where Jung uses the terms *Gott* (God), *Götter* (Gods), *Gottesbild* (God image), and many others of a similar kind.
2 Evil defined as "the absence of good."
3 Jung, 1937, para. 140.

References

Cambray, J. (2004). 'Synchronicity as emergence'. In *Analytical Psychology: Contemporary Perspectives in Jungian Analysi*, edited by Joseph Cambray and Linda Carter. Hove and New York: Brunner-Routledge.
Cambray, J. (2010). 'Emergence of the self'. In *Jungian Psychoanalysis*, edited by Murray Stein. Chicago: Open Court.

Donati, M. (2004). 'Beyond synchronicity: The worldview of Carl Gustav Jung and Wolfgang Pauli'. *Journal of Analytical Psychology*, 49, 5, 707–728.

Dourley, J. (2007). 'The Jung-White dialogue and why it couldn't work and won't go away'. *The Journal of Analytical Psychology*, 53, 3, 275–295.

Euler, W. (2004). 'Christ and the knowledge of God.' In *Nicholas of Cusa: A Guide to a Renaissance Man*, edited by Christopher Bellitto, Thomas Izbicki, and Gerald Christianson. New York and Mahwah, NJ: Paulist Press.

Hogenson, G. (2006). 'The self, the symbolic, and synchronicity: Virtual realities and the emergence of the psyche'. In *Edges of Experience: Memory and Emergence*. Einsiedeln: Daimon Verlag.

Jung, C.G. (1934). 'The practical use of dream-analysis'. *CW* 16.

Jung, C.G. (1940). 'Psychology and religion'. *CW* 11.

Jung, C.G. (1946). 'The psychology of the transference'. *CW* 16.

Jung, C.G. (1947/1954). 'On the nature of the psyche'. *CW* 8.

Jung, C.G. (1948/1953). 'The spirit Mercurius'. *CW* 13.

Jung, C.G. (1951). 'Aion'. *CW* 9/2.

Jung, C.G. (1952a). 'Synchronicity: An acausal connecting principle'. *CW* 8.

Jung, C.G. (1952b). 'Religion and psychology: A reply to Martin Buber'. *CW* 18.

Jung, C.G. (1952c). 'Answer to Job'. *CW* 11.

Jung, C.G. (1954). 'Archetypes of the collective unconscious'. *CW* 9/1.

Jung, C.G. (1955/56). *Mysterium Coniunctionis*. GW 14. (*CW* 14).

Jung, C.G. (1963). *Memories, Dreams, Reflections*. New York: Random House.

Knox, J. (2003). *Archetype, Attachment, Analysis: Jungian Psychology and the Emergent Mind*. Hove and New York: Brunner-Routledge.

Lammers, A. and Cunningham, A. (2007). *The Jung-White Letters*. London and New York: Routledge.

Urban, E. (2005). 'Fordham, Jung and the self: A re-examination of Fordham's Contribution to Jung's conceptualization of the self'. *Journal of Analytical Psychology*, 50, 5, 571–594.

Wilkinson, M.A. (2006). *Coming into Mind. The Mind-Brain Relationship: A Jungian Clinical Perspective*. Hove and New York: Brunner-Routledge.

Chapter 13

Mary Watkins

Born in Texas in 1950, I grew up on Long Island, New York, in a completely Southern white Memphian family. Learning to interrogate the stark differences between the public schools' version of the history of slavery and the Civil War and my grandmother's racist rendition was a crash course in the constructed nature of histories and the importance of ascertaining who and what each version serves. This was underscored when, at the height of the Vietnam War, I attended a Quaker high school while living in a Republican family. Slavery, civil rights, pacifism, and social justice were on my mind as an adolescent, but so were struggles to understand my mother's psychology, as well as my own.

I decided to study psychology in college and was soon disappointed by the mainstream offerings, engulfed in positivism and behaviorism. I turned to anthropology, religion, and the work of Jung. In Jung's active imagination, I found a description of the kind of waking dreams that were beginning to overtake me, as I struggled with the onset of a depression at 19. For my senior thesis at Princeton University, I researched directed and undirected daydreaming, a work that later became *Waking Dreams*. During this period, I awoke at dawn one morning and experienced light and a voice suffusing my bedroom: "To love is to listen; to listen is to love" repeated over and over again and then receded. This became my orienting koan.

Inspired by the work of Laing to help create alternative community living situations for people undergoing psychotic breaks, upon graduation I began to volunteer and live at such a place and worked nights at a psychiatric inpatient unit. One night, as I checked on people, I discovered a teacher trying to kill herself. It deeply affected me. My Jungian analyst suggested that I read James Hillman's *Suicide and the Soul*. I was very moved by his honoring of the difficult images that are suffered in the midst of suicidal periods. Hillman was teaching at the Jung Institute in Zürich, and I decided to study there.

During my year at the Institute, 1973–1974, I was fortunate to be able to listen to Hillman's lectures that became *Re-Visioning Psychology* and *The Dream and the Underworld*, to join the early group of archetypal psychologists, and to have some of my writing published in *Spring Journal*. I also studied the work of another Zürich analyst, Medard Boss, who was bringing Heidegger's ideas into

DOI: 10.4324/9781003148982-14

his work. I decided that I also wanted to study further afield from Jung and left to study phenomenological and existential psychology at Duquesne University, the first graduate school in the United States to teach qualitative methodologies. I took to Amedeo Giorgi's phenomenological approach to research, a cousin of which—critical phenomenology—I still teach today.

I then decided to study developmental and clinical psychology with Bernard Kaplan at Clark University. Bernie, like Hillman, was extremely generous and encouraging to budding female scholars, not a common occurrence at that time. I took a deep dive into object relations theories, which began to ground my clinical practice with children and adults. Kaplan allowed me to write my dissertation on imaginal dialogues, how they had been treated in various cultures, and why they were so derided and confined to childhood in American psychology. This work became *Invisible Guests: The Development of Imaginal Dialogues*.

Once free from graduate school, I continued to practice, teach, and write. But my life was divided between social and psychological issues. Then, in the early 1980s, I began to experience a series of nightmares about nuclear war. The social broke through into the imaginal. The Australian physician Helen Caldecott was establishing Physicians for Social Responsibility in Cambridge, where I lived, and I began to work with them. Part of my week was spent in clinical sessions in which people spoke intimately about their interior lives, families, and friends. The other part was spent working along with other social activists on a variety of social issues. I was deeply struck by how many of the latters' intense feelings and images concerned social justice situations, whereas my middle- and upper-class clients rarely reflected on politics, economics, and injustice in their sessions. I came to understand how depth psychologies of that time had come to define the psychological as apart from the social, the cultural, the political, and the ecological. Slowly, I saw that the underlying paradigm of individualism was distorting our understandings, and I began to theorize and work from an interdependent paradigm.

In 1985, while preparing to adopt my first daughter from Northeast Brazil, I encountered the work of Paulo Freire, a Brazilian liberatory pedagogist. I experienced his work as the missing half of depth psychology. It led me to the work of Frantz Fanon and Ignacio Martín-Baró and the evolving work being done in liberation psychology, centering psychology in the service of justice. This helped me to cross a bridge into more community-based participatory and dialogical approaches (see *Toward Psychologies of Liberation*).

Once teaching at Pacifica Graduate Institute, my life as a mother of four daughters and my life as a teacher became a daily balancing act, punctuated by maternal joy. I developed a community and ecological fieldwork and research component of the Depth Psychology Program that I co-founded in 1996. In 2009, I co-founded a doctoral specialization in Community, Liberation, Indigenous, and Eco-Psychologies. Here students and faculty are involved in what I call the "public" practice of psychology in a wide variety of settings, as they attempt to understand the effects of coloniality and dream and act to create decolonial realities. My own work over the last 15 years has been centered on forced migration, the US-Mexico border, and the plight of asylum seekers in detention prisons in the US (see *Up Against the Wall: Re-Imagining the U.S.-Mexico Border*).

My life now is not as divided as it was in my 30s. The false separations that one learns have given way. A deep desire to learn with others remains a daily companion, a sustaining joy. Lewis Hyde (2007) said that the "ego's firmness has its virtues, but at some point we seek the slow dilation . . . in which the ego enjoys a widening give-and-take with the world" (p. 21). I feel this deeply.

Seeing From "the South"
Using Liberation Psychology to Reorient the Vision, Theory, and Practice of Depth Psychology

This was an invited keynote address to the Society for Theoretical and Philosophical Psychology, Division 24, of the American Psychological Association, March 2, 2019, Vanderbilt University upon receiving the 2019 Award for Distinguished Theoretical and Philosophical Contributions to Psychology.

Like most of you, my readers, I am on a long journey with the theories and practice of depth psychologies. The Euro-American discipline of psychology is one of my life partners. For a very short period, early in my life, I idealized it. I have been both educated and disappointed by it. At times it has flooded me with excitement, and, at others, suffused me with shame. Bidden and unbidden, it is a source of abiding interest, but also of my continuing resistance and defection.

My formal education in psychology was based in the northeast of the United States and in Zürich, Switzerland. My informal psychological education was based in the south of the United States. Although I grew up in New York, I did so in a completely southern, white, Memphis family. My formal education rooted me in phenomenology, depth psychologies, developmental psychology, and the clinical paradigm. My informal education rooted me in a felt sense of the profound racial injustice around me, an injustice that clearly affected individuals and also families, schools, neighborhoods, towns, and institutions; an injustice that not only oppressed victims of racism but that psychically and interpersonally deformed perpetrators of it.

Issues of social and environmental justice were absent from my study of phenomenological psychology at Duquesne University (Pittsburgh, PA) in the 1970s and very rarely evident in the developmental and clinical psychology I studied at Clark University (Worcester, MA), also in the 1970s. By the time I completed graduate school in 1982, my library was noticeably divided: social justice, ecological, and spiritual issues on one set of shelves in my bedroom, and psychology on other shelves in my office.

In the early 1980s, fresh from graduate school, my work weeks were as divided as my library: individual clinical work with children and adults on weekdays and group social action work in the evenings and on weekends. Each operated in its own register of emotion and concern, rarely intersecting. It seemed like both psychotherapists and clients had learned to draw a tight circle around what was defined as problematic psychologically and worked assiduously to keep within the local confines of the individual and the immediate family. I began to reflect on how I colluded with this circumscription, enabling me to slowly understand and then challenge individualism as an adequate underlying paradigm for psychological theory and practice (Watkins, 1992) and proposing instead a shift to interdependence.

I was deeply uncomfortable with the split I was living. I learned as much as I could from authors like Fromm, Horney, Laing, Sullivan, and Szasz about how to heal this divide, but it was an unexpected turn to the south—to Brazil—that gifted me with the glimmerings of the perspective I needed to understand and address the split. I was adopting my first daughter from northeast Brazil, and I began to immerse myself in all things from the *Nor'este* of Brazil: music, poetry, food, history, and the work of Paulo Freire. As I read Freire's *Pedagogy of the Oppressed* in 1984, I witnessed a scholar-activist who understood the deep interpenetration of the psychological and the cultural, seeing both from the perspectives of the history of colonialism and the pressing social needs it spawned. I began to understand that to the extent that psychological theories turned a blind eye to the underlying paradigm of individualism, they had made it difficult for me to deeply grasp that the psychological unfolds within history, that psychology itself was bound to be affected by the 500 years of colonialism that was at its apex in the first part of the 20th century and that has since morphed into neoliberalism and transnational capitalism. I have a very specific body memory from the first day I deeply entered the pages of *Pedagogy of the Oppressed*. I realized I had been looking for a missing half of Euro-American depth psychologies. Suddenly there was the promise of it.

Freire had to learn to reorient himself to create his form of liberatory pedagogy, a group method of developing critical understanding of the sociocultural roots of psychological and social misery. He reflected on some of his own lessons in moving from the position of teaching others to learning with them. His work was inflected with the values of liberation theology, particularly its shift to a preferential option for the poor. One night he was asked to speak with a roomful of workers, and he shared with them how he understood the situation they were in and what he thought they should do. On the drive home, he noticed that his wife, Elsa, was distant and he inquired why. She confronted him, "Look, Paulo, it does not work like this." Freire says he answered, "What did I do? I spoke serious about serious things." She said, "Yes, of course. All you said is right, but did you ask them whether they were interested in listening to you speak about that? You gave them the answers *and* the questions" (Horton & Freire, 1990, p. 65). He realized he had failed to listen to them or to understand what they knew about the situation, what kinds of transformation they deeply desired, and what they were willing to work for together.

According to Freire, this moment marked the beginning of his most important contribution to liberatory education, the process of conscientization, *conscientização*, a problem-posing group methodology that seeks to bring into awareness and dialogue what people know about their struggles and their dreams for themselves and their communities so that they can together act to transform their shared oppressive circumstances. This kind of experience helped Freire to decenter and deprivilege his own knowledge, enabling him to be a partner in dialogue, not as an expert but as an accompanist. Due to his own exposure to fascist groups, Jung did not believe groups to be a likely place to build consciousness. Freirean methodology shows clearly the conditions under which groups are extremely effective in building critical understanding.

As a clinician, Freire's work tutored me in posing generative questions to assist individuals and small groups to gain insight into the relationships between their intimate psychological symptoms and struggles and the historical, sociocultural contexts of their lives. Like Jung's approach to the amplification of images, this form of sociocultural amplification also assists individuals to feel less isolated and to understand that others also shoulder versions of their difficulties because of their common roots. Conscientization helps to transmute the burden of feelings of personal failure and defectiveness into sociocultural insights that can fuel transformations.

As one develops a critical consciousness of a particular situation, one understands how the situation has been constructed and created. One can denounce the destructive aspects. The work does not stop, however, with denunciation. Denunciation opens the path for what Freire called annunciation or prophetic imagination. Freire activated creative imagination by recognizing the possibility for creation inherent in all impasses. In his language, limit situations, where we at first seem unable to imagine how things could be otherwise, are the very locations where the most intense experiences of prophetic imagination can occur, unlocking transformative potentials. The path from Freire led me to the work of Frantz Fanon, Ignacio Martín-Baró, Virgilio Enriquez, and Marie Langer, further portals into key concepts and practices in liberation psychology.

In his short life, Martinican psychiatrist and liberation fighter Frantz Fanon (1967), with his cogent grasp of the work of Merleau-Ponty, Lacan, and Sartre, eloquently laid out how psychology not only left out the experiences of people of color but how psychiatry was used against them in North Africa. In his resignation as director of the Blida-Joinville Psychiatric Hospital in Algeria, Fanon rejected the use of psychiatry to help individuals make personal accommodations to unjust and destructive social environments. In his writings, he worked to place phenomenological inquiry into the service of sociopolitical and psychological liberation. His work prefigured what is now called decolonial or critical phenomenology.

Fanon (1967) critiqued Jung's understandings of the collective unconscious as arising from "cerebral heredity" and of the "myths and archetypes" as "permanent enneagrams of the race" (p. 188). He argued that the contents of the collective unconscious are not collective but "the result of . . . the unreflected imposition of a culture" (Ibid., 1967, p. 191). "The collective unconscious is cultural, which means acquired;" "it is the sum of prejudices, myths, collective attitudes of a given group" (p. 188). He cites Jung's innovation of wanting to go back to the "childhood of the world" (p. 190). But, Fanon said, "he made a remarkable mistake: He went back only to the childhood of Europe" (p. 190). Fanon points out that the Indigenous people that Jung knew had all had traumatic contacts with the white man (p. 187) and that Jung failed to adequately take into account the effects of colonialism on them and their cultures.

These critiques made it clear that Jung's work was predominantly about the white, largely privileged, European psyche that was central to the perpetrating and sustaining of colonialism. These critiques enabled me to see more clearly that some of the shifts Jung was encouraging in his patients could be understood as treatments to redress the colonial or imperial ego of white European colonialists, what James Hillman later termed the heroic ego. Both men were acutely aware of how efforts to dominate and control, both oneself and others, led to overidentification with the ego and the persona and to destructive relationships (Watkins, 2014).

Spanish-born Jesuit and social psychologist Ignacio Martín-Baró (1994) brought the insights and commitments of liberation theology into dialogue with psychology, naming this orientation from the south "liberation psychology." From his perspective in El Salvador in the 1980s, psychological trauma was not only an individual affliction but the shared suffering of whole communities struggling with violence, poverty, and oppression. He introduced the term "psychosocial trauma," also understood as collective trauma. His understanding of psychosocial trauma throws light on the ways in which Western trauma theory failed to adequately include people of color in its theorizing and practices.

As a psychologist, Martín-Baró accompanied the oppressed as they sought to stop the injustices saturating their lives. In addition, he used his role as a psychologist to create research that informed the wider world of the violence being inflicted on the Salvadoran people. By collecting and publishing anonymous narratives and composite polls, he was able to provide a completely different portrait of what the Salvadoran people were enduring than the government's version, saturated with propaganda. He was targeted by the Salvadoran military along with five of his fellow Jesuits and assassinated in 1989 by a U.S.-trained death squad.

Filipino psychologist Virgilio Enriquez (1992), like Martín-Baró, came to reject the naïve deployment of American psychology in the Philippines. Both men studied psychology in the United States, but when they went to use North American psychology in the south, they discovered its limits. Enriquez came to realize that Filipinos enjoyed their own forms of Indigenous psychology that were unrecognized and endangered by the universalism and imperialism of U.S. psychology. His work decisively linked liberation psychology to Indigenous psychology, rejecting what Freire called cultural invasion—interpretations and interventions imposed from outside a given culture. This decentering of Western epistemology presaged the present decolonial emphasis on pluriversal understandings (Escobar, 2018). By virtue of this decentering, we can come closer to claiming various depth psychological approaches as themselves indigenous to particular peoples at a particular set of historical moments. Once we understand this, our study of depth psychologies can more clearly educate us about the primarily white, upper-middle and upper classes. As Fanon suggested, we can sort the concepts that may be useful in another particular context, while critiquing the universalism and racism where it is harbored in theories. Enriquez's turn from transplanting American psychology onto Filipino soil to understanding and further articulating Indigenous psychologies in the Philippines has now been deployed in many places, including the Māori & Psychology Research Unit at the University of Waikato in New Zealand, which is indigenizing liberation psychology (Rua et al., 2021).

Marie Langer (1989), author of *From Vienna to Managua: Journey of a Psychoanalyst*, offered a model for cultural synthesis in psychoanalytic work. In cultural synthesis, Freire offered, people "do not come to *teach* or *transmit* or *give* anything, but rather to learn, with the people, about the people's world" (Freire, 2000, p. 180)—there is a synthesis of worlds through efforts of mutual understanding. Langer learned to move fluidly between the direct service of providing psychotherapeutic accompaniment to refugees fleeing state terror to work on co-constructing a national mental health system for Nicaraguans deeply affected by losses from a civil war and by centuries of colonial exploitation.

Like the liberation theologians' challenge to priests who supported exploitative elites, Langer directly critiqued her colleagues in the Argentine Psychoanalytic Association, which she had founded. During the "Dirty War" (1973–1983), she called out those psychoanalysts who were colluding with a repressive class system, profiting from their treatment of elites, and separating mental health issues from the pernicious psychosocial effects of class struggle. She urged psychoanalysts to use their knowledge to facilitate rather than to oppose progressive social movements (Hollander, 1997; Langer, 1971).

Her vocal human rights activism, denunciation of atrocities, and advocacy to democratize mental health care led to her placement on a death squad list in 1974, causing her to seek asylum in Mexico. There she treated refugee survivors of the brutal military dictatorships in Central and Latin America and helped to create The Committee on Solidarity with the Argentine People, which helped new refugees with housing, clothes, work, and psychological care, while working to document the human rights abuses they had suffered in Argentina (Hollander, 2010). It is important to note her clear understanding that at times treatment is less important than working to provide the necessities of daily life, upon which psychological well-being is also dependent.

In 1981, she joined with twelve psychologists and medical doctors with psychoanalytic training to form the Internationalist Team of Mental Health Workers, Mexico-Nicaragua. They accompanied Sandinistas in Nicaragua as they created their first national mental health system, one with universal access and a focus on prevention (Hollander, 1991). I see such efforts as a decommodification of psychology, a giving away of what others may find useful in a given context, even if this undermines the economic security of professionalized practice.

"Accompaniment" is a term sprinkled throughout the literature of liberation theology and liberation psychology. It has compelled my attention for the last 15 years. As I began to track it, I found it used in arenas as diverse as social medicine, peace activism, human rights, pastoral support, social psychology, animal rights, and liberation psychology (Watkins, 2015, 2019). The concept is used when speaking of accompanying the ill who are also poor (Farmer, 2011), those caught in prison and detention systems (Lykes, Hershberg, & Brabeck, 2011), political dissidents (Romero, 2001), refugees (Jesuit Refugee Service), those suffering under occupation (Ecumenical Accompaniment Programme in Palestine), victims of torture and other forms of violence, those forcibly displaced (Sacipa-Rodríguez, Vidales, Galindo, & Tovar, 2007), those suffering from human rights violations (Mahoney & Eguren, 1997), and those attempting to live peacefully in the face of paramilitary and military violence (such as the peace communities in Colombia). In Latin America, "psychosocial accompaniment" has arisen as a role that is distinct from that of psychotherapist or psychological researcher, though it may include elements of each. In countless other situations of human and environmental duress, accompaniment is engaged in without recourse to the term.

Paul Farmer, the co-founder of Partners in Health, describes accompaniment:

> To accompany someone is to go somewhere with him or her, to break bread together, to be present on a journey with a beginning and an end. There's an element of mystery, of openness, of trust, in accompaniment. The companion, the accompagnateur, says: "I'll go with you and support you on your journey wherever it leads. I'll share your fate for a while—and by "a while," I don't mean a little while. Accompaniment is about sticking with a task until it's deemed completed—not by the accompagnateur, but by the person being accompanied.
> (Farmer, 2013, p. 234)

Indeed, accompaniment conveys the relational horizontality and the solidarity that can emerge through committed co-presence. When "psychosocial" is added as an adjective, accompaniment gains a dimensionality that is resonant with conscientization, inclusive of understanding the historical and sociocultural context and engaging in transformative action.

Through these vignettes I have outlined some key compass points for reorienting depth psychological theory and practice to liberatory ends: liberatory pedagogy, conscientization, annunciation or prophetic imagination, decolonial phenomenology, an interdependent paradigm, collective or psychosocial trauma, the preferential option for the poor and the marginalized, the Indigenization of psychology, cultural synthesis, and psychosocial accompaniment (Watkins & Lorenz, 2008).

As my own reorientation was taking place, an opportunity arose to explore what psychological work might look like if it were released from the clinical paradigm while being inflected by depth psychologies and deeply influenced by the insights, social justice aims, and practices of liberation psychology. In a graduate program that I co-founded in 1996—the M.A./Ph.D. Depth Psychology Program at Pacifica Graduate Institute—many of our students and fieldwork faculty engaged in this reorientation from the south and nourished the community and ecological fieldwork we were doing with the insights and practices of liberation psychology. Some colleagues argued vehemently that this was not psychology at all and certainly not depth psychology—but maybe sociology or perhaps social work. As I defended to depth psychologists the logic of linking individual and community well-being, I discovered it had already been—historically speaking— at the roots and heart of psychoanalytic practice.

It would be difficult to tell from much of the contemporary mainstream practice of depth psychologies in the United States that psychoanalysis was conceived in an atmosphere of acute consciousness of social inequalities and their impact on mental health. In *Freud's Free Clinics: Psychoanalysis and Social Justice, 1918–1938,* Elizabeth Danto (2005) chronicles this now rarely considered early history of the psychoanalytic movement, forged in the aftermath of the economic and social devastation of World War I.

Many early psychoanalytic practitioners were engaged Marxists, socialists, or social democrats, whose practice of depth psychology issued from hopes of liberation on social and psychological fronts, fronts that were seen as inextricably intertwined. In the early period of psychoanalysis, forged in Red Vienna, psychoanalysts were deeply involved in initiatives to create and staff free clinics for psychoanalytic treatment, free clinics for reproductive health care and education for women, initiatives to help women struggle against various forms of domination, abuse, and control, experimental schools for inner-city children, school-based treatment centers for children traumatized by war and poverty, settlement house psychology classes for workers, the first child guidance clinics, suicide prevention centers, They worked to build conditions for peace and stability in Austria and Europe and supported the kindergarten movement and architectural initiatives for public housing that would help to build urban families' sense of community, a sense understood to undergird psychological health (Danto, 2005). For these analysts, there was not a strict divide between their work in private practice and their work in what I call "public practice."

In 1918, Freud gave a speech in Budapest on awakening the conscience of society. He expressed that suffering was not evenly distributed in a society but was "imposed unfairly and largely according to economic status and position" (Danto, 2005, p. 19). In this talk, Freud reversed his earlier assertion that low or no fees compromised psychoanalytic treatment in the eyes of the patient, and he retracted his image of the psychoanalyst as a medical entrepreneur. From this point forward, Freud became an advocate for free psychoanalytic clinics, flexible fees, and lay analysis. He worked to wrestle psychoanalytic practice from the medical establishment and attempted, with his colleagues, to expand the circle of those who could benefit from psychoanalytic treatment to include the poor. The first psychoanalytic free clinic was in Berlin. It adopted the practice of performing initial intake evaluations that were blind to one's capacity to pay. Analysts who were part of the international society agreed to donate their time one day a week to provide psychoanalytic care to those who could not afford it or to contribute the equivalent in funds for the clinics.

Psychoanalytic understanding of the effects of culture grew dimmer as psychoanalysis was transplanted from Europe to America during and after World War II. Many Jewish émigré analysts sought refuge in America. Russell Jacoby (1983) argues that the transplanted analysts suppressed their history of social and political engagement in Europe to avoid delays in the U.S. naturalization process. Many felt this suppression continued to be necessary because of the political climate in America as the Cold War deepened and McCarthyism erupted. Those with allegiances to Marxism and socialism were afraid they would be seen as communists or traitors. Émigré analysts sought economic security by flight from the kinds of public and socialist initiatives popular in Vienna to private practice models that uncritically embraced capitalism's brutal divisions in the provision of health care. Psychoanalysis became relatively indifferent to racial and cultural issues and insufficiently reflective of its own cultural location within a multicultural society (Altman, 1995).

As psychoanalysis retreated from interest in and commitment to social justice, it took refuge in disease models that undergird a perceived need for individual treatment. Lay analysis was outlawed in America against Freud's wishes. This pushed psychoanalysis away from cultural criticism and public practice toward medicalized practice. Economic stresses on the health-care system forced a wide adoption of the disease model, locating pathology almost entirely within individuals, requiring a diagnosis of psychopathology, and systematizing interventions in order to gain payment from third party insurance.

Once the consulting room and the therapist were segregated from the community, the daily lives of the people who consulted them, and the community life beyond their view, the office became not only a quiet and hopefully safe place for the client to work on their private and psychological life but a place and a practice that segregated the psychologist from the life of the community and those caught in what sociologist Saskia Sassen (2014) calls "elementary brutalities." The consulting room can be seen as a place of refuge from grappling more directly with issues of social, economic, and environmental justice. It can be a place of defense that makes it less likely we will be working alongside people who feel the brunt of neoliberalism and coloniality. If we live in economically, racially, and ethnically segregated neighborhoods, and if we practice our spirituality in a homogeneous group, our segregation is compounded. As our privilege increases and is more solidified with advanced professionalization, without great effort we can find ourselves increasingly separated from others whose experiences are quite different from our own.

Fourteen years ago, an opportunity arose to use curricular space at Pacifica Graduate Institute to create a doctoral depth psychology specialization that emphasizes the integration of critical community psychology, liberation psychology, Indigenous psychologies, and environmental justice. During these years, community and ecological fieldwork and research at Pacifica have deepened and profited from coursework that supports insight into moving away from coloniality toward decoloniality, Indigenous approaches to research, and serious attention to anti-racism work. Over 700 examples of community and ecological fieldwork and research have emerged over 24 years of community and ecological fieldwork and research at Pacifica, many oriented by liberation psychology. Each year, students and I study phenomenologically the fieldworkers' experiences and the outcomes, difficulties, and joys of their work. We have tried to discern some of the points of orientation of ecopsychosocial accompaniment that have been useful. In the following, I will try to give a sense of how mutual accompaniment can unfold, using these points of orientation. To do so, I will draw on aspects of my own field-work experience with forced migration and the U.S.-Mexico border over the last 18 years, in concert with others', to exemplify some of the principles of this work.

First Point of Orientation: Discern "the call" you experience and reflect on its relationship to your own autobiography and positionality. We ask ourselves to be aware of the issues that are compelling our attention and to work to become aware of how they intersect with our lives, discerning our own complex positionality in relation to them.

I am a relative newcomer to the southwest, having spent the first 45 years of my life in New York and Boston. When I moved west, I began to try to understand my new city: Santa Barbara, a city of 38% Mexican and Mexican Americans and the rest predominantly white Anglos. In 2002, I had the opportunity to travel with a group of young Quakers to an autonomous community, Maclovio Rojas near Tijuana, Mexico, to accompany Maclovians at their request during a period when the government was trying to displace the members of the community in order to sell the land to transnational companies that were building *maquiladores*, large industrial plants. On the way there, we stopped at Friendship Park, where Tijuana and the most southern part of the U.S. meet at the edge of the Pacific Ocean. There I first encountered the U.S. border wall. I had a sickening feeling when I first saw it. A wall between two friendly peoples, a wall to keep out people who are struggling to feed themselves and their families when the U.S. has created policies that worsen this struggle in their home country, a wall in the middle of historically bicultural communities, a wall that separates family members and that marks an unjust conquest of land. My attempt to understand my own community in Santa Barbara, where so many live in the shadow of this wall, strengthened my sense that I should commit to border studies and action. From my own autobiography, it resonated with my informal education in U.S. racism.

The border crystallizes many of the profound social problems of our time. It is indeed a wound, as Gloria Anzaldúa (2007) described it, *una herida*, a scar across the land. It permits the free flow of consumer goods but makes unfree the passage of human beings. The wall is not aimed at keeping people out or guns in. What it does achieve is to make immigrant labor cheap and laborers afraid and disenfranchised, without any path to citizenship and voting. Those who fail in crossing are swallowed as cheap labor by the vast *maquiladores* at the border. Many who succeed in crossing the border never get past the multiple checkpoints and become entrapped in the abandonment zones of the *colonias* in Texas.

The border is a place where Americans must grapple with what it means to shut the door on people who are fleeing unlivable and violent conditions, conditions created in part by our own country and our ways of living.

Second Point of Orientation: Guard against cultural invasion by seeking invitation and by your own patient immersion, listening, and learning. An awareness of psychology's history of cultural invasion has led to fieldwork where fieldworkers are not bringing interventions to places they do not know and who do not know them. This does not mean that they do not have skills and theories in their backpacks, but it does mean that if they are entering a situation or community as an outsider, that they do so only with invitation and that their first and abiding work is listening, learning, immersing themselves, and building relationships. This takes time and patience, but it yields understanding of and respect for local knowledge and approaches. It creates the groundwork for potential solidarity.

Over the next several years (2002–2006), I took advantage of several invitations for immersion at the border: through Borderlinks, an organization in Tucson that helps groups travel to both sides of the border in Arizona, speaking to Border Patrol agents, migrants, maquiladora workers, humanitarian organizations that provide food and water in the desert, and those sustaining the sanctuary movement; through Global Xchange, which focuses on human rights issues at the border in Tijuana and surrounding the Zapatista communities in Chiapas; and through language study. I spoke with migrants and with people assisting them, and I helped to place water in the desert for people crossing in extremely high temperatures, a practice that has fought criminalization by the U.S. government.

Third Point of Orientation: Join into the ongoing work of the community. Psychologists have a lot to learn from cultural workers who have been engaged in community-based initiatives, most often outside the academy. With a better understanding of migration from Mexico, I located a Latino organization, PUEBLO, in Santa Barbara that was working on issues of immigration and that welcomed my Anglo presence. I faithfully attended their meetings, got to know members, and helped with whatever was needed. While I felt out of place and was unable to understand much of what was said in Spanish, I began to grasp what those without documents were enduring in my community. One year into this, a young member said she had a dream of creating an oral history of the undocumented community in Santa Barbara, but she was unsure of how to go about this and wondered if any people wanted to help.

Fourth Point of Orientation: Engage in participatory and dialogical inquiry with community members. This initiated my participation in an oral history research project for several years with a small group of young adult immigrants without immigration documents. They interviewed community members without documents, translated these interviews, worked together to identify themes, organized a book, and then introduced it to the community (Pueblo Immigration Committee, 2008). This created a forum for people without documents to speak to citizen neighbors about their lives and challenges. It enabled topics like racism, economic inequality, poor housing, harassment by the police, and seizure of cars at police checkpoints to become community topics. The psychological sequelae of these stresses were often broached.

Fifth Point of Orientation: Forego expertism and practice horizontality and shared leadership. Initially, many of the young people looked to me as an older, white, educationally privileged professional for direction. While providing background about creating oral history, I tried as much as possible to move into a more horizontal and off-center position, supporting other members of the group to assume leadership. At the same time, there were opportunities for speaking and sharing their work that I could access through my professional privilege, such as their speaking at a Grand Rounds at the local hospital. Now with feet in both Anglo and Mexican communities, it was possible to use my positionality to create bridges between communities that are too rarely in meaningful contact, while being careful not to usurp the leadership of young people of color.

This occurred when the so-called Secure Communities Act swung into place, striking terror into the hearts of immigrant families, while Anglo community members barely noticed. BorderLinks announced that increased dangers at the Arizona-Mexico border were making their border immersion delegations unsafe. They proposed instead to create border immersion programs in our own communities. In Santa Barbara, we invited representatives of immigrant groups to educate a largely Anglo audience about their concerns and struggles. We also included representatives from the police department, the county jail, and Border Patrol so that attendees could gain a fuller picture of the issues from multiple viewpoints.

Sixth Point of Orientation: Understand history critically and engage in ongoing efforts of conscientization. Our psychological well-being, as well as the well-being of our communities, is inextricably linked to our interdependent histories. These histories are crucial to developing a deepened understanding of ourselves and others and to the work before us to build more beloved communities.

For a year, I spent some of my free time each week in the history archives of my city, trying to piece together how Santa Barbara, a Mexican town that was more important than Los Angeles in 1860, had become a wealthy Anglo enclave, oblivious to its history of creating an internal colony of Mexicans and Mexican Americans. For instance, in 1930 people of Mexican descent—U.S. citizens included—were lied to in order for Anglos to expel them. At the behest of the city government, social workers promised them land and tools in Baja, Mexico. They were gathered onto railway cattle cars. Once in Baja, they discovered the hoax. In adjacent Carpinteria, CA, children of Mexican descent suffered educational and social segregation until after World War II: separate and unequal schools, and even differential access to areas of the beach and the movie theater. I was able to bring forward many aspects of this extruded history at gatherings, in the newspaper, and in a book (Casey & Watkins, 2015). A local movement to include such history in ethnic studies classes in the public schools has finally succeeded.

Seventh Point of Orientation: Engage in border crossing, reverse osmosis.
As I got to know families affected and afflicted by detention and deportation, the
emerging American gulag of detention centers began to come into focus for me. To
deport almost half a million people a year, the Obama administration had to expand
detention facilities. Our country is now laced not only by prisons but by 200 detention centers, imprisoning 39,000 migrants a day (Detention Watch Network, 2016).

For accompanists from the outside, those who have not grown up in or as a
part of the community with which they are working, accompaniment often entails
reverse border crossing; what I call reverse osmosis (Watkins, 2021). While others attempt to avoid prisons and detention facilities, for example, those practicing
reverse osmosis seek to provide witness and accompaniment there.

New Sanctuary Coalition in New York City requests accompaniment from citizens for immigrants needing to report to Federal Plaza for immigration check-ins
and immigration hearings. Often family members cannot attend to provide support
because they do not have documents and are afraid of being apprehended. If a
person is detained, someone needs to be present who is knowledgeable to contact
family members so they will know where their loved one is. As you wait for the
hearing to begin, people share their stories and their fears of being uprooted. After
hearing about some of their stories of being detained, I volunteered for Sojourners,
which helps to support First Friends in New Jersey. It is a visitation program that
pairs an accompanier with a detainee. The accompanier visits regularly until the
detainee is released or deported. To enter a detention center in the United States is
to enter into a dark awareness of the warehousing of human lives in which our government is engaged. Our country detains more people than any other in the world.

During the Trump administration, I retooled myself to provide pro bono foren-
sic reports for asylum seekers, for female migrants without documents who are
caught in domestic violence here, and for those fighting their deportation due to
the extreme hardship it would cause to their citizen or permanent resident family
members. Fewer than 50% of asylum applicants are granted asylum. Without a
lawyer, one's chances are practically zero. If one's case is presented in places like
Atlanta, regardless of the merit of the case, it is likely to be denied.

Even if one wins asylum, the path to creating a life in the United States is
extremely hard for people without English skills, financial means, or families.
Accompanying asylees during their resettlement can make a decisive difference
in the outcome. Psychologist Mary Pipher (2003) realized that refugees arriving
to her private practice in Loncohn, Nebraska often needed a very different kind
of relationship and set of experiences than those of psychotherapy. This requires
the clinicians among us to leave our offices and to practice border crossing and
reverse osmosis, leaving behind whatever measure of familiarity and authority we
enjoy in our more circumscribed offices.

For the past 18 years, a group of Colombian social, political, and clinical psychologists from Pontifical Javeriana University have done just this as they accompany families who were forcibly displaced by paramilitaries from the countryside
to the capital of Bogatá. Many of these displaced persons have experienced acute

and chronic violence and often the loss of family members (Sacipa-Rodríguez, Vidales, Galindo, & Tovar, 2007). The accompanists were seeking to construct a daily practice that was consistent with their understanding of social commitment (Sacipa-Rodriguez & Montero, 2014). The members of this group—Social Bonds and Peace Culture—committed themselves to resist the trivialization of death and the rampant depersonalization of others that characterized daily reality in a society that has been torn for decades by armed conflict.

Stella Sacipa-Rodriguez describes her team's perspective on psychosocial accompaniment:

> [W]e conceive psychosocial accompaniment as a way of offering displaced people support and providing spaces for expressing and recognizing the emotional impact these violent events have had on them. . . .
>
> Psychosocial accompaniment is a process marked by respect, acknowledgment of the human dignity of the person who has suffered displacement, a process which seeks to establish bonds and bridges for the renewal of confidence in a work of successive, respectful rapprochement, aimed at opening up the psychosocial relationship, to reach the heart of others from within oneself, through mutual recognition in everyday dialogue, in active listening and in shared work and play.
>
> We believe that accompaniment should be directed toward the affirmation of displaced persons as subjects in their own stories and the reconstruction of the social fabric of the community.
>
> (2014, p. 67)

Eighth Point of Orientation: Open yourself to learn what is needed rather than supplying what you already know. The psychologists found that, in accompaniment, one is often faced with needs about which the accompanist has very little knowledge. Together they must learn new skills or gather resources to meet these needs. For instance, many of the displaced families wanted it to be clear in public records and in memory that their loved ones were falsely assumed to be guerillas. They also wanted to know where their loved ones' remains were so that proper burials could be conducted. Honoring these deep desires, the psychologists needed to become knowledgeable about and effective in interfacing with relevant judicial and public authorities and processes.

Ninth Point of Orientation: Commit to working across levels of organization. The Colombian psychologists, like Fanon before them, emphasize that a fuller recovery from such psychosocial suffering requires societal circumstances that make meaningful work, peace, and a dignified life possible. For the psychosocial reconstruction of a community to ultimately be effective, it must be part of a holistic approach that includes changes in the social, economic, and political life of the country. For these reasons, at a systems level, the psychologists have also been exploring their possible contributions as psychologists to creating cultures of peace in Colombia. They embrace UNESCO's call for cultures of peace founded on "solidarity, active nonviolence, pluralism, and an active posture against exclusion and structural violence." To be able to pivot from the "private" practice of psychology to a community-oriented or "public" practice entails ongoing learning about how to nimbly work across levels of organization.

Let us place these principles into dynamic relationship with one another: Of all the forms of psychological research, participatory action research (PAR) is one of the most compatible with the practice of accompaniment. In PAR, a researcher partners with a group or community to offer research support for the questions to which they are seeking answers. Instead of participants serving the research agenda of someone outside of their community, the researcher partners agree to serve the research needs of the community. The researcher may or may not be a member of the community. Community members formulate research questions, conduct research conversations, analyze data, and discern meaningful ways of disseminating findings that assist in the achievement of shared goals.

Liberation psychologist M. Brinton Lykes's work over three decades offers an inspiring example of participatory action research as accompaniment. Lykes accompanied Mayan women in Guatemala as they suffered genocide, struggled to give testimony, and worked together to make the genocide known internationally (2001). More recently, through the Post-Deportation Human Rights Project (PDHRP), Lykes has been collaborating with human rights lawyers, immigrant community groups in the U.S., deportees, and families without immigration documents to explore the effects of current U.S. detention and deportation policies on Salvadoran and Guatemalan families residing in the northeast United States. A major goal "is to reintroduce legal predictability, proportionality, compassion, and respect for family unity into the deportation laws in the U.S. through successfully defending individual deportees, thereby setting new precedents and creating a new area of legal representation" (Lykes, Hershberg, & Brabeck, 2011, p. 26). Through her long-standing accompaniment of Guatemalans who suffered genocide, Lykes is intimately aware of the need of many to migrate to the U.S. due to poverty and ongoing violence, the conditions of precarity they suffer in the U.S. without legal documents, their lack of representation during deportation proceedings, and the family fragmentation that results both from forced migration and forcible deportation. Her team has interviewed family members who were separated due to forced migration and returning deportees and has "create[d] collaborative spaces for bridging the growing chasms between citizens and non-citizens and for deepening a shared understanding of and response to injustices that immigrant families (many of which include U.S.-born citizen children) face" (Lykes, Hershberg, & Brabeck, 2011, p. 24).

Lykes honestly acknowledges that accompanists who hold social privilege must question the paradox of personally benefiting from the colonial power they are seeking to disrupt and transform. Accompaniment can easily go awry if the colonial framework of "helping," "charity," and "being of service" are not thematized and deconstructed. Too often, humanitarian, community, and psychosocial work occurs within the same structure of colonial relations that gives rise to a community's suffering in the first place. Hierarchical relations are mindlessly reproduced, ignoring or denigrating the knowledge of community members. Ameliorative actions (Prilleltensky & Nelson, 2005) can neglect the deeper causes of distress, particularly those of systemic injustice.

Mutuality of Accompaniment

There is no doubt that I entered the study of psychology with a simplistic and naïve desire to "help" people, largely ignorant of the implications of my own positionality and the wider sociocultural and historical contexts of eco-psychosocial suffering. Only in time have I come to understand the wisdom articulated by an aboriginal activist group in Queensland, Australia, in the 1970s:

> If you come here to help me,
> you are wasting your time.
> If you come because your liberation is bound up with mine,
> then let us work together.

Now I place the word "mutual" in front of eco-psychosocial accompaniment to underscore this interdependence of one person's liberation with another's, one community's with others'—inclusive of ecosystems and other-than-human animal communities.

Walsh and Gokani (2014) help us to confront the reality that if our own social, economic, and professional standing is enhanced by neoliberal capitalism, it is likely that our work will at best be reformist and at worse be collusive with the very status quo that manufactures these disorders. We need to struggle to extricate ourselves as much as possible from those structures that have negative consequences and find ways to improvise liberatory eco-psychosocial work apart from the models dictated by a capitalist service economy.

The compass points of Western psychology as a whole will never be those of liberation psychology, because psychology as a Euro-American discipline has multiple and conflicting teloi. But for those who actively seek a more just and peaceful world, a world where, as Freire (2008) says, it will be easier to love, the reorientation of depth psychology by liberation psychology from the south offers important coordinates to orient our theorizing and practice.

References

Altman, N. (1995). *The analyst in the inner city: Race, class, and culture through a psychoanalytic lens*. Analytic Press.

Anzaldúa, G. (2007). *Borderlands/La Frontera: The new mestizaje*. San Aunt Lute Books.

Casey, E. & Watkins, M. (2015). *Up against the wall: Re-imagining the U.S.-Mexico border*. Austin, TX: University of Texas Press.

Danto, E. (2005). *Freud's free clinics: Psychoanalysis and social justice, 1918–1938*. New York, NY: Columbia University Press.

Detention Watch Network (2016). Immigration detention 101. Retrieved 8/30/20 from https://www.detentionwatchnetwork.org/issues/detention-101

Enriquez, V. (1992). *From colonial to liberation psychology: The Philippine experience*. Quezon City, Philippines: University of the Philippines Press.

Escobar, A. (2018). *Designs for the pluriverse: Radical interdependence, autonomy, and the making of worlds*. Durham, NC: Duke University Press.

Fanon, F. (1967). *Black skin, white masks*. New York, NY: Grove Press.

Farmer, P. (2011). *Re-imagining accompaniment: Global health and liberation theology conversation between Paul Farmer and Father Gustavo Gutiérrez (10/24/2011)*. Ford Family Series, South Bend, IN: Notre Dame University.

Farmer, P. (2013). *To repair the world: Paul Farmer speaks to the next generation*. Berkeley, CA: University of California Press.

Freire, P. (2008). *Pedagogy of the oppressed*. New York, NY: Continuum.

Hollander, N. (1991). Introduction. In Marie Langer (Ed.), *From Vienna to Managua: Journey of a psychoanalyst*. London, UK: Free Association Books.

Hollander, N. (1997). *Love in a time of hate: Liberation psychology in Latin America*. Brunswick, NJ: Rutgers University Press.

Hollander, N. (2010). *Uprooted minds: Surviving the politics of terror in the Americas*. Routledge.

Horton, M. & Freire, P. (1990). *We make the road by walking: Conversations on education and social change*. Philadelphia, PA: Temple University Press.

Jacoby, R. (1983). *The repression of psychoanalysis: Otto Fenichel and the political Freudians*. Chicago, IL: University of Chicago Press.

Langer, M. (1971). Psicoanálisis y/o revolucion social. In M. Langer (Ed.), *Cuestionamos*. Buenos Ares, AR: Granica Editor.

Langer, M. (1989). *From Vienna to Managua: Journey of a psychoanalyst*. London, UK: Free Association Books.

Lykes, M. B. (2001). Activist participatory research and the arts with rural Mayan women: Interculturality and situated meaning making. In D. Tolman & M. Brydon-Miller (Eds.), *From subjects to subjectivities: A handbook of interpretive and participatory methods* (pp. 183–199). New York, NY: New York University Press.

Lykes, M. B., Hershberg, R. & Brabeck, K. M. (2011). Methodological challenges in participatory action research with undocumented Central American migrants. *Journal for Social Action in Counseling and Psychology*, 3 (2). Users/marywatkins/Downloads/425-Article%20Text-381-1-10-20180730.pdf

Mahoney, L. & Eguren, L. E. (1997). *Unarmed bodyguards: International accompaniment for the protection of human rights*. West Hartford, CT: Kumarian Press.

Martín-Baró, I. (1994). *Writings for a liberation psychology*. Cambridge, MA: Harvard University Press.

Pipher, M. (2003). *The middle of everywhere: Helping refugees enter the American community*. New York, NY: Houghton Mifflin.

Prilleltensky, I. & Nelson, G. (2005). *Community psychology: In pursuit of liberation and well-being*. New York, NY: Palgrave Macmillan.

Pueblo Immigration Committee (2008). *In the shadows of paradise: Testimonies from the undocumented community in Santa Barbara/ En las sombras del paraíso: Testimonios de la comunidad de inmigrantes indocumentados en Santa Barbara*. Santa Barbara, CA: Pueblo Education Fund.

Romero, O. (2001). Fourth pastoral letter: Misión de la iglesia en medio de la crisis del país. In J. Sobrino, I. Martín-Baró, & R. Cardenal (Eds.), *La voz de los sin voz: La palabra viva de Monseñor Romero* (pp. 123–172). San Salvador, ELSL: UCA Editores.

Rua, M., Groot, S., Hodgetts, D., Waimarie Nikora, L., Masters-Awatere, B., King, P., Karapu, R. & Robertson, N. (2021). Decoloniality in being Māori and community psychologists: Advancing an evolving and culturally-situated approach. In G. Stevens & C. Sonn (Eds.), *Decoloniality and epistemic injustice in contemporary community psychology* (pp. 177–192). New York, NY: Springer.

Sacipa-Rodriguez, S. (2014). To feel and to re-signify forced displacement in Colombia. In S. Sacipa-Rodríguez & M. Montero (Eds.), *Psychosocial approaches to peacebuilding in Colombia* (pp. 59–74). New York, NY: Springer.

Sacipa-Rodriguez, S. & Montero, M. (Eds.) (2014). *Psychosocial approaches to peacebuilding in Colombia*. New York, NY: Springer.

Sacipa-Rodríguez, S. R., Vidales, R., Galindo, L. & Tovar, C. (2007). Psychosocial accompaniment to liberate the suffering associated with the experience of forced displacement. *Universitas Psychológica Bogatá,* 6 (3), 589–600. http://www.scielo.org.co/pdf/rups/v6n3/v6n3a11.pdf

Sassen, S. (2014). *Expulsions: Brutality and complexity in the global economy*. Cambridge, MA: Harvard University Press.

Walsh, R. T. G. & Gokani, R. (2014). The personal and political economy of psychologists' desires for social justice. *Journal of Theoretical and Philosophical Psychology,* 34 (1), 41–55.

Watkins, M. (1992). From individualism to interdependence: Changing paradigms in psychotherapy. *Psychological Perspectives,* 27, 52–69.

Watkins, M. (2014). Hillman and Freire: Intellectual accompaniment by two fathers. In J. Selig & C. Ghorayeb (Eds.), *A tribute to James Hillman: Reflections on a renegade psychologist*. Sacramento, CA: Mandorla Books.

Watkins, M. (2015). Psychosocial Accompaniment. *Journal of Social and Political Psychology,* 3, 1. http://jspp.psychopen.eu/article/view/103/html

Watkins, M. (2019). *Mutual accompaniment and the creation of the commons*. New Haven, CT: Yale University Press.

Watkins, M. (2021). Toward a decolonial approach to accompaniment from the "outside". In G. Stevens & C. Sonn (Eds.), *Decoloniality, knowledge production and epistemic justice in contemporary community psychology*. New York, NY: Springer.

Watkins, M. & Lorenz, H. (2008). *Toward psychologies of liberation*. New York, NY: Palgrave Macmillan.

Chapter 14

Luigi Zoja

I did not have a linear trajectory. Despite having always attended Catholic schools, or perhaps because of it, a vocation in the church was not for me. As my father ran the family firm that had been founded by my great-grandfather, I decided to study business at Italy's most prestigious university (Università Bocconi). However, on graduating all I knew was that I had no interest in business. In 1967–1968, I instead moved into sociology and participated in the rise of the protest movements. But at one demonstration, when I heard the slogan "Masters, bourgeois, a few more months," I walked away: I thought my father was a good person, even if he was bourgeois. In fact, I realized that I was also bourgeois – and at only 24 I was not happy to think I had only a few months left. That also marked my departure from sociology, and I found myself reading more and more books about psychoanalysis. So off I went ("running away" I told myself) to the C.G. Jung Institute in Zürich. After completing my analytical training, I worked for a few years at the Klinik am Zürichberg before returning to Milan, where I worked mainly in private practice. At the time, I said that one of the reasons I wanted to be an analyst was because I found groups awkward and preferred talking to one person at a time. I would probably still say the same today if I'm perfectly honest.

Following a stint as president of the International Association of Jungian Analysts (IAAP) and some teaching activity at university level and the Jung Institute in Zürich, my next move was to New York. I was there just in time to witness the aftermath of the Twin Towers' collapse and to observe and study the collective paranoia that abounded, in terrorists and in the average American public. Paranoia eventually became the subject of my longest book. It seemed to me that humans have an inextricable need for enemies, even more than for friends. Perhaps that explains why wars are started even when it is clear that both sides will have more to lose than to gain: perhaps having an enemy is the hardest thing to give up.

Upon my return to Italy, I continued to work as an analyst but also devoted more time to writing. There is no one common theme to my work; the variety in my books is the result of my curiosity about a multitude of topics. One area that still interests me, despite my youthful rejection of the subject, is economics and above all its absurd core. Why, according to economics, must "needs" – and therefore the market – continue to grow, when the resources of the earth on which

DOI: 10.4324/9781003148982-15

we live are exhausted? What about life – does it also have a finite limit? These twentieth-century questions are, it seems to me, also the most important issues of the twenty-first century. They concern both psychology and economics; indeed it is impossible to separate them.

In short, my economic, political, social, and psychological reflections are an attempt to express respect and even gratitude for the lives I have not lived.

The Clash of Civilizations?
A Struggle Between Identity
and Functionalism

Originally presented as a paper at the "E' Scontro di Civiltà?" conference in Milan, Italy on October 23, 2007.

Among several disconcerting titles by Elias Canetti is *Die gespaltene Zukunft* (1972). The schizoid or "dissociated future" of which Canetti speaks refers to both a psychic and a cultural condition. His text sounds the following keynote:

> The times now approaching us are unprecedented. They are coming at us faster, and we are more conscious of making them happen. Their dangers and hopes are our own doing. The future is split, into destruction and a better life. Both of these tendencies are in train, whether in the world or in us.

Canetti identified two branches of civilization which collide, but already in 1972 he said that they stem from the same trunk, and that the outcome of the battle depends on Western man and globalization.

Why do problems become inextricably political and psychological? Because the times speed up not only urgency but also complexity. They call for increasingly decisive solutions but also ever more complex mediations. This contradiction proves to be more intractable than the agony of our environment, and the temptation of mental escape simply mounts. Hypermodernity, as Canetti remarks, compresses events as well as mental processes; the mind suffocates beneath urgency, even if that feeling is not necessarily conscious. And whoever is suffocating, of course, thinks only of the next breath. Far-reaching problems fall into neglect, separated from the subject and fobbed off onto an adversary. These processes of flight and projection correspond to those forms of psychopathology known as *mania* and *paranoia*.

Complexities, however, are increasing far more rapidly than conflicts.[1] It is our need for flight from new complexities that simplifies them, presenting them as *clashes*. A good example might be the fact that the population of New York City, a concentration of American hegemonic power,[2] will soon be only one quarter white and perhaps only 10–15% WASP.

Maniacal flight from and paranoid projection of responsibility are of interest to psychiatry only in extreme cases. In history, however, they are the stuff of daily life and the roots of most human conflicts. In the primitive scapegoat ritual, a group designates as evil one of its members or an animal (often a goat), who is cast out and sacrificed. According to René Girard (1986), this practice of purification seamlessly splices the tribal world with European history. What we fear most deeply is not diversity but its opposite, the indefinite. We want to define difference in order to fight it and expel it. To single out a symbolic carrier of evil is to *reinforce our identity* (we shall return to this problem presently). This archaic group self-therapy is paradoxically essential in our own day, because frantic economic and social changes—and the conversion of human relationships[3] into virtual phantasms by new technology—feed anxiety about identity, and this drives people to seek out a goat. The current fashion, which believes itself to be infinitely removed from tribal paranoia as well as its perverse Hitlerian and Stalinist reductions, in reality sustains it daily in a soft version (for example, in "reality" show TV).[4]

About the concepts of culture and civilization, James Hillman (1982) has remarked, "Culture flowers, Civilization works."[5] *Culture*, from the Latin, points to cultivation, by way of continuity with and growth of roots. Therefore, it pays due respect to natural cycles, such as the growing season. It holds to values that live in its past (the soil) and aims to conserve them in the future. Culture cannot indulge in mania because it must confer *identity* by remaining stable through time. Civilization, by contrast, is instrumental and neutral. Like technology but unlike nature, it is able to make leaps, and by leaping it wounds the roots of identity. Civilization gives us *functionalism*. It heeds utility, not values. This clash, inside us and out, is perhaps the profoundest and truest opposition with which we must deal.

The continual increase in functional demands coming our way instills panic; we fear losing our identity forever, but we do so unconsciously, limiting ourselves to rearranging the cyclone of the moment. Without making ourselves responsible over the long term, we insure that anxiety becomes permanent. To free ourselves from these demands, we speed up the processes of maniacal escape and paranoid projection. This reactivity in its turn is functional, for it serves no purpose other than to banish responsibility into the provinces of space and time.

In the view of analytical psychology, the psyche functions through pairs of opposites. The negation magnified by one aspect of a polarity (for example, between masculine and feminine) is unable to simplify the dyad of which it is part and sooner or later leads to the return of the repressed in a pathological form. When the West too firmly excluded the feminine from its values, it was reborn in the hideous fantasy of the witch.

The disturbance that psychiatry calls manic-depression matches up with the dissociation between two absolutely natural psychic functions (as long as they remain balanced): activity and reflection. The word *mania* derives from an

Indo-European root that simply means mental activity and that stands behind any number of modern terms, such as the English *mind*. But the Western mind nevertheless is tempted to run to excess, and so these terms can also mean runaway thinking (in ancient Greek *maìnomai*) and agitation (*exmania*). This characteristic swerve of the West with respect to the East implies a mentality that prefers external objects, overrides intervals of rest, and fills up free time. Not only do external events come at us more quickly, as Canetti has said, but these very psychic processes accelerate themselves. The Western mind also suffers from juvenility, because the young are quick and older minds require deliberation. Therefore, in our communication media the world goes on presenting itself as young, even though we know from statistics that the average age in the West is the oldest since the birth of humanity.

Paranoia, in turn, is the *moral expression* of maniacal hurry. The mind makes no allowance for periods of doubt and so preventively assigns to others either specific evils or imagined wicked intentions. One consequence is that this mentality would immediately attack them to head off their "intentions."

At the pole opposite mania stands depression. Its most notable cultural expression has been melancholy. For centuries, melancholy has nourished visual art, music, and poetry. But the postmodern world, obsessed with instant responses in real time, sees depression and melancholy above all as diseases. Their typical mental spaces frame progressions in slow rhythm, are introverted, and are given to doubt and various shades of guilt. To eliminate these as being dysfunctional and unproductive is to reject one's responsibility for oneself and, in a vicious circle, to enhance paranoia.

By worshipping haste and refusing those feelings of responsibility which are born from doubt, we have irreversibly broken up the bipolar equilibrium between two psychologies, the manic-paranoid and the depressive-reflective. This European contagion, through imperialism, colonialism, and globalization, has infected the whole world.

At the origins of Western thought, the Greeks, being reflective, practiced the art of self-limitation. Aristotle (2013) criticized those who would enlarge the state;[6] its optimal population size was never to exceed the number that could be reached by a public speaker's voice. Anything larger would result in people not knowing each other as well and weaken their common life. The unlimited growth of the state—our own condition today—is a function of power inimical to identity. Giving in to the temptation of growth, the state swells with foreigners. We may also interpret Aristotle's concern symbolically: with inordinate growth, not only does a country fill itself with immigrants but the collective mentality accumulates too many new contents. The foreigner inevitably becomes the otherness internal to a country's workings, just as a suspect notion inevitably turns into the mind's other; in this way, identity (which the foreign presence places in doubt) and functionalism (which population growth enhances) oppose each other. Aristotle obviously did not invoke the scapegoat, but he would have found himself in agreement with Girard. Sooner or later the contrast will be projected onto some neighboring country or onto a different culture and driven out, activating on a local scale the "clash of civilizations."

In the 5th century BCE, the respect for limits was already infected by its opposite; the Greeks defeated the grandiosity of the Persian Empire, but then, following suit, they began to feel grandiose themselves. First Athens, then Macedonia, and then Rome changed over to an expansive mentality, which reached them from the barbarian and Eastern tribes. The seeds of mania and paranoia came to be scattered throughout the world.

Something analogous happened with religion. A maniacal expansiveness (evident in the hyperactive Paul of Tarsus) shattered the equilibrium of psychic opposites. Christianity invented mission efforts and proselytism aimed at increasing the demographics of the faithful. A few hundred years later, another new branch of Hebraic monotheism showed up on the Arabian peninsula and sought expansion. In this perspective, the greater part of the historical conflicts between Islam and Christianity are intramural Western affairs, stemming from expansive tendencies established long since. Obviously the two World Wars, also known as "Europe's civil wars," were purely internal to our psychic equilibrium, as was the Cold War.

We are talking, therefore, about the Western world in the largest sense. Likewise the duel between Christianity and Islam—the "civil war of monotheism"—and those between left and right and between capitalism and communism (if communism ever existed: many have maintained that it has not been tried, because after World War Two very few countries so-called were actually communist societies) are tendencies *internal* to this secular swerve toward mania and paranoia.

Naturally, an alternative mental model has always existed, which Democritus anticipated with his dictum, "It is better to correct one's own errors than those of others" (Diels & Kranz, 1952, p. 60). Bertrand Russell (1930) diagnosed the Western malady as a "Byronic unhappiness," which is to say a frenzy condemned to permanent dissatisfaction. A background chorus of wisdom supports this view, but in the West these insights have never constituted a mass culture. This reflective attitude, in the modern epoch, has had to look to the Enlightenment and to psychology for reinforcement. Paradoxically, however, in the last few decades, the self-assumed responsibility for sustaining psychic equilibrium seems to have regressed due to the effects of mass merchandizing and mass communication; both of these agencies habituate people only to external objects and to ready access and assimilation.

To be sure, it is not possible to reduce history to a conflict between a maniacal, expansive West and a reflective rest of the world. China, for example, was constantly tempted by grandiosity. Seventy-five years before the discovery of America, Admiral Zheng He already had at his disposal a fleet of several hundred ships and tens of thousands of sailors, which he aimed westward. Columbus commanded less than a hundred men and three caravels, the smallest of which was as long as the Chinese flagship's rudder. It is interesting to observe that, although Western writers note (Menzies, 2002) that such expeditions could have initiated world conquest, the Chinese themselves say (Zhang, 2004) they served above all to strengthen the honor and prestige of the empire.

All the same, while Zheng He was under sail, back at the court in Peking the Mandarin faction, in every sense representing culture and national identity (these high functionaries achieved their positions through difficult examinations in classical literature, not in administrative matters), defeated the Eunuch faction (the party of activism, functionality, and immediate results). Lightning started large fires in the Forbidden City, and this precipitated a round of contentious and arcane debates; presumably heaven was not in full harmony with emperor Zhu Di, perhaps because he had engaged in too many cyclopean undertakings. When the emperor died, his successors adopted policies that forcefully closed China. Naturally merchants suffered (foreign trade was straightaway reduced to piracy), but they were not the priority. China sealed its borders.

What happened in Europe also cannot be simplified too readily. In the following century, the greatest theological battle of all time developed in Spain. The conquest of the Americas set off a contest between an imperialistic theology (according to which the natives did not have souls or were naturally inferior) and a nativist theology (by Bartolomeo de Las Casas and Francisco de Vitoria), according to which the native peoples were the equals of Europeans. Nativist theologians won the debates and laid out the legislative basis for relations with the colonies, anticipating modern international law. While discussion was taking place in Spain, however, and affirming its abstractions—those "useless passions" of the Europeans—in America the first and greatest genocide in history was carried out. Europe already lacked the equilibrium of the East; utilitarian expansion—civilization, ho!—proved to be far stronger than affiliation with a culture and its values.

When it turns back on itself, therefore, our postmodern viewpoint can observe a dramatic contest between identity (the Mandarins defending China, or the great theologians Las Casas and Vitoria standing up for native peoples) and functionalism, which, dispensing with values, gives absolute precedence to conquest, an accumulation of means that still have not settled on the problem of their ends. As we know, over time values grow weak; in the epoch we have surveyed, military, economic, and technical developments have imposed themselves on morals. Spanish law declared natives the equals of Europeans, but in the colonies, a few friars were faced with an ever growing number of adventurers and immigrants and an immense array of commercial interests.

China, along with the Japan that closed its borders 200 years later, succeeded in barricading its identity for a long time, but today they are mounting a maniacal Western relay race.

In the final decade of the last century, Francis Fukuyama (1992) defined the fall of the Berlin Wall and the end of the Cold War in *The End of History*. While the history that has followed has lodged its dissent, it remains true that the 1990s were a privileged period exceptionally free of paranoia. The projection of evil onto an absolute enemy no longer prevailed. Conflicts seemed to migrate back along the dry branches of geography and history into the Balkans or Africa; it seemed that the era was busy selling them off like out-of-date goods on the counters at supermarkets. A transatlantic collective unconscious saw them by that time as postmodern versions of Kipling's (1989) white man's burden: not as mortal challenges to the West but as confirmations of its superiority, for which only a small price had to be paid.

It was a unique period during which, in the absence of major challenges, the West would have been able directly to assume global responsibility for the environment, disarmament, and the defense of cultural identity. That is, attention could have focused not on partial disputes and their brief intervals but on chronic themes, which call for unrelenting self-criticism: the depressive but profound psychology of Cronus.

If the 1990s were "easy" from the viewpoint of international economics and politics, they were none the less psychologically difficult for the West, constrained as it was to an equilibrium extraneous to its workings. Our mentality is accustomed to a maniacal rhythm and tempo and to the projection of responsibility; a pause for reflection can seem to fall like some chance obstacle on the street down which we are running. Unconsciously, we look for some new scapegoat and some new enemy to hunt down.

The collective unconscious imagination therefore heaved a sigh of relief with the arrival of 11 September 2001. The mass media in the new century have been able to galvanize into life once again all of the old mental reaction patterns of the Cold War, transformed into the *Clash of Civilizations* that Samuel Huntington (1993) has erected as a counterfaçade to Fukuyama's *The End of History*, to the point where we might call his manifesto "the restoration of history." Altogether it amounts to a return of history with ideology; the media rolled out the political manifesto drafted long before in the 1990s by the right-wing Republican Project for a New American Century (PNAC), which proposed American supremacy as its program.[7]

The vision of the future promoted in this document adopts the mental perspectives of the past, overlooking two fundamental facts: (1) The radical attack on "American civilization" is symbolic and media-framed, not military. It would call, first of all, for a commitment to the psychology of symbols and only secondarily for a strengthened military role. (2) The struggle no longer pits the United States against a revolutionary movement or an "Empire of Evil," which was easily identified with what was beyond the Iron Curtain, but (if these distinctions have any meaning) against a reactionary religious vision bent on restoring a mythical past and a theocratic society scattered like the leopard's spots across the globe. Today the battle is asymmetrical in both time and space. This second aspect combines with the first. From the pharaohs to Bush Junior,[8] no theocracy has been subdued solely by military means. The Aztec Empire, for example, which was far stronger militarily than the invading Spaniards, crumbled when Montezuma was no longer able to feel his divine status and was shot by his own subjects.

In essence, the American government (and in its wake the entire media system of the West) has failed to take into account either factor. Through sheer inertia, the United States continues to lay out the greatest military expenditure of any government of all time. After 12 September 2001 it has only increased, and by now it totals nearly half of all military outlays in the world (or, as has been noted, around

30 times the amount that would meet the challenge of world hunger). In this diz-zying number shines the absence of any attention to psychology.

If we adopt a psychological perspective, 12 September 2001 is more interest-ing than the 11th. If the 11th is symbol, the 12th is panic, revealing our fear of that symbol, our estrangement from symbols, and the paranoid reaction and anti-psychological attitude of the principal actors. With 12 September 2001, the real encounter swims to the surface and is entirely internal to Western civilization. Its stark contrast comes forth, between the unconscious, inflicting itself purely in the form of collective fantasies and the rationality that sets out in lockstep to colonize the new century.

If we believe that a "Clash of Civilizations" has taken the West by surprise, then we also would have to ask why it might be surprised by anything at all, when marketing was entirely ready for it. In fact, however, the West has actually been accustomed to such collisions for a long time. The first description of a clash of civilizations comes in the 5th century BCE. The writer is known as Herodotus of Halicarnassus, and the book is called *The Histories* (1972). The first page of the initial episode (Book I.1–5) already tells how the contrasts between East and West came about, attributing them to artificial exaggeration. And on the second page, Herodotus shakes his head over the futility of the conflict; in fact, the whole thing comes down to a series of kidnappings of women, the second woman being named, significantly, Europa.

> Abducting young women, in their opinion, is not, indeed, a lawful act; but it is stupid after the event to make a fuss about it. The only sensible thing is to take no notice; for it is obvious that no young woman allows herself to be abducted if she does not wish to be.
>
> (Herodotus, 1972, p. 4)

The father of history, besides establishing that misogyny is as old as history itself, demonstrates that history is a paranoid psychic contagion. It consists of coming down with a fever brought on by the "original paranoid event," from which eve-rything else follows.

If I pin psychic error on an adversary, I am able to avoid confronting my own contradictions and evils; as their subject I simply assign them to an external *object* (Latin *ob-iiectare*, against-throw). Thus does one denounce the crimes of a neigh-bor. This behavior changes the counterpart not only into a criminal but also into a *permanent enemy*. It gives the appearance that dealing with evil is a moral task, but in substance it corrupts us in turn. We must confess that crime is more seduc-tive than any other psychic principle, because we so readily make it our own. So long as we commit an evil act in response, it is good. But we also need to increase the dosage of evil, for now that the guilty party is also an enemy, one must obtain *not only justification but victory*. Throughout the chapters of Book One, Hero-dotus identifies the virus of historical process as *tsisis* or retributive, vengeful justice. The individual psychic infection circulating in society and in history becomes collective and permanent, just as an individual bacterial infection can mutate into epidemic and then endemic conditions. In this way, Herodotus wrote, Asia and Europe began to invest their energies in successive campaigns of self-ruination, instead of enjoying the civilizations that they had already brought to flower. Within one generation, the ugly practice of rape had become so contagious that one Eastern prince, Paris of Troy, loaded Helen with his baggage, confident that he would get away with it just as the Greeks had done (Book I.3); instead, he brought on the most famous conflict of all time, the Trojan War.

Continental battles—the most intense eruptions of this volcano—run through our history from Herodotus to Huntington with a clear response, the simplest one. Even when brushed by catastrophe, Europe managed to exercise overwhelming military superiority. In 490 BCE, when the Persians attacked Athens and met the hoplite infantry spears of the Greek militia, they lost 33 times more men than did the Greeks. Twenty-two centuries later, in 1683, the Polish cavalry of King Jan Sobieski smashed the siege of Vienna and the secular expansion of the Ottoman Turks with one stroke, killing around 15,000 troops in a few hours.

The West has won all of these historic encounters but, as Nietzsche and then Spengler have warned, it is as if the West lost a decisive battle with its victory. Gradually in recent generations, and at a dizzying pace in the last few years, society has become unbalanced by history. For the first time it has conquered hunger, but also for the first time it grows sick from too much food. Its citizens are not afraid, or are only marginally so, of external enemies who would take their lives, but there are now more who would take their own lives. The civilization that has subdued the hazards of the natural environment is the same that has turned itself, unnaturally so, into the greatest of hazards for the survival of the environment.

The dilemma that is perfectly clear to psychology and anthropology is almost impossible to translate into the language of the mass media. The theoretical catch-phrase "clash of civilizations" simplifies it, rendering it visible and exiling it for as long as possible to the outside, like the longed-for goat. It is no longer the traditional duel between neighboring countries but one between distant civilizations, separated by geography as well as developmental age and spurred into flight by every kind of anxiety because *they are too close*. The whole matter is a continuation of the Western tradition of exporting its internal problems in the form of colonialist enterprise.

In the collective imagination of the West, the clash of civilizations is a narrative continuation of the conflict between Asia and Europe framed by Herodotus: an archaic fact that, like certain childhood nightmares, traumatically returns at the prompting of certain surface details. What is new in all of this, with acknowledgment to Huntington, is its *systematic and eschatological arrangement*: the media mobilization of the public through menacing shocks delivered to the global masses. In sum, the new thing is not the clash of civilizations but the cultivation of clashes.

The narrative of 12 September—namely, the crusade and revenge of the West—was there all along, pre-existent in the unconscious and gathering force and autonomous dynamism. It absorbed these elements from centuries and millennia of our culture, and a fact of this nature cannot subsist without having consequences. The myths of vengeance, set aside by official culture, do not simply disappear; quite simply, they show up as pathological irruptions, more or less in the manner of a dormant volcano that sometimes turns active. In the terms that the mass media render banal, two very different things—the clash of civilizations and *the narrative of 12 September*—are identified with each other. The date of 11 September 2001 is *that of a calamitous event, but not of a new civilizational conflict.* Instead, a new narrative gets underway[9] that has no small consequences: to mention only one among many, an altered relationship between the two continents flanking the North Atlantic.

In the global scenario, the paranoid style of fear has agreed to declare war against not an enemy but an abstraction (*the war on terror*) and an invisible adversary (*faceless enemy*). On the inner plane, the scapegoat is the immigrant group (attracted by a business community that seeks cheap labor, but that also might finance right-wing movements that demand the expulsion of immigrants). Naturally the perfect synthesis is achieved when immigrant and terrorist become one and the same.

We can almost formulate it axiomatically: any idea can be sold, in paranoid terms, if mass media successfully reduce the adversary's attitude to a threat to identity. The populace trains its eyes on the scapegoat, forgetting that the same brand went on fire sale many years earlier simply to maintain the semblance of ever-growing vitality. In Switzerland, which thanks to prosperity has been flooded with guest-worker immigrants for decades, Max Frisch (1965) was the first to observe sarcastically: "What a terrible thing! We called for workers, and instead we got people!"

Let us return to "Canetti's dilemma." As for the continual erosion of self-criticism in a society gripped by haste and consumerism, we reject with increasing force any conflict among the alternatives that are possible *to us.* We project our psychological dilemmas into conflicts outside ourselves, leaving ourselves to stand for what is right. To return to the example quoted earlier, we do not look at the potential conflicts internal to ethnic groups in New York City, but at the clash of Islam with the West. Making our daily concessions to functionalism, we renew the Faustian bargain of the soul in a postmodern way. This blindness comes at a tremendous cost and makes us accomplices to globalization, which by now affects every country.

Let us take an example: hunger is age-old whether in India or Brazil (in treating quite different countries, we would do well to approach certain problems as common ones). A new economic development is now supporting many people on many fewer calories. But, just as this premodern problem finds resolution, a postmodern one explodes, with no ability on the part of statistics to pigeonhole it: tens of millions of citizens of India and Brazil already are overweight. Without having had time to escape famine, we are already prisoners of overeating. Because it is children above all who are affected, in a few years obesity will strike like a cultural form of AIDS. In these same countries, too, consumption has already swollen beyond actual need.

The availability of food, unfortunately, grows through *functional* means that operate at the expense of *identity*. The excesses of functionalism, in turn, are part and parcel of maniacal *hubris* without either object or end, truly a psychic infection that emerging nations import from the West. The industrialization of agriculture eliminates the family farm and accelerates the disappearance of tasks related to agriculture as well as their communities. Culture (both senses of the word intended) is vanishing, and nothing is arising to replace it. To produce food and to live from that practice were always both ritual and culture, that is, they have always constituted values and identity in themselves. The raising of calories without culture—without sowing seed, protecting growing plants, and celebrating the rituals of harvest—starves the human psyche.

Let me close with another example, this time pertaining to the West.

The American Medical Association (AMA) has taken a stand on the interrogations of detainees at Guantàánamo (the modern American statue of anti-liberty). Whatever they are called—whether the word *torture* is used or not—they cause suffering and therefore violate the Hippocratic Oath. The Association defends the millennial cultural identity of the physician, with no concessions whatsoever made to *functionalism*. By contrast, the American Psychological Association or APA has broken apart over the question. The "psychological technique of interrogation," with all of its attendant torments, has seemed to many in this group a neutral business,[10] something that should manage to reach its goal of defending America and its values. Instead, the country's own historical identity, represented by the Constitution (its Fourth, Fifth, and Sixth Amendments) has come to be sacrificed, like a scapegoat, to the Golem of functionalism.

The suspension of law in order to more quickly reach political objectives had already extinguished the comet that burned across the 20th century, the one named Communism. If the triumph of the West amounts to the triumph of maniacal functionalism and the rejection of responsibility, then the real struggle has already been lost, even for the liberal democracies. It is significant that their prototype, the United States of America, is defined predominantly not in state form but as an activity: *the American way of life*. That operational definition does not propose a goal or a purpose, but a way, a road,[11] a function, a means: just as a *war* (*on terror*) or a *clash* (*of civilizations*) is only a movement, not a destination.

By worshipping success as such (regardless of whether it be economic or military), the West has also mistaken a means for an end. But the West, in accepting the continual change that comes with utilitarianism, feels untrue to itself and chips away at its own identity. In this way, it condemns itself to always seek out new conflicts as screens onto which to project its bad faith.

Notes

1 From 1910 to 2000, that is, in only 90 years, the white population of New York City has declined from 98% to only 35% (see the tables published in *The New York Times*, Section B, pp. 6–7, for 16 March 2001). In the second decade of the 21st century, it

should decline to approximately one-quarter of the whole. This genuine revolution is accompanied by social problems, not by cultural or ethnic clashes.

2 James Hillman's definition, employed at the same conference.

3 In psychotherapeutic relationships, for example, where the question is if the transference survives sessions that are carried out via teleconferencing or on a chatline.

4 See a sociological analysis of this problem in Zygmunt Bauman, *Society under Siege* (2002). I have touched on this theme in *La morte del prossimo* (2009a).

5 Hillmann, J. "On Culture and Chronic Disorder," the inaugural lecture at the Dallas Institute of Humanities and Culture, 1981, published in the Institute Newsletter, 1.2, Dallas 1982.

6 Aristotle, *Politics VII.4*, 1326ab.

7 For the PNAC document, see www.newamericancentury.org. As for the chronology between Fukuyama and Huntington, whereas Fukuyama's text was written after the fall of the Berlin Wall, in 1992, Huntington published under this title for the first time in 1993 in the journal *Foreign Affairs*, in response to Fukuyama (following suit in 1996 with a book). Therefore, we are dealing with an original rather than a specialized analysis, which subsequently was rolled out on new wheels in response to the attacks on the Twin Towers and the Pentagon.

8 George W. Bush, the 43rd president of the United States (served from 2001 to 2009).

9 For such a complex problem, it is possible to use only simple examples. In one of his most memorable speeches—for its contribution to fueling global anti-Americanism—George W. Bush spoke of a crusade against Islamic threats. Naturally he immediately tried to rectify the situation, so as not to offer the impression that he wished to revive the conflict between Islam and the West that began in the preceding millennium. The incident closed as if it were an unwitting mistake, helped along by the president's proverbial ignorance. But Freud has shown us that the personal unconscious does not make casual mistakes. In their turn, too, the collective unconscious and its narratives exist prior to any individual expressions of them.

10 It is interesting to reconstruct how psychologists came to find themselves in the torture chamber. For some time the CIA had run the approved programs of SERE (Survival, Evasion, Resistance, and Escape), in which military personnel were taught how, if captured by an enemy, to resist treatment that violated the Geneva Conventions pertaining to combatants. But, in terms of technique, why not turn this approach upside down and use the experience to deal with prisoners who, by happy chance, were not protected by the Geneva Conventions? The magical notion is to do a bit of reverse engineering, inverting technology, just as with a mechanism that one can run in one direction or the other. Naturally, if interrogation is morally neutral, then it may also be put out on contract. And so it happened that reductive subcontracting assigned these interrogations to private agencies (security firms) run by psychologists.

11 See my article "Violent Hearts" in *Violence in History, Culture, and the Psyche*, *Spring Journal*, 2009b.

References

Aristotle. (2013). *Aristotle's Politics*. 2nd edn, transl. and with an Introduction, Notes and Glossary by Carnes Lord. Chicago and London: The University of Chicago Press.

Bauman, Z. (2002). *Society under Siege*. Cambridge: Polity Press.

Canetti, E. (1972). *Die gespaltene Zukunft: Aufsätze und Gespräche*. München: Carl Hanser.

Diels, H. & Kranz, W. (1952). *The Presocratic Fragments*. Berlin: Weidmann.

Frisch, M. (1965). 'Vorwort', in Seiler, A. *Siamo Italiani. Die Italiener. Gespräche mit italienischen Arbeitern in der Schweiz*. Zürich: EVZ-Verlag.

Fukuyama, F. (1992). *The End of History*. London: Hamish Hamilton.

Girard, R. (1986). *The Scapegoat*. Baltimore, MD: Johns Hopkins University Press. [Or. ed. (1982). *Le bouc émissaire*, Paris: Grasset].

Herodotus. (1972). *The Histories*. London and New York: Penguin

Hillmann, J. (1982). 'On Culture and Chronic Disorder'. *The Institute Newsletter*, 1.2, Dallas.

Huntington, S. (1993). 'The Clash of Civilizations?'. *Foreign Affairs*, vol. 72, n° 73, Summer.

Kipling, R. (1989). '*The White Man* Burden'. *The Times*, 4 February 1899.

Menzies, G. (2002). *1421: The Year China Discovered America*. London: Bantam Press.

Russell, B. (1930). *The Conquest of Happiness*. London: George Allen & Unwin.

The New York Times in section B, pp. 6–7, 16 March 2001.

Zhang, Q. (2004). *Traditional Chinese Culture*. Beijing: Foreign Languages Press.

Zoja, L. (2009a). *La morte del prossimo*. Torino: Einaudi.

Zoja, L. (2009b). *Violence in History, Culture, and the Psyche*. New Orleans: Spring Journal [Or. ed. *Contro Ismene*, Torino: Bollati Boringhieri].

Contributors

Paul Bishop, Ph.D., is the William Jacks Chair of Modern Languages at the University of Glasgow, Scotland. His books examine the history of ideas and the histories of psychoanalysis and analytical psychology, with particular emphasis on Goethe, Schiller, Nietzsche, C.G. Jung and Ludwig Klages. He has edited companion volumes on Goethe's *Faust* and on Nietzsche's life and works; written a "critical life" of Jung; and authored an introductory "toolkit" on the thought of Klages. His most recent publications include *German Political Thought and the Discourse of Platonism: Finding the Way out of the Cave* (2019).

Ann Casement, LP, is a London-based Jungian psychoanalyst and a senior member of the British Jungian Analytic Association. She worked in psychiatry for several years beginning in the late 1970s, chaired the UK Council for Psychotherapy (1997–2001), and served on the executive committee of the International Association for Analytical Psychology (IAAP, 2001–2007). She has lectured, supervised and taught in many countries around the world, and she contributes to *The Economist* and to psychoanalytic journals worldwide and is on the editorial boards of several of them. She served on the Gradiva Awards Committee (New York) in 2013.

Her published books include (among others) *Post-Jungians Today* (Routledge, 1998), *Carl Gustav Jung* (Sage, 2001), *Who Owns Psychoanalysis?* (Karnac, 2004), which was nominated for the 2005 Gradiva Award, and *Who Owns Jung?* (Karnac, 2007).

James Hollis, Ph.D., was born in Springfield, IL, and graduated from Manchester University, Indiana in 1962 and Drew University, Madison, NJ, in 1967. He taught humanities for 26 years in various colleges and universities before retraining as a Jungian analyst at the Jung Institute of Zürich, Switzerland (1977–1982). He served as executive director of the Jung Educational Center in Houston, TX, for many years, was executive director of the Jung Society of Washington until 2019, and now serves on their board of directors. He is a retired senior training analyst for the Inter-Regional Society of Jungian Analysts, was the first director of training for the Philadelphia Jung Institute, and is vice-president emeritus of the Philemon Foundation. Additionally, he is a professor of Jungian Studies for Saybrook University of San Francisco and Houston.

Verena Kast, Dr. Phil., studied psychology at the Universities of Basel and Zürich, Switzerland, and trained as a psychoanalyst at the C.G. Jung Institute Zürich. From 1973 to 2008 she taught at the University of Zürich. She has lectured internationally and at the C.G. Jung Institute Zürich. She is past president of the Swiss Society for Analytical Psychology and past president of the IAAP. She was chairwoman of the International Society for Depth Psychology, co-director of the Lindau Psychotherapy Weeks and president of the C.G. Jung Institute. She has written in the fields of emotions, attachment and separation, and also symbolism. She loves the imagination and its development.

Stanton Marlan, Ph.D., ABPP, FABP, LP, is a Jungian analyst and clinical psychologist in private practice in Pittsburgh, PA, and an adjunct clinical professor of psychology at Duquesne University in Pittsburgh. He is a training and supervising analyst with the Inter-Regional Society of Jungian Analysts and president of the Pittsburgh Society of Jungian Analysts. He is a director of the American Board and Academy of Psychoanalysis (ABAPsa) and its past president. Dr. Marlan has published numerous articles on Jungian psychology and is the editor of four books, including *Archetypal Psychologies: Reflections in Honor of James Hillman*. He was a Fay lecturer at Texas A&M, College Station, TX, and is the author of *The Black Sun: The Alchemy and Art of Darkness*.

Renos K. Papadopoulos, Ph.D., is Professor of Analytical Psychology and Director of the Centre for Trauma, Asylum and Refugees, a member of the Human Rights Centre, the Transitional Justice Network and the Armed Conflict and Crisis Hub, all at the University of Essex UK, and Honorary Clinical Psychologist and Systemic Family Psychotherapist at the Tavistock Clinic, UK. He is a practising clinical psychologist, family therapist and Jungian psychoanalyst. He served on the executive committee of the IAAP, was responsible for setting up the Academic Section and the Developing Groups within IAAP, and organised the first IAAP Academic Conference (in 2002). He was editor of *Harvest: International Journal for Jungian Studies* for 14 years, founding editor of the *International Journal of Jungian Studies* and co-founder of the International Association for Jungian Studies. His four-volume work *C.G. Jung: Critical Assessments* (1992) remains the lengthiest book on Jung (1750 pages).

Denise G. Ramos, Ph.D. is a clinical psychologist and Jungian analyst and member and former director of the Brazilian Society of Analytical Psychology (IAAP). She was a Fulbright recipient at New School for Social Research in New York City. She is Full Professor in the graduate program in Clinical Psychology at the Catholic University of São Paulo, Brazil, and chair of the Center of Jungian Studies. Her current fields of interest are psychosomatic phenomena and cultural complexes as the bases of social pathologies, especially corruption, and racial and gender prejudice. She has been politically active in the Jungian community, having been a member of the executive committee and vice president of the IAAP and the International Society of Sandplay Therapy (ISST) for several years. In Brazil, she was elected member of the Academia of Psychology of Sao Paulo, chair 27.

Susan Rowland, Ph.D., is Chair of the Engaged Humanities and the Creative Life MA at Pacifica Graduate Institute, Carpinteria, CA. She earned her Ph.D. from the University of Newcastle, UK, and her M.A.s from the University of London and Oxford University, UK. She was the first chair of the International Association of Jungian Studies (IAJS). She is the author of many studies on Jung, literary theory and gender, including *C.G. Jung and Literary Theory* (1999), *Jung: A Feminist Revision* (2002), and *Jung as a Writer* (2005), and she also edited *Psyche and the Arts* (2008). Professor Rowland's work is not so much "about" Jung as an attempt to develop his special insights into myth, technology, the feminine, nature and the numinous for today's wounded world.

Sonu Shamdasani, Ph.D., is a London-based author, editor, and professor at University College London. His research and writings focus on Carl Gustav Jung and cover the history of psychiatry and psychology from the mid-nineteenth century to current times. Professor Shamdasani edited the first publication of Jung's *Liber Novus, The Red Book*. He is also the editor of Jung's *Black Books* (2020).

Heyong Shen, Ph.D., is a professor of psychology at the City University of Macao and South China Normal University, Guangzhou. He is a Jungian analyst (IAAP member), Sandplay therapist (ISST), and president of the China Society for Analytical Psychology (CSAP) and the China Society for Sandplay Therapy (CSST). He was a speaker at the Eranos East and West Round Table Conferences (1997, 2007 and 2019), the main organizer of the International Conference of Analytical Psychology and Chinese Culture (1998–2018), and founding member of the Garden of the Heart & Soul project. He is the author of *Psychology of the Heart* (Fay Lecture), *C.G. Jung and Chinese Culture, Chinese Culture Psychology* and numerous articles on the interface between analytical psychology and Chinese culture.

Thomas (Tom) Singer, MD, is a psychiatrist and Jungian psychoanalyst who lives and practices in the San Francisco Bay Area, CA. He has written and edited many books, including *Who's the Patient Here?*, *A Fan's Guide to Baseball Fever*, *The Cultural Complex*, *Ancient Greece/Modern Psyche*, *The Vision Thing*, *Psyche and the City: A Soul's Guide to the Modern City*, *Initiation: The Living Reality of An Archetype* and, most recently, *Placing Psyche: Exploring Cultural Complexes in Australia*.

Murray Stein, Ph.D., is a training and supervising analyst at the International School of Analytical Psychology Zürich (ISAP-ZÜRICH). He was president of the International Association for Analytical Psychology (IAAP) from 2001 to 2004 and president of ISAP-ZÜRICH from 2008 to 2012. He has lectured internationally and is the editor of *Jungian Psychoanalysis* and the author of *Jung's Treatment of Christianity, In MidLife, Jung's Map of the Soul, Minding the Self, Outside Inside and All Around* and *The Bible as Dream*. The first volume of his collected writings, titled *Individuation*, has recently been published. He lives in Switzerland and has a private practice in Zürich.

Mary Watkins, Ph.D., chairs the M.A./Ph.D. Depth Psychology Program at Pacifica Graduate Institute, Carpinteria, CA. She is co-founder and co-chair of its specialization in Community, Liberation, Indigenous, and Eco-Psychologies and founding coordinator of community and ecological fieldwork and research at Pacifica. She is the author of *Mutual Accompaniment and the Creation of the Commons, Waking Dreams* and *Invisible Guests: The Development of Imaginal Dialogues*. She is co-author of *Toward Psychologies of Liberation*. She has worked as a clinical psychologist with adults, children and families and has also worked with small and large groups around issues of immigration, peace, alternatives to violence, envisioning the future, diversity, vocation and social justice. In 2019 she received the award for Distinguished Theoretical and Philosophical Contributions to Psychology from the Society for Philosophical and Theoretical Psychology (Division 24, American Psychological Association).

Luigi Zoja, Ph.D., is past president of CIPA and past president of IAAP. He has taught at the School of Psychiatry of the Faculty of Medicine, State University of Palermo, Italy, the University of Insubria, Italy, and the University of Macao, China. His publications in English include *Drugs, Addiction and Initiation* (1989/2000); *Growth and Guilt* (1995); *The Father* (Gradiva Award 2001); *The Global Nightmare. Jungian Perspectives on September 11* (2002); *Cultivating the Soul* (2005); *Ethics and Analysis* (2007); *Violence in History, Culture and the Psyche* (2009); and *Paranoia. The Madness that Makes History* (2017).

Index

Page numbers in *italics* indicate a figure.

Ingram Content Group UK Ltd.
Milton Keynes UK
UKHW020033170323
418718UK00007B/46